Controversy in

CARDIOLOGY

The Practical Clinical Approach

Edited by

Edward K. Chung

With Contributions by
G. E. Burch · L. S. Chung · R. L. DeJoseph · J. E. Doherty
D. J. W. Escher · S. M. Fox · T. Giles · R. Gottlieb
A. D. Hagan · W. D. Johnson · R. I. Levy · M. Luxton
M. T. Monroe · L. A. Papa · T. Peter · L. Pordy · B. M. Rifkind
W. C. Roberts · A. Rosenthal · N. Ruggiero · R. T. Shore
G. Sloman · C. L. Weisberger · D. P. Zipes

With 99 Figures

Springer-Verlag
New York Heidelberg Berlin 1976

EDWARD K. CHUNG, M.D.
Professor of Medicine Jefferson Medical College of Thomas Jefferson University and Director of the Heart Station Thomas Jefferson University Hospital Philadelphia, PA. 19107

ISBN 978-3-642-86002-7 ISBN 978-3-642-86000-3 (eBook)
DOI 10.1007/978-3-642-86000-3

Library of Congress Cataloging in Publication Data. Main entry under title: Controversy in cardiology: the practical clinical approach. 1. Cardiology—Addresses, essays, lectures. I. Chung, Edward K. [DNLM: 1. Heart diseases. WG200 C764] RC681.C69 616.1'2 75-22026

Softcover reprint of the hardcover 1st edition 1976

Typesetting by William Clowes & Sons Ltd., Colchester, England

To My Wife, Lisa and
To Linda and Christopher

Preface

The purpose of this book is not to discuss in depth various topics in medicine nor to describe in detail all possible controversial subjects in cardiology. The primary intention is to describe common cardiac problems with significant controversial viewpoints frequently encountered in our daily practice.

This book presents 19 chapters, including the Coronary Arteries in Fatal Coronary Events, Prophylactic Antiarrhythmic Therapy in Acute Myocardial Infarction, Mobile Coronary Care—Is It Really Needed?, The Use of Artificial Pacemakers in Acute Myocardial Infarction, Treatment of Cardiogenic Shock, Serum Digitalis Level—Practical Value, Factors Modifying the Efficacy of Digitalis, Hyperlipidemia and Vascular Disease, Antianginal Agents for Coronary Heart Disease, Anticoagulation Therapy for Coronary Heart Disease, When to Operate on Congenital Heart Diseases, Indications for Coronary Artery Surgery and Patient Selection, Cardiomyopathy: Diagnostic Criteria and Classification, Therapeutic Approach to Idiopathic Hypertrophic Subaortic Stenosis, Current Concepts of Hemiblocks, Physical Activity and Coronary Heart Disease, His Bundle Electrocardiography—Its Clinical Value, Computerized Electrocardiography—Its Practical Value, and Echocardiography—Its Practical Value.

As the title of the book indicates, the "pro and con" viewpoints are described in each chapter, and the authors final conclusions are expressed at the end of each. It is hoped that the book will be provocative as well as educational and practical.

The contents are intended to be clinical, concise, and practical, so that this book will provide all physicians with up-to-date materials that will assist them directly in the daily care of their patients with common cardiac problems.

The book will be extremely valuable to all practicing physicians with various backgrounds, particularly internists, cardiologists, and family physicians. In addition, house staff, cardiology fellows, medical students, and coronary care unit nurses will also benefit by reading this book.

I am sincerely grateful to all authors for their valuable contributions to *Controversy in Cardiology*. I also wish to thank my personal secretary, Miss Theresa McAnally, for her devoted and cheerful secretarial assistance. She has been most valuable in handling correspondence to all contributors in addition to typing several chapters of mine for this book.

Philadelphia, Summer 1975

EDWARD K. CHUNG, M.D.

Contents

List of Contributors

GEORGE E. BURCH, M.D., F.A.C.P., M.A.C.P., F.A.C.C., Professor of Medicine, Tulane University School of Medicine, 1430 Tulane Avenue, New Orleans, La. 70118.

EDWARD K. CHUNG, M.D., F.A.C.P., F.A.C.C., Professor of Medicine, Jefferson Medical College of Thomas Jefferson University, and Director of the Heart Station, Thomas Jefferson University Hospital, Philadelphia, PA. 19107.

LISA S. CHUNG, M.D., Medical Director and Chief Medical Officer, U.S. Public Health Service, Philadelphia, PA.

ROBERT L. DEJOSEPH, M.D., Assistant Professor of Medicine, The Milton S. Hershey Medical Center, Pennsylvania State University, University Drive, Hershey, PA. 17033.

JAMES E. DOHERTY, M.D., F.A.C.P., F.A.C.C., Professor of Medicine and Pharmacology, University of Arkansas School of Medicine, Director, Division of Cardiology, VA—UAMC Hospitals, Little Rock, Arkansas 72206.

DORIS J. W. ESCHER, M.D., F.A.C.C., Associate Professor of Medicine, Albert Einstein College of Medicine, Chief, Cardiac Catheterization Laboratory, Montefiore Hospital and Medical Center, 111 East 210th Street, Bronx, N.Y. 10467.

SAMUEL M. FOX, III, M.D., F.A.C.P., F.A.C.C., Professor of Medicine, Director of the Office of Continuing Education, and Director of Cardiology Exercise Laboratory, Georgetown University School of Medicine, Washington, D.C. 20007.

THOMAS GILES, M.D., F.A.C.C., Clinical Associate Professor of Medicine, Tulane University School of Medicine, 1430 Tulane Avenue, New Orleans, La. 70118.

RONALD GOTTLIEB, M.D., Assistant Professor of Medicine, Co-Director, Cardiac Catheterization Laboratory, Thomas Jefferson University, Philadelphia, PA. 19107.

ARTHUR D. HAGAN, M.D., F.A.C.C., CAPT., MC., USN., Associate Clinical Professor of Medicine, University of California, San Diego, and Head of Cardiology, Department of the Navy, Navy Regional Medical Center, San Diego, Calif. 92134.

W. DUDLEY JOHNSON, M.D., F.A.C.S., F.A.C.C., Associate Clinical Professor of Surgery, Medical College of Wisconsin, Milwaukee, Wisconsin.

ROBERT I. LEVY, M.D., F.A.C.C., Director, Division of Heart & Vascular Disease, National Heart & Lung Institute, National Institutes of Health, Bethesda, Maryland 20014.

MICHAEL LUXTON, M.B., M.R.A.C.P., Cardiology Registrar, Royal Melbourne Hospital, Victoria, 3050, Australia.

MATTHEW T. MONROE, M.D., Ph.D., Fellow in Cardiology, Thomas Jefferson University, Philadelphia, PA. 19107.

LOUIS A. PAPA, D.O., Fellow in Cardiology, Thomas Jefferson University, Philadelphia, PA. 19107.

THOMAS PETER, M.D., Dreyfus Medical Foundation Research Fellow, Royal Melbourne Hospital, Victoria, 3050, Australia.

LEON PORDY, M.D., F.A.C.C., Associate Clinical Professor of Medicine, The Mount Sinai School of Medicine, New York, N.Y. 10028.

BASIL M. RIFKIND, M.D., F.R.C.P., Chief, Lipid Metabolism Branch, National Heart & Lung Institute, National Institute of Health, Bethesda, Maryland 20014.

WILLIAM C. ROBERTS, M.D., F.A.C.C., Chief, Section of Pathology, National Heart & Lung Institute, National Institutes of Health, Bethesda Maryland 20014, and Clinical Professor of Pathology and Medicine (Cardiology), Georgetown University School of Medicine, Washington, D.C.

AMNON ROSENTHAL, M.D., F.A.A.P., Associate Professor of Pediatrics, Harvard Medical School, and Senior Associate in Cardiology, Children's Hospital Medical Center, 300 Longwood Avenue, Boston, Mass. 02114.

NICHOLAS RUGGIERO, M.D., Fellow in Cardiology, Thomas Jefferson University, Philadelphia, PA. 19107.

RICHARD T. SHORE, M.D., Cardiovascular Surgeon, Saint Luke's, St. Mary's Hospitals, Milwaukee, Wisconsin.

GRAEME SLOMAN, M.D., F.R.C.P. (Ed.), F.R.A.C.P., M.R.C.P., (Lond.), F.A.C.C., Director, Cardiology Laboratory, Royal Melbourne Hospital, Victoria, 3050, Australia.

CALVIN WEISBERGER, M.D., Fellow in Cardiology, Thomas Jefferson University, Philadelphia, PA. 19107.

DOUGLAS P. ZIPES, M.D., F.A.C.P., F.A.C.C.,* Associate Professor of Medicine, Indiana University School of Medicine, and Senior Research Associate, Krannert Institute of Cardiology, Indianapolis, Indiana 46202.

* *Office Address*:

LEON PORDY, M.D., F.A.C.C., 150 Park Avenue, New York, NY. 10028.

DOUGLAS P. ZIPES, M.D., F.A.C.P., F.A.C.C., Associate Professor of Medicine, Indiana University School of Medicine, 1100 West Michigan Street, Indianapolis, Indiana 46202.

Chapter 1 The Coronary Arteries in Fatal Coronary Events

WILLIAM C. ROBERTS, M.D.

General Considerations

Coronary or ischemic heart disease (IHD) represents an imbalance between coronary blood flow and myocardial oxygen requirements. Although coronary luminal narrowing from atherosclerosis is the usual cause of inadequate myocardial oxygenation, symptoms of IHD are attributed not to the coronary narrowing but to inadequate myocardial oxygenation. Thus, the myocardium is the *responder* and the coronary artery, the *activator*. The myocardium, however, responds quite differently, both functionally and anatomically, to similar degrees of coronary arterial luminal narrowing: one patient with severe coronary disease, for example, may have "pure" angina pectoris and another with similar degrees of coronary narrowing may have acute myocardial infarction without angina; similarly, a patient with severe coronary narrowing by atherosclerosis may have extensive myocardial scarring, whereas another with apparently similar degrees of coronary narrowing will have no myocardial scarring at all. Since the culprit of IHD resides in the coronary artery and not in the myocardium, this report will focus on the status of these arteries in this condition.

Postmortem Findings of Epicardial Coronary Arteries with Fatal Ischemic Heart Disease

Certain characteristic changes in the epicardial coronary arteries are present at necropsy in patients with fatal ischemic heart disease and these changes will be summarized (2, 6, 17–22) (Table 1-1).

1. *The coronary arteries are diffusely involved by atherosclerotic plaques.* Virtually no segments of any of the major (right, left anterior descending and left circumflex) extramural coronary arteries are free of atherosclerotic plaques. Although the lumens of some segments are narrowed more severely than others, *all portions* of the extramural coronary tree are involved by the atherosclerotic process.

2. *In fatal ischemic heart disease, with rare exception (8, 22) at least one and usually two of the three major coronary arteries are narrowed > 75 percent by old atherosclerotic plaques (Figures 1-1 to 1-3).* The 75-percent demarcation point is useful because it separates normal and abnormal flow. Flow of a fluid (blood) through a tube (coronary artery) is not decreased until at least 75 percent of the lumen is obliterated. Thus a major challenge is not to eliminate coronary

Table 1-1. Status of the Coronary Arteries and Myocardium in Fatal Ischemic Heart Disease

	SCD	AMI		AP
		TM	SE	
Major Coronary Arteries				
Diffuse atherosclerosis	+	+	+	+
Luminal narrowing > 75% of 2 of 3 by atherosclerotic plaques	+	+	+	+
Thrombus	10%	60%	0	0
Hemorrhage into plaque	25%	25%	25%	25%
Left Ventricular Myocardium				
Necrosis	0	+	+	0
Fibrosis (TM or SE)	50%	50%	50%	50%

Abbreviations: AMI = acute myocardial infarction; AP = angina pectoris; SCD = sudden coronary death; SE = subendocardial; TM = transmural

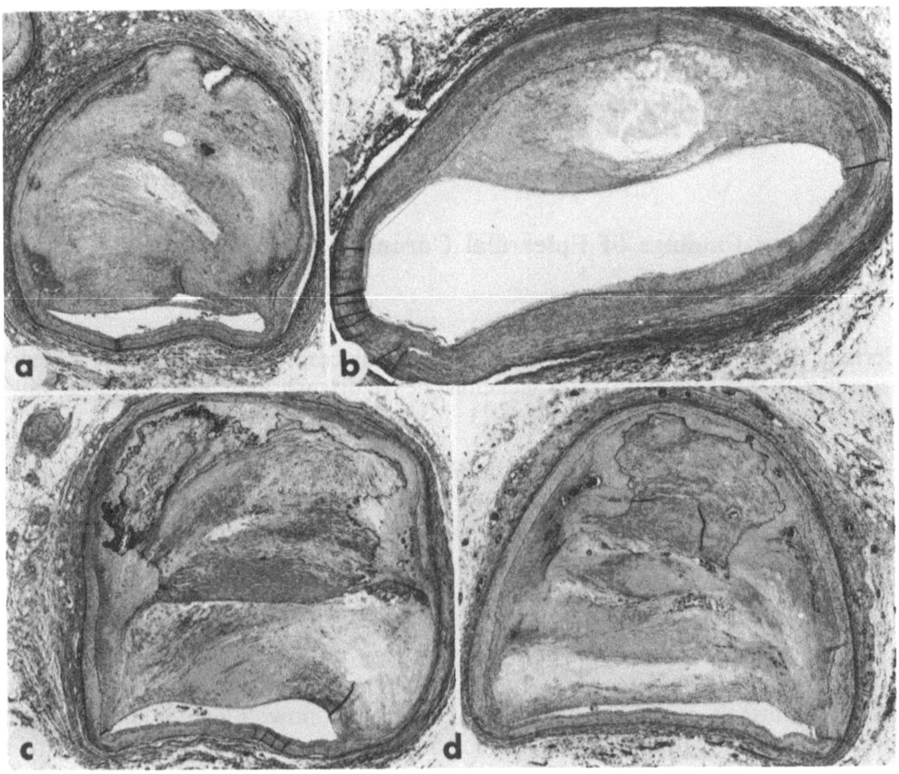

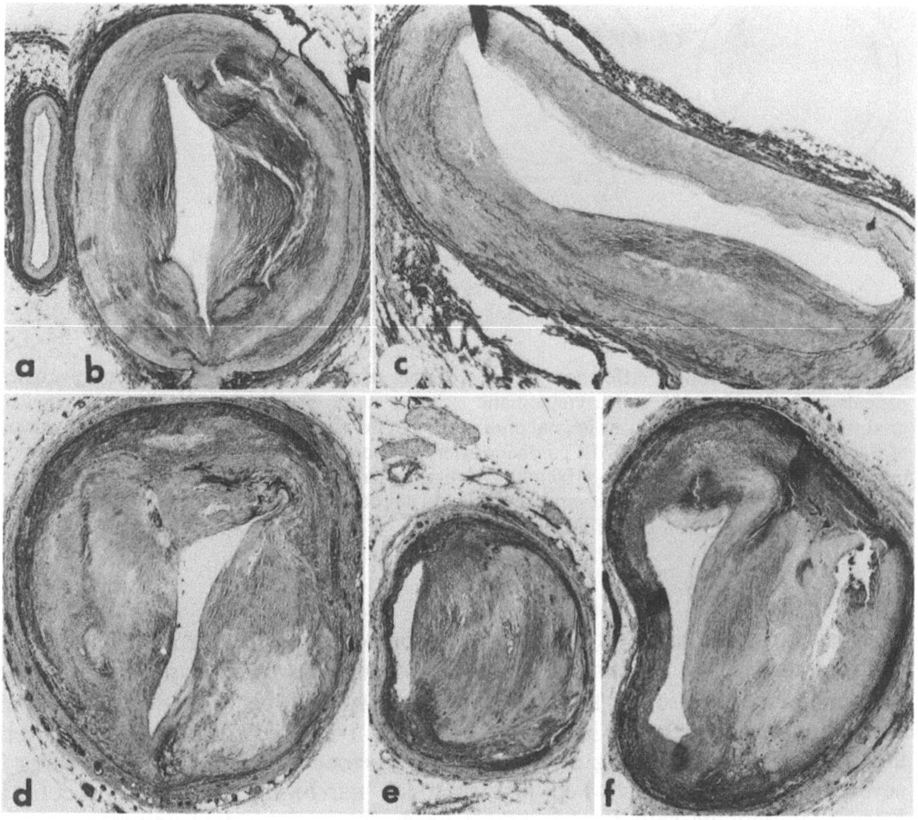

Fig. 1-2. Extramural coronary arteries at sites of maximal narrowing in a 41-year-old man who died suddenly and unexpectedly at home (sudden death). He apparently had no previous symptoms of cardiac disease. At necropsy, the heart weighed 430 g and all major coronary arteries were narrowed > 75 percent by old atherosclerotic plaques. No coronary thrombi or hemorrhages were observed. **(a)** posterior descending branch. It is unusual to find a branch of a major coronary artery normal, and this one is, when the major vessels are severely diseased. **(b)** right, **(c)** left main, **(d)** left circumflex, **(e)** left marginal, and **(f)** left anterior descending coronary arteries (Movat stains, each ×20).

◁

Fig. 1-1. Major extramural coronary arteries at sites of maximal narrowing in a 54-year-old man who died of acute subendocardial myocardial necrosis 12 hours after the onset of chest pain. The patient had angina pectoris and adult onset diabetes mellitus but never suffered congestive heart failure or shock. The heart (weight, 430 g) was severely scarred; left ventricular fibrosis was mainly subendocardial and virtually circumferential from apex to base; rarely, a focus of transmural fibrosis was present. No thrombi or hemorrhages were present in the coronary arteries. **(a)** right, **(b)** left main, **(c)** left circumflex, and **(d)** left anterior descending coronary arteries. All three major coronary arteries were narrowed > 75 percent by old atherosclerotic plaques. The coronary arteries were heavily calcified, a common observation in patients with diabetes mellitus (Movat stains, each ×21).

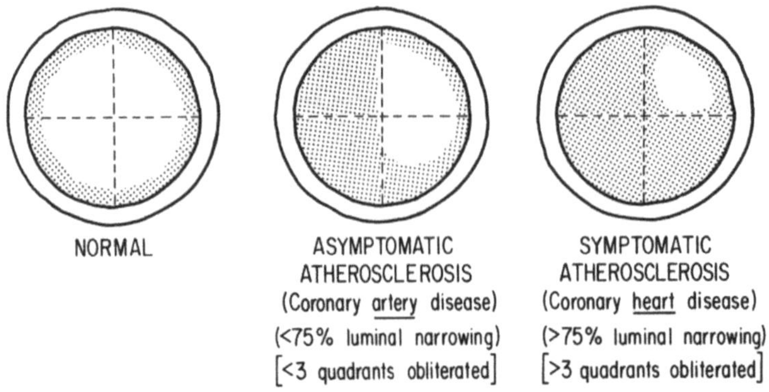

Fig. 1-3. Diagram showing differences between degrees of luminal narrowing of coronary arteries in patients with symptomatic and asymptomatic ischemic heart disease. By age 20, in all population groups worldwide, there is fibrous intimal proliferation in the coronary arteries about equal in thickness to the thickness of the media of the coronary artery. In population groups with hypercholesterolemia (serum cholesterol levels > 200 mg/100 ml) this intimal proliferative process generally continues. Symptoms of myocardial ischemia, with rare exception, do not occur, however, until the intimal proliferative process obliterates > 75% of the lumen.

atherosclerosis but simply to limit to < 75 percent luminal narrowing. Not only is > 75 percent of the lumen of the coronary artery narrowed in patients with fatal ischemic heart disease but this degree of narrowing probably is present in patients with symptomatic ischemic heart disease (Figure 1-3). Study of the coronary arteries in patients who died during or shortly after aortocoronary bypass procedures for severe angina pectoris showed just as much narrowing of the major coronary arteries as patients with fatal ischemic heart disease who died naturally.

3. *The atherosclerotic process is limited to the epicardial coronary arteries*, i.e., the major trunks and their near right-angle branches, and *spares the intramural (intramyocardial) coronary arteries* (Figures 1-4 and 1-5).

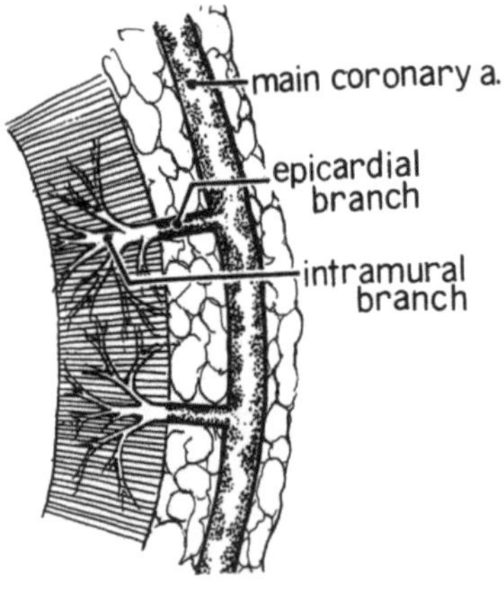

Fig. 1-4. Diagram of a main epicardial coronary artery, its epicardial branches, and the intramural branches. The atherosclerotic process is limited to the epicardial arteries and spares the intramural portions.

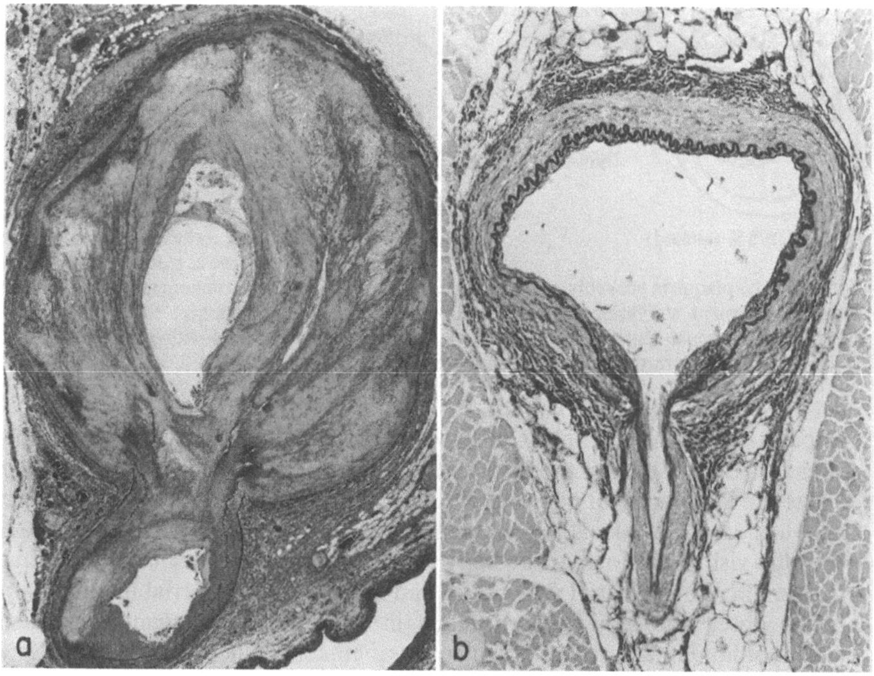

Fig. 1-5. Extramural (epicardial) (a) and intramural (b) coronary arteries in each of 2 patients, both of whom had severe atherosclerosis of the major epicardial trunks and their near right-angle epicardial branches, as shown in **(a)**, but their intramural coronary arteries, as shown in **(b)**, were entirely normal. Atherosclerosis affects the epicardial arteries and spares the intramural coronary arteries (Movat stain **(a)**, ×20; elastic van Gieson stain **(b)**, ×100).

4. *Certain portions of the coronary tree tend to develop larger atherosclerotic plaques, and, therefore, more narrowed lumens, than other portions.* The most severe narrowing of the left anterior descending and left circumflex branches is usually within 2 cm of the bifurcation of the left main; in contrast, the distal third of the right coronary artery usually is more narrowed than the proximal or middle third. The left main coronary artery is narrowed > 75 percent in about 25 percent of patients with fatal ischemic heart disease and the degree of narrowing is indicative of particularly severe diffuse coronary atherosclerosis (all three major coronary arteries > 75 percent narrowed) (3).

5. *Of the so-called three types of atherosclerotic plaques, i.e., lipid, fibrous, and complicated* (7), *only the complicated plaque is responsible for significant* (>75 *percent narrowing) of the lumens of the coronary arteries.* Lipid and fibrous plaques are worldwide in their distribution. The complicated plaque, i.e., those containing calcific deposits, cholesterol clefts, pultaceous debris, and so forth, are found only in populations that develop ischemic heart disease. The major component of even the complicated plaque is fibrous tissue (collagen). It is likely that the fibrous component of the atherosclerotic plaque is irreversible or nondissolvable. In contrast, the lipid component, at least experimentally, is reversible (dissolvable) (1). Whether or not low-lipid diets or lipid-lowering drugs will cause depletion of lipids in complicated

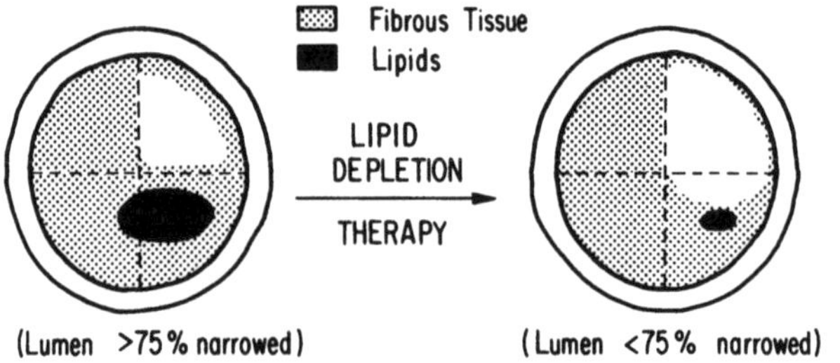

Fig. 1.6. Composition of atherosclerotic plaque in symptomatic coronary disease and the possible effect of lipid lowering or lipid withdrawal, on its composition and luminal size. Although the dominant component of atherosclerotic plaques is fibrous tissue, lipid deposits, usually extracellular, form a portion of most plaques. The fibrous component of the plaque is probably nonreversible. In contrast, the lipid component may well be reversible. Possibly, transient starvation may cause the size of the lipid component to diminish and possibly decrease the luminal narrowing from >75% (the amount associated with symptoms, Figure 5), to <75% (an amount rarely associated with symptoms).

symptom-producing coronary atherosclerotic plaques is uncertain. Although fat stores in the body consist predominantly of triglycerides, and atherosclerotic plaques consist predominantly of cholesterol esters, the latter, nevertheless, might decrease in size when caloric intake is low enough to cause a decrease in the size of fat deposits in readily visible portions of the body (anterior panniculus, for example). Emaciated prisoners in World War II apparently had little coronary arterial luminal narrowing. Similar observations have been made in victims of malignant neoplasms. The amount of lipid in atherosclerotic plaques of emaciated necropsy patients appears to be less than that observed in nonemaciated necropsy patients.

Transient starvation may well be a neglected but beneficial form of therapy (possibly also a form of prevention) for symptomatic ischemic heart disease. If the

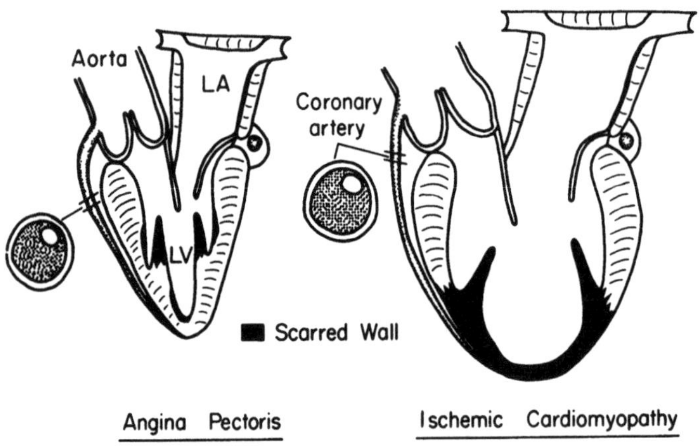

	Angina Pectoris	Ischemic Cardiomyopathy
CHF	0	Severe
LV cavity	Normal size	Very dilated
LV scarring	Subendocardial	Transmural
Coronary atherosclerosis	Severe	Severe
LV aneurysm	0	Usually

Fig. 1-7. The spectrum of ischemic heart disease. **CHF** = congestive heart failure; **LA** = left atrium; **LV** = left ventricle.

lumen of a coronary artery is obliterated 90 percent by atherosclerotic plaques, for example, generally about 25 percent of the plaque consists of lipid deposits, the depletion of which would allow the lumen to narrow < 75 percent; there is no decrease in the amount of flow through a tube (artery) until it is narrowed > 75 percent (Figure 1-6). As long as the lumen of a coronary artery is < 75 percent narrowed, symptoms of myocardial ischemia rarely occur (Figure 1-3).

6. *The degree of coronary arterial luminal narrowing by atherosclerotic plaques and the extensiveness of plaquing are similar in patients with fatal IHD irrespective of the type of fatal coronary event* (*Table 1-1*). No significant differences in the amount of coronary atherosclerotic plaquing have been observed in patients dying of angina pectoris (without clinically apparent acute myocardial infarction at any time), either subendocardial or transmural acute myocardial infarction, progressive congestive cardiac failure after healing of an acute myocardial infarct or a sudden arrhythmia (sudden coronary death) (23) (Figure 1-7). Although the degree of coronary luminal narrowing by atherosclerotic plaques is similar in each of the above coronary events, the myocardial reaction obviously is quite different. Patients who died suddenly from severe coronary atherosclerosis and those with severe fatal angina pectoris infrequently have severe congestive cardiac failure (Figure 1-8). The reason for the differences in myocardial response to apparently similar degrees of coronary atherosclerosis is uncertain.

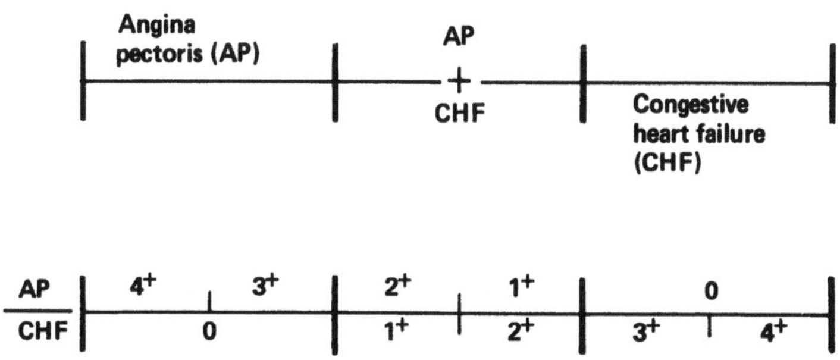

Fig. 1-8. Spectrum of angina pectoris and congestive cardiac failure in ischemic heart disease.

7. *The composition of coronary atherosclerotic plaques and the degree of coronary arterial luminal narrowing in patients with fatal IHD appears similar, irrespective of whether or not the blood lipoprotein pattern is normal or abnormal* (24) (Figures 1-9 and 1-10). Patients with types II, III, or IV hyperlipoproteinemia clearly have accelerated atherosclerosis as compared to persons of similar age and sex with normal lipoprotein patterns. However, hyperlipoproteinemia is not a prerequisite for premature development of severe atherosclerosis (24). Severe narrowing of the left main coronary artery is more common in patients with type II hyperlipoproteinemia than in patients with type III or IV hyperlipoproteinemia or in persons with normal lipoprotein patterns (3). Furthermore, atherosclerosis of the ascending aorta may be prominent in patients with type 2 hyperlipoproteinemia; this is especially true if the hyperlipoproteinemia is of the homozygous rather than the

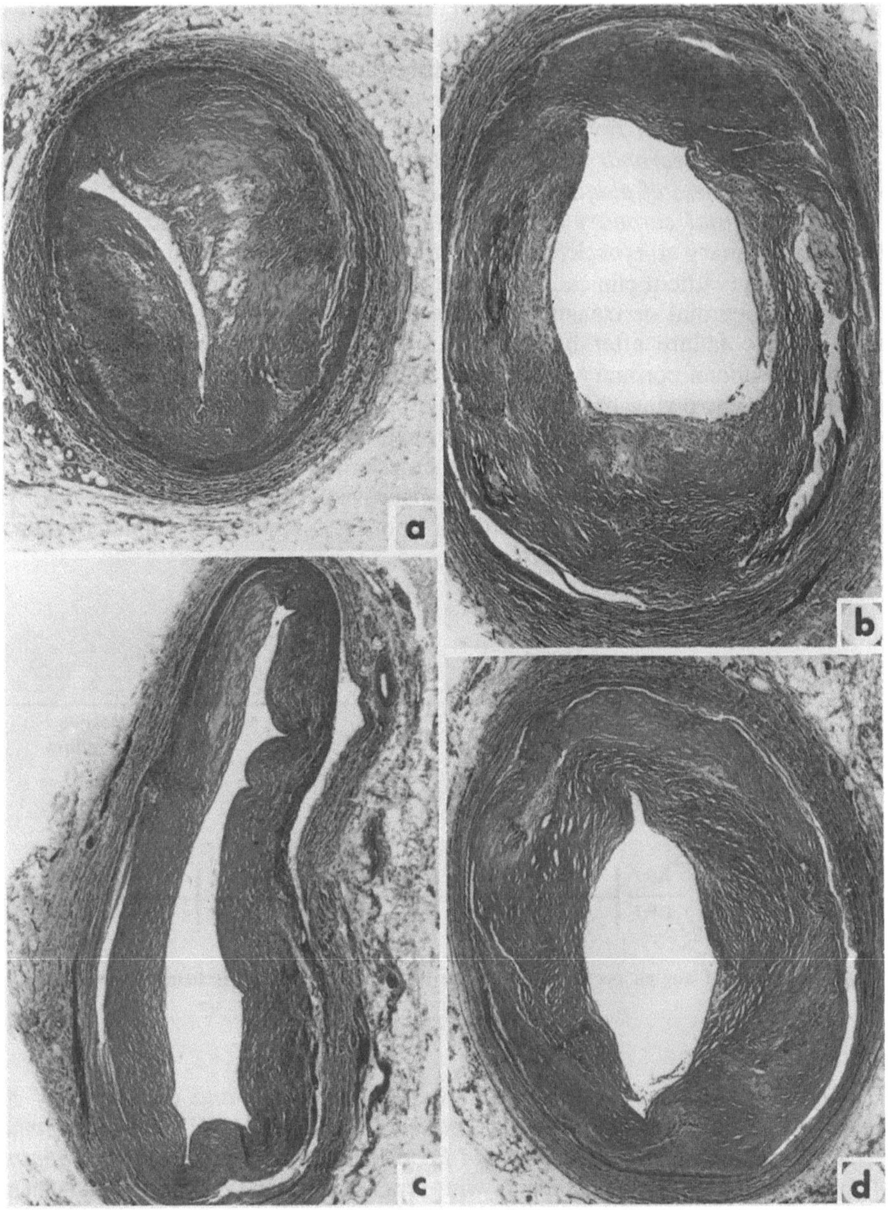
a
b
c
d

Fig. 1-9. Major extramural coronary arteries in a 29-year-old woman with heterozygous type II hyperlipoproteinemia. She had had angina pectoris for 4 years and died suddenly. The atherosclerotic plaques consist primarily of fibrous tissue despite very elevated serum cholesterol levels. Shown is right **(a)**, left main **(b)**, left anterior descending **(c)**, and left circumflex **(d)** coronary arteries (Hematoxylin-eosin stains, each ×33).

◁

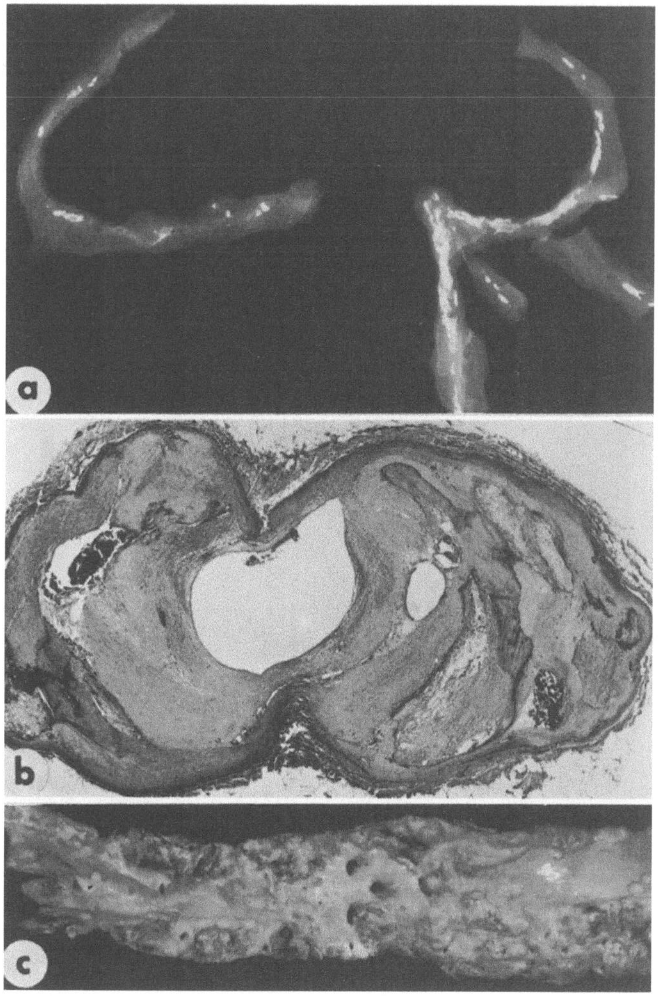

Fig. 1-10. Coronary arteries **(a** and **b)** and aorta **(c)** in a 47-year-old man with type II hyperlipoproteinemia. He died suddenly. He had had angina pectoris for 2 years but never had clinical evidence of acute myocardial infarction or congestive cardiac failure. **(a)** There are heavy calcific deposits in the more proximal portions of the left coronary artery, but few calcific deposits in the right coronary artery. (b) Photomicrograph at bifurcation of the left main into the left anterior descending and left circumflex coronary arteries. The left main coronary artery as well as the proximal portions of both left anterior descending and left circumflex coronary arteries are severely narrowed. **(c)** Extensive atherosclerotic plaquing in the aorta; the abdominal portion is shown here (Movat stain **(b)**, × 15).

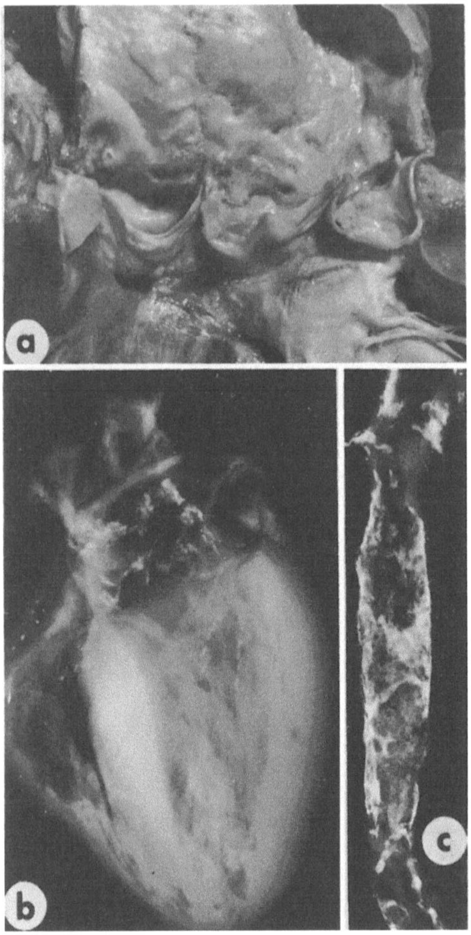

Fig. 1-11. Heart and aorta in a 51-year-old man with heterozygous type II hyperlipoproteinemia. During life he had a grade 2/6 systolic ejection murmur interpreted as evidence of "aortic stenosis." At necropsy, there were small calcific deposits present on the aortic aspects of each cusp, but the cusps were freely mobile and the valve orifice was not stenotic. **(a)** Opened ascending aorta, aortic valve, and left ventricle. Although extensive atherosclerotic plaquing is present in the ascending aorta, the degree is far less than that observed in the patient with homozygous Type II hyperlipoproteinemia (Figure 16). **(b)** Radiograph of heart specimen disclosing calcific deposits in the aortic valve, root of aorta, and coronary arteries. **(c)** Radiograph of abdominal aorta showing extensive calcific deposits.

heterozygous variety (24) (Figure 1-11). Also, in the homozygous form, the coronary ostia may be narrowed severely by aortic atherosclerosis, which also may involve the aortic valve cusps directly.

8. *The shapes of lumens of atherosclerotic coronary arteries are quite variable* (Figure 1-12). The residual lumen may be located centrally or peripherally and its shape may be circular, oval, slit-like or half-moon. The slit-like lumen which extends from one side of the artery to the other may appear as a normal-sized orifice on angiography.

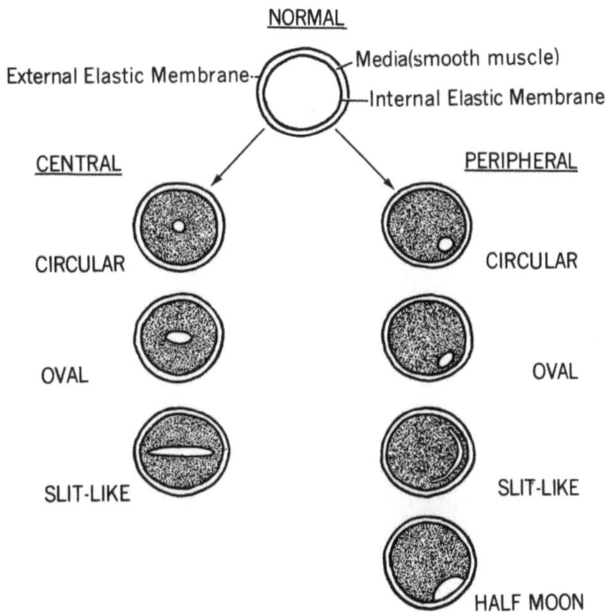

Fig. 1-12. Diagram showing various shapes and locations of lumens in narrowed coronary arteries.

9. *Although the number one risk factor to development of symptomatic atherosclerosis in the Western World is advanced age, it does not necessarily indicate the presence of severe coronary atherosclerosis.* Shown in Figure 1-13 are sections of coronary arteries at sites of maximal luminal narrowing in a 100-year-old woman who died of a noncardiovascular condition. Actually, acute myocardial infarction is infrequent in patients over 90 years of age. The explanation probably lies in the fact that these arteries dilate as the years progress (Figure 1-14), unless extensive atherosclerotic plaques develop within them, and then the plaques prevent this "normal" dilatation. Obviously, the greater the dilatation, the wider the lumen.

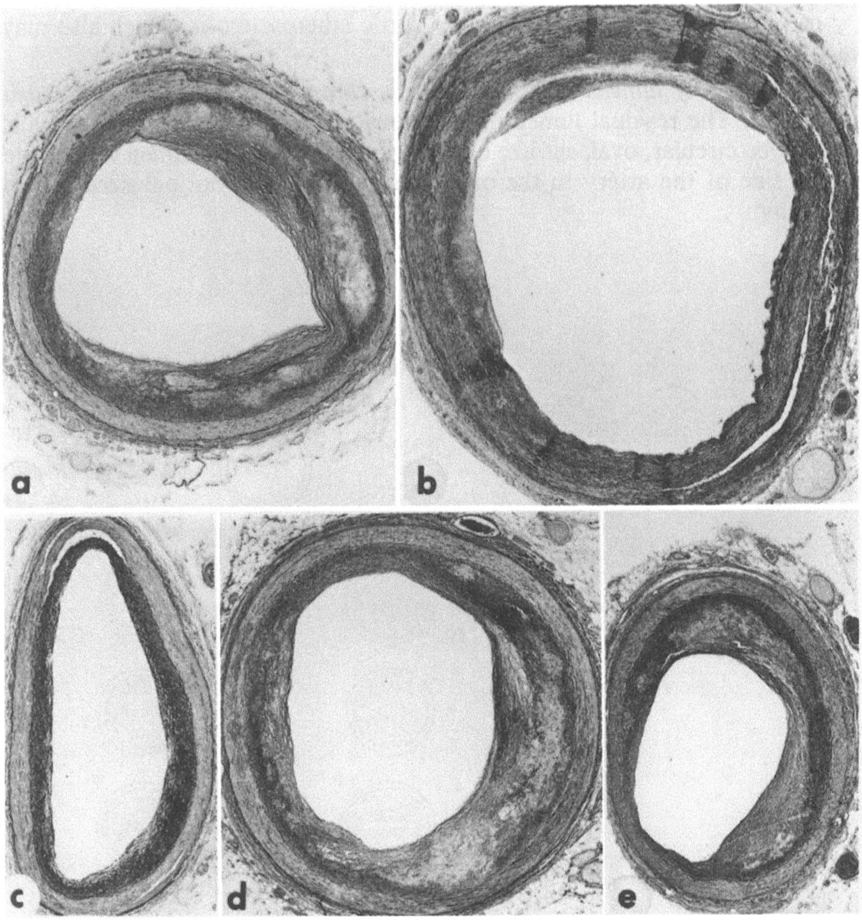

Fig. 1-13. Major extramural coronary arteries at sites of maximal narrowing in a 100-year-old woman who died of a noncardiac condition. Although each artery contains some atherosclerotic plaques, the vessels are actually dilated and the lumens, wide open. Severe atherosclerosis, in other words, is not necessarily a consequence of advanced age. Shown are right **(a)**, left main **(b)**, left circumflex **(c)**, left anterior descending **(d)**, and left diagonal **(e)** coronary arteries, each at the same magnification (×16). Elastic van Gieson stains on each.

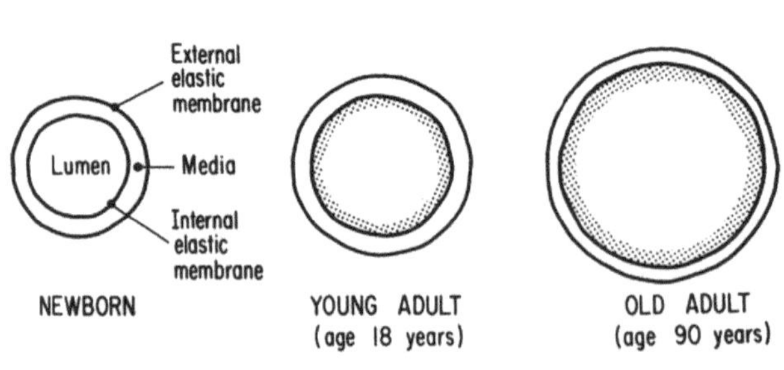

Fig. 1-14. Diagram showing relative size of coronary arteries at various ages. The intimal lesion (**hatched areas**) represent fibromuscular proliferation, presumably a response to the intraarterial pressure and not a form of atherosclerosis.

Postmortem Findings of Acute or Recent Lesions in Major Coronary Arteries with Fatal Ischemic Heart Disease

Some observations on acute or recent lesions in major coronary arteries of patients with fatal acute ischemic heart disease are summarized as follows:

1. *Among patients with fatal ischemic heart disease thrombi are infrequent (about 10 percent) in patients who die suddenly and in those in whom necrosis is limited to the subendocardium* (*22*) (*Table 1-1*). (*Sudden coronary death* is defined herein as that occurring within 6 hours after the onset of symptoms of myocardial ischemia and unassociated with histologic evidence of myocardial necrosis; subendocardium, as the inner one-half of the myocardial wall.)

2. *Thrombus is found in a coronary artery in about 60 percent of patients with fatal transmural acute myocardial infarction* (*22*). In about 80 percent the thrombus is occlusive, i.e., it obliterates the residual lumen entirely; in the other 20 percent it is mural, usually causing no significant additional luminal narrowing.

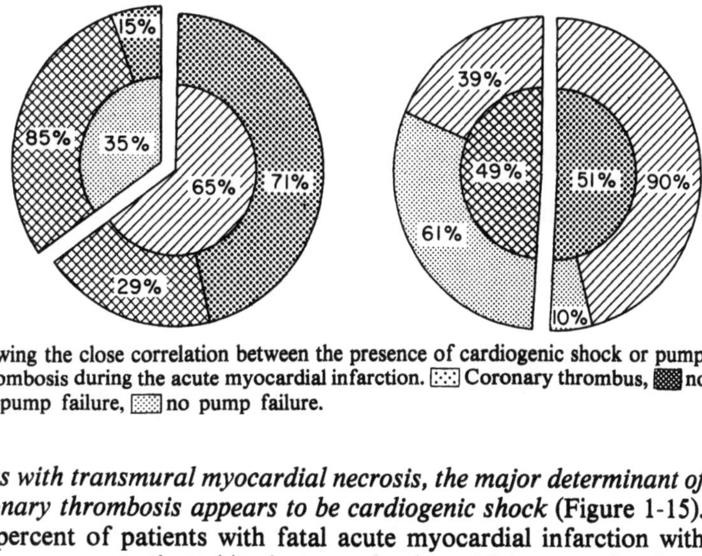

Fig. 1-15. Diagram showing the close correlation between the presence of cardiogenic shock or pump failure and coronary thrombosis during the acute myocardial infarction. [dotted] Coronary thrombus, [dark] no coronary thrombus, [hatched] pump failure, [stippled] no pump failure.

3. *Among patients with transmural myocardial necrosis, the major determinant of the presence of coronary thrombosis appears to be cardiogenic shock* (Figure 1-15). At necropsy > 70 percent of patients with fatal acute myocardial infarction with cardiogenic shock have coronary thrombi, whereas only about 15 percent of patients without the power failure syndrome associated with fatal acute myocardial infarction have coronary thrombi (27). Tissue necrosis itself, especially in a shock situation, also appears to increase blood coagulability.

4. *The larger the area of myocardial necrosis, the greater the likelihood of coronary thrombosis.* The larger the infarcted area, however, the greater the likelihood of cardiogenic shock. The latter generally indicates that > 40 percent of the left ventricular wall is either necrotic, or fibrotic, or both, whereas shock is infrequently associated with infarcts or scars involving < 40 percent of the ventricular wall (16).

5. *When coronary thrombosis is associated with acute myocardial infarction, the thrombus is always located in the artery responsible for perfusing the area of myocardial necrosis* (*22*). Thus in anterior wall infarction a thrombus, if present, will be located in the left anterior descending coronary artery.

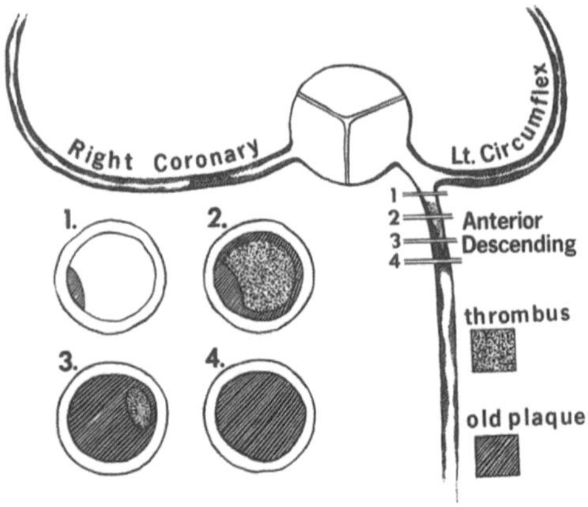

Fig. 1-16. Diagram illustrating the diffuse nature of coronary atherosclerosis and the usual status of a vessel at and distal to a thrombus. At level 2, in the anterior descending artery, the lumen is obstructed primarily by a thrombus. At level 3, however, the major percent of narrowing is the result of old atherosclerotic plaquing and just distal to the thrombus, the lumen is severely narrowed (>75%) or totally obstructed by old plaque only.

6. *In fatal ischemic heart disease thrombi occur in coronary arteries already severely narrowed by old atherosclerotic plaques* (Figures 1-16 and 1-17). At the distal site of attachment of the thrombus, or just distal to this site, the lumen of the coronary artery is nearly always > 75 percent narrowed by old atherosclerotic plaques. Not infrequently, a thrombus may occur in an area between two sites of severe narrowing, like in a valley between two mountains.

7. *Coronary thrombi in fatal acute myocardial infarction are usually (90 percent) single, occlusive (80 percent), short (<2 cm long), and located entirely in the major trunks* (as opposed to their near right-angle branches or intramural coronary arteries). The thrombus, when only a few hours old, may consist nearly entirely of

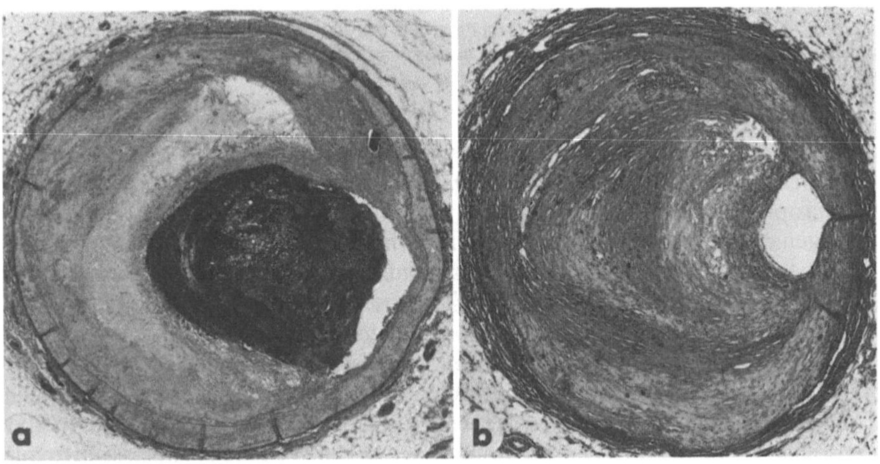

Fig. 1-17. Coronary artery thrombosis and the artery most distal to the thrombus in a patient with fatal acute transmural myocardial infarction (**a and b**). Left circumflex coronary artery in a 57-year-old woman who died 4 days after onset of myocardial necrosis. **(a)** At site where the thrombus is large, **(b)** just distal to the distal site of attachment of the thrombus (Movat stains, each ×21).

platelets, but thereafter is composed primarily of fibrin. By definition, the thrombus is *adherent* to the surface of the arterial wall bordering the lumen. The most "downstream" portion of the thrombus may differ in composition from the most "upstream" portions: the former contains more platelets or later may consist entirely of fibrin; the latter may contain no platelets but many erythrocytes and this portion may not be adherent to the inner lining of the atherosclerotic plaque. Almost surely, the thrombus enlarges by growing backwards or toward the coronary ostia.

Since 1912 when Herrick first described the often dramatic clinical event characterized at necropsy by necrosis of portions of the left ventricular wall, it has been assumed that the usual cause of acute myocardial infarction is coronary thrombosis (12, 13). Two factors implicate coronary thrombosis as the *precipitating cause* of acute myocardial infarction: (a) coronary arterial thrombi in many patients with fatal acute myocardial infarction and (b) the location of the thrombus in the coronary artery responsible for supplying the area of myocardial necrosis. Five factors, however, tend to indicate that coronary thrombosis is a consequence rather than the precipitating cause of acute myocardial infarction: (a) the very low frequency of thrombi in patients who died suddenly, with or without previous evidence of cardiac disease, (b) the increasing frequency of thrombi with increasing intervals between onset of symptoms of acute myocardial infarction and death; (c) the absence of thrombi nearly as often as they are present in fatal transmural acute myocardial infarction; (d) the near absence of thrombi in fatal subendocardial acute myocardial infarction; and (e) a high percentage of thrombi only in patients in cardiogenic shock, most of whom have large transmural infarcts.

The key to coronary thrombosis, as to thrombosis anywhere in the body, is *slow blood flow,* or relative stasis and sufficient time for the thrombus to form. The absence of these two factors may explain the absence of coronary thrombosis in cases of sudden death, and the increasing frequency of thrombosis as the interval from onset of symptoms of myocardial ischemia to death increases (25, 26). Blood flow in the coronary artery responsible for supplying the area of myocardial infarction is markedly reduced. This observation was made in dogs after acute myocardial infarction was induced and the animals had normal, i.e., widely patent vessels (11). In fatal acute myocardial infarction in humans, the thrombus is always located in an artery already containing considerable atherosclerotic plaques, and, therefore, the infarct-induced relative coronary stasis is probably even greater. Cardiogenic shock must further diminish coronary flow.

The type of activity experienced by patients at the time of onset of acute myocardial infarction may reflect slowed blood flow. In nearly 75 percent of patients with acute myocardial infarction the onset of chest pain occurs during sleep, rest, or mild activity (14). Although inactivity may cause a slight diminution in coronary blood flow, considerable stasis of blood (infarction induced plus cardiogenic shock) is usually necessary for a thrombus to form. In contrast to fatal acute myocardial infarction, coronary thrombosis is rarely observed in fatal angina pectoris. Evidence of thrombus formation is nearly always observed in arteries implanted into the left ventricular myocardium, but if the implant is allowed to drain into the right ventricular cavity, no thrombus occurs (28). Thus, it appears that a period of diminished coronary blood flow is necessary for a thrombus to form in a coronary artery. Shock, congestive cardiac failure, and inactivity all decrease coronary flow and, with time, may allow thrombosis.

Further support for the concept that coronary thrombosis is a consequence of rather than a precipitating cause of acute myocardial infarction was supplied recently by Erhardt and associates (9) who observed radioactivity at necropsy in coronary arterial thrombi in patients with acute myocardial infarction who had been given radioactive [^{125}I] labeled fibrinogen after admission. This finding implicated coronary thrombosis as a secondary event, occurring sometime after the infarction.

Thus there is substantial evidence that acute thrombus formation does not precipitate acute fatal ischemic heart disease. The major problem is diffuse generalized coronary atherosclerosis with severe (>75 percent) luminal narrowing (at least two of the three major coronary arteries).

Acute Lesions Other than Thrombi in Coronary Arteries Postmortem

Acute lesions other than thrombi in coronary arteries are summarized below:

1. *Hemorrhage into an old atherosclerotic plaque* (Figure 1-18). Hemorrhages into coronary atherosclerotic plaques are observed in about 25 percent of patients with fatal ischemic heart disease (22). Even when hemorrhage into plaques occur, however, the lumen of the coronary artery is not further narrowed. Plaque hemorrhages have no relationship to the site of myocardial necrosis; when a thrombus is observed in a coronary artery, it corresponds to the site of necrosis. When the infarction is in the anterior wall and a coronary thrombus occurs, the latter is located

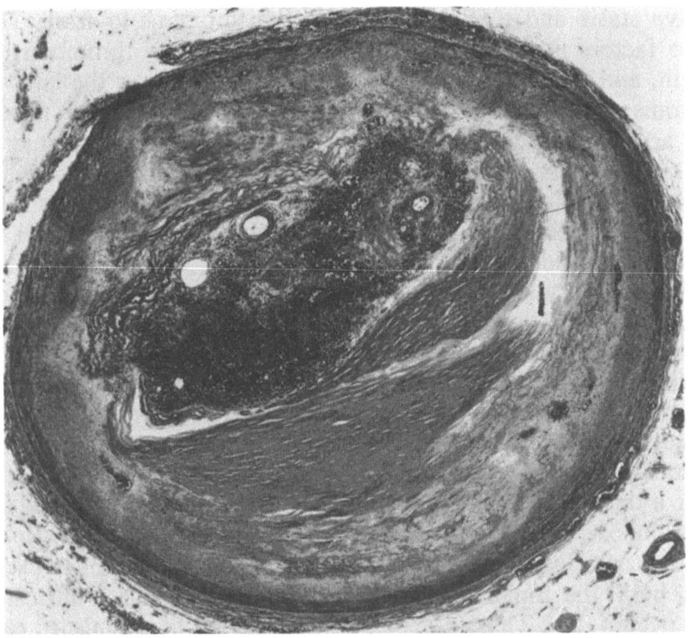

Fig. 1-18. Hemorrhage into an atherosclerotic plaque. Shown are photomicrographs of the left circumflex coronary artery in a 63-year-old hypertensive man who died suddenly and unexpectedly. The above artery is severely narrowed and three small channels are present in the plaque in the area of the hemorrhage, which does not appear to further narrow the lumen (Hematoxylin-eosin stain, ×27).

in the left anterior descending coronary artery. Except in rare instances, other thrombi are not found in the right or left circumflex coronary arteries. In contrast, when hemorrhages occur into atherosclerotic plaques they bear no relation to the site of myocardial necrosis. The anterior wall may be the site of infarction, but the hemorrhage may involve a plaque in the right coronary artery, all three coronary arteries, or multiple sites in a single coronary artery. It is possible that plaque hemorrhages occur throughout the adult life of patients with and without symptomatic ischemic heart disease. Although there are dissenting views, it appears unlikely that plaque hemorrhages are responsible for precipitating acute myocardial

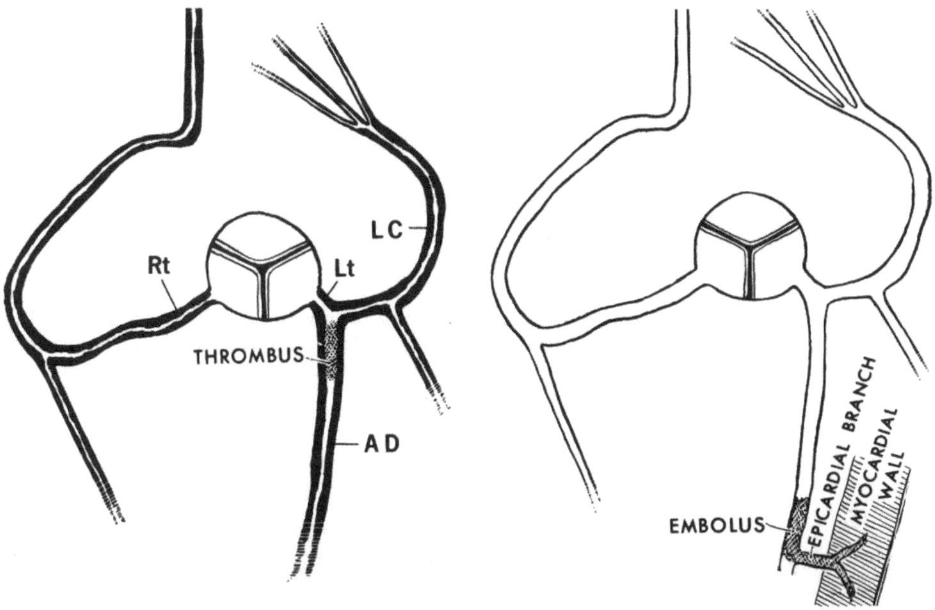

Fig. 1-19. Diagram depicting differences between coronary arterial thrombosis and embolism. The thrombus is usually proximal and superimposed on old atherosclerotic plaques. The thrombus does not extend into intramural coronary arteries. The embolus is distal and usually extends into an intramural artery. The embolus usually occurs in a coronary tree devoid of significant old atherosclerotic plaques.

ischemia because they do not narrow the lumen and they are not necessarily related to sites of myocardial necrosis. The frequency of hemorrhages into plaques is not increased by the use of anticoagulants.

2. *Coronary arterial embolism* (Figures 1-19 to 1-22). This is a rare cause of fatal ischemic heart disease. Diagnosis of embolism requires identification of the site from which the embolus dislodged or at least a condition predisposing to the development of embolism, such as infective endocarditis, intracardiac mural thrombus, cardiac catheterization or operation, or a coagulopathy. Embolism is extremely difficult to recognize when superimposed on an extensively atherosclerotic coronary arterial tree. Thus, diagnosis of embolism usually requires the presence of a clot in a coronary tree devoid of heavy atherosclerotic plaques. Furthermore, in contrast to coronary thrombosis, which never involves the intramural coronary arteries and infre-

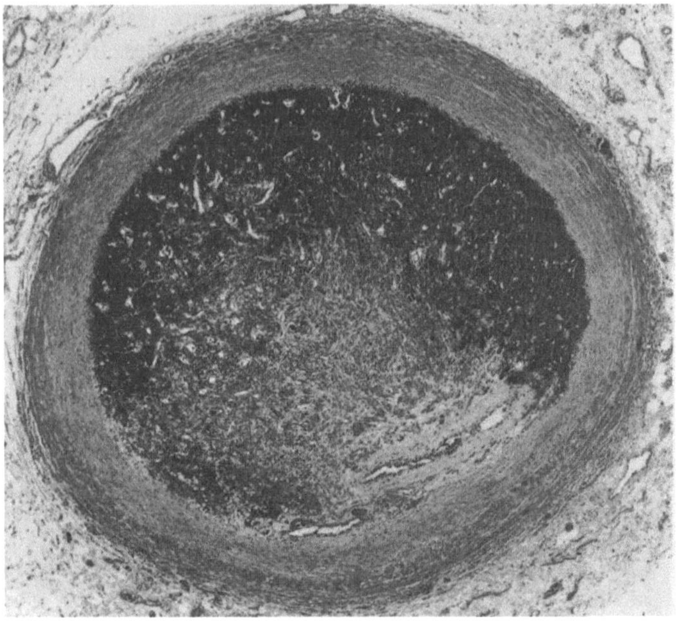

Fig. 1-20. Occluded distal right coronary artery by embolus in a 56-year-old man who died 31 days after onset of acute myocardial infarction, which began during cardiac catheterization, performed because of severe mitral regurgitation. This embolus fills the entire lumen and there is no underlying atherosclerosis (Hematoxylin-eosin stain, ×25).

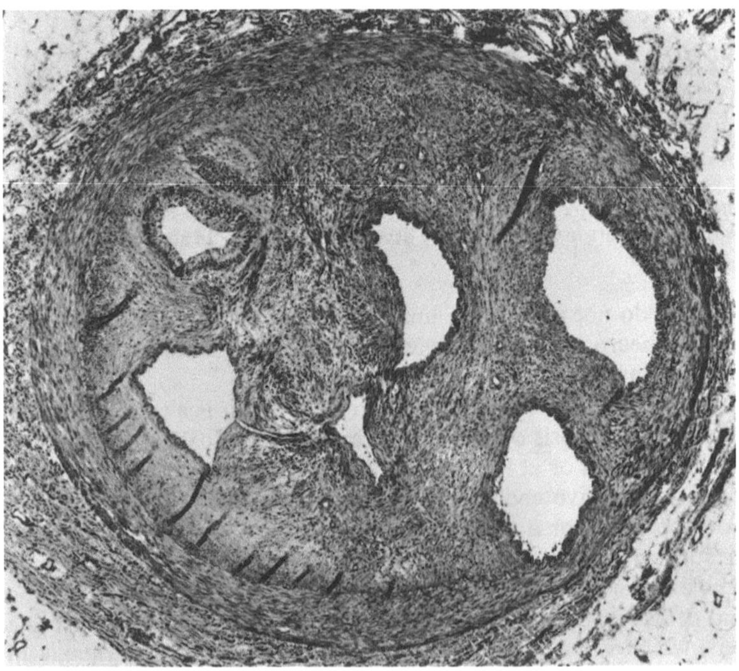

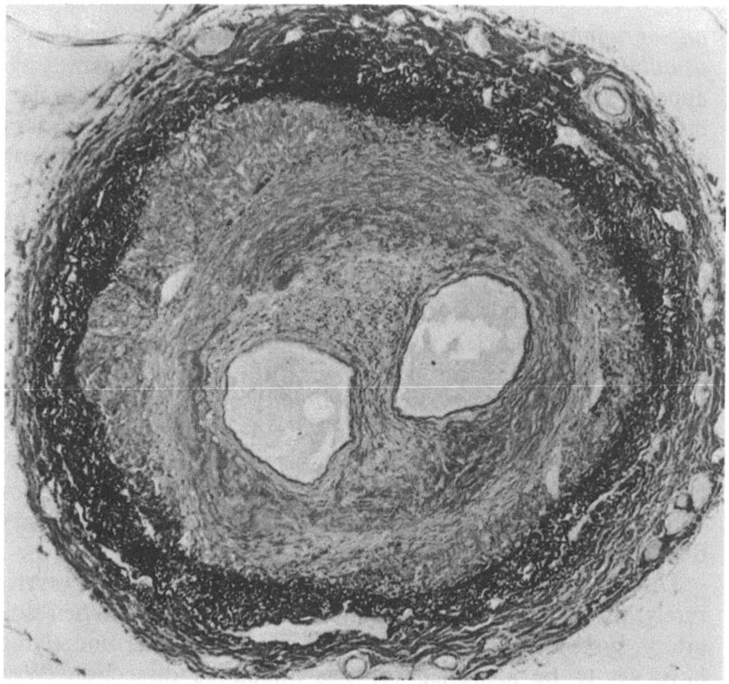

Fig. 1-22. Most often multiple luminal channels are observed in coronary trees which show severe luminal narrowing in other areas with only a single channel. Shown here is a section of left circumflex coronary artery in a 58-year-old man who had had an acute myocardial infarct at age 54 and the onset of another one about 1 hour before death. Multiple luminal channels are present. The occurrence of multiple luminal channels suggests organization of clot—either thrombus or embolus (Elastic van Gieson stain, ×20).

quently involves the distal portions of the extramural coronary arteries, embolism generally involves both the intra- and extramural arteries, usually the distal portions of the latter.

In recent years a number of publications described patients with "myocardial infarction and angiographically normal coronary arteries" (10, 15). Despite clinical papers on this subject, there have been no necropsy studies, to our knowledge, on patients with this clinical combination unassociated with an additional cardiac disorder, such as valvular aortic stenosis or hypertrophic cardiomyopathy. It is essential to keep in mind that normal coronary arteries in this circumstance means *angiographically normal,* not necessary anatomically normal, and that

---

◁

Fig. 1-21. Recanalized embolus in distal anterior descending coronary artery of a 26-year-old man who developed a massive anterior wall acute myocardial infarct 3 years earlier at the time he had infective endocarditis of the aortic valve. This process clearly resulted from organization of fibrin-platelet-erythrocyte-leukeocyte clot, almost surely embolus, and similar lesions are found in patients with extensive coronary arterial atherosclerosis. Note that each recanalized channel has developed its own internal elastic membrane and smooth muscle medial wall (Hematoxylin-eosin stain, ×46).

angiographic studies were not done at the time of the acute myocardial infarction but usually several months later, at which time the patient was again asymptomatic. It appears unlikely that all major coronary arteries were normal at the time of the acute myocardial infarction. Indeed there are no reports demonstrating normal coronary arteries angiographically at the time of acute myocardial infarction. It is unlikely that spasm of a normal coronary artery can produce sufficient narrowing to cause myocardial necrosis. The most reasonable explanation for myocardial infarction with normal coronary is coronary embolism. Such occlusion of a previously normal extramural coronary artery by a clot virtually always produces acute myocardial infarction. The embolus organizes, most likely by developing large channels within it (recanalized channels), which on angiography some time later appear as normal vessels.

3. *Dissecting aneurysm (hematoma) of a coronary artery with and without associated dissection of aorta* (Figure 1-23). Dissection of one or both coronary arteries, causing luminal narrowing, is commonly associated with dissection of the aorta. The resulting myocardial ischemia in this circumstance may be fatal. Virtually all patients with aortic dissecting aneurysm, with or without associated dissection of the coronary arteries, have systemic hypertension.

Dissection of one or more major coronary arteries, however, may occur, although rarely, in the absence of dissection of the aorta (5). When isolated to the coronary artery, systemic hypertension is infrequent but other underlying precipitating causes have yet to be identified for this idiopathic dissection. Women are more often affected than men; death is usually sudden and there is no histologic evidence of

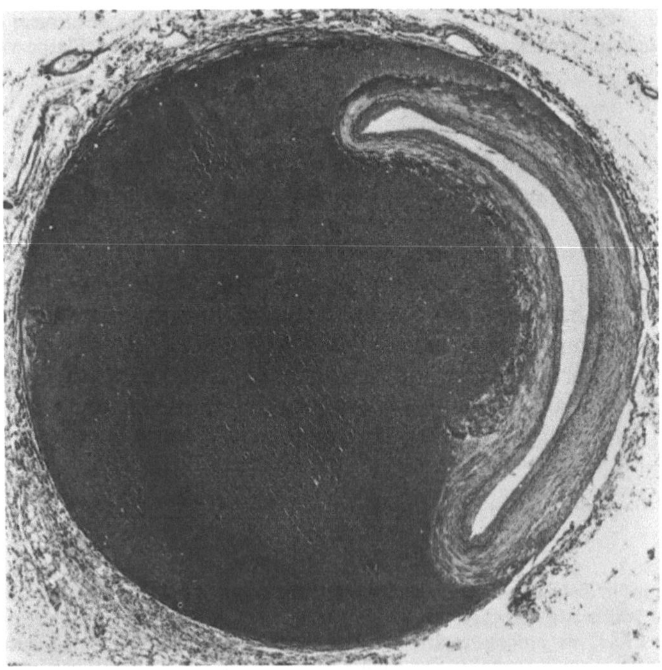

Fig. 1-23. Isolated coronary arterial dissection (hematoma) in a 66-year-old woman. The dissection of the left anterior descending coronary artery caused instantaneous death.

myocardial necrosis. In addition to the idiopathic variety, isolated coronary dissection may be iatrogenic in origin: a result of coronary angiography coronary bypass operations (4), or cardiac massage.

Summary

In fatal ischemic heart disease the coronary arteries may be characterized as follows: (a) atherosclerosis is diffuse, not focal; (b) usually the lumens of two of the three major coronary arteries are narrowed > 75 percent by old atherosclerotic plaques; (c) the atherosclerotic process is limited to the epicardial arteries, and spares the intramural arteries; (d) certain portions develop more severe atherosclerosis than do others; (e) of the three types of atherosclerotic plaques, only the complicated ones cause significant (>75 percent) luminal narrowing; (f) the degree of luminal narrowing by atherosclerotic plaques is similar irrespective of the type of fatal coronary event; (g) the composition of the atherosclerotic plaque and the degree of luminal narrowing appears similar irrespective of whether the blood lipoprotein pattern had been normal or abnormal; and (h) advanced age does not necessarily indicate the presence of severe atherosclerosis.

Certain observations regarding coronary thrombosis in fatal ischemic heart disease are becoming established: (a) thrombi are infrequent (about 10 percent) in patients who die suddenly and in those in whom myocardial necrosis is limited to the subendocardium; (b) a thrombus is found in the coronary artery in about 60 percent of patients with fatal transmural acute myocardial infarction; (c) in transmural acute myocardial infarction, the major determinant of coronary thrombosis is cardiogenic shock; (d) the larger the area of myocardial necrosis, the greater the likelihood of coronary thrombosis; (e) a coronary thrombus is always located in the artery responsible for perfusing the area of myocardial necrosis; (f) thrombi occur in coronary arteries already severely narrowed by atherosclerotic plaques; (g) coronary thrombi are usually (90 percent) single, usually (80 percent) occlusive, short (< 2 cm long), and located entirely in the major epicardial trunks (as opposed to their near right-angle branches or intramural coronary arteries); and (h) coronary emboli may be distinguished from thrombi by their distal occurrence in arteries relatively free of atherosclerotic plaques.

References

1. Armstrong, M. L. and Megan, M. B. Lipid depletion in atheromatous coronary arteries in Rhesus monkeys after regression diets. Circ. Res., 30:675, 1972.
2. Buja, L. M. and Roberts, W. C. The coronary arteries and myocardium in acute myocardial infarction and shock. In Gunnar, R. M., Loeb, H. S., and Rahimtoola, S. H. eds. Shock in Myocardial Infarction. New York, Grune and Stratton, 1974, p. 1.
3. Bulkley, B. H. and Roberts, W. C. Severe (>75%) narrowing of left main coronary artery: an indication of generalized severe coronary atherosclerosis. Circulation, 49 and 50: Suppl. 3:150, 1974.
4. ——— Isolated coronary arterial dissection. A complication of cardiac operations. J. Thorac. Cardiovasc. Surg., 67:148, 1974.
5. ——— Dissecting aneurysm (hematomal) limited to coronary artery. A clinicopathologic study of six patients. Am J. Med., 55:747, 1973.

6. Chandler, A. B., Chapman, I., Erhardt, L. R., Roberts, W. C., Schwartz, C. J., Sinapius, D., Spain, D. M., Sherry, S., Ness, P. M., and Simon, T. L. Coronary thrombosis in myocardial infarction. Report of a workshop on the role of coronary thrombosis in the pathogenesis of acute myocardial infarction. Am. J. Cardiol., 34:823, 1974.
7. Classification of atherosclerosis lesions. Reports of a study group. W.H.O. Tech. Rep. Ser. 143, 1958.
8. Eliot, R. S., Baroldi, G., and Leone, A. Necropsy studies in myocardial infarction with minimal or no coronary luminal reduction due to atherosclerosis. Circulation, 49:1127, 1974.
9. Erhardt, L. R., Lundman, T., and Mellstedt, H. Incorporation of ^{125}I-labelled fibrinogen into coronary arterial thrombi in acute myocardial infarction in man. Lancet, 1:387, 1973.
10. Glancy, D. L., Marcus, M. L., and Epstein, S. E. Myocardial infarction in young women with normal coronary arteriograms. Circulation, 44:495, 1971.
11. Hellstrom, H. R. Coronary artery stasis after induced myocardial infarction in the dog. Cardiovasc. Res., 5:371, 1971.
12. Herrick, J. B. Thrombosis of the coronary arteries. J.A.M.A., 72:387, 1919.
13. —— Clinical features of sudden obstruction of the coronary arteries. J.A.M.A., 59:2015, 1912.
14. Master, A. M., Dack, S., and Jaffe, H. L. Activities associated with the onset of acute coronary artery occlusion. Am. Heart J., 18:434, 1939.
15. O'Reilly, R. J. and Spellberg, R. D. Rapid resolution of coronary arterial emboli. Myocardial infarction and subsequent normal coronary arteriograms. Ann. Intern. Med., 81:348, 1974.
16. Page, D. L., Caulfield, J. B., Kastor, J. A., DeSanctis, R. W., and Sanders, C. A. Myocardial changes associated with cardiogenic shock. N. Engl. J. Med., 285:133, 1971.
17. Roberts, W. C. Coronary thrombosis and fatal myocardial ischemia. Circulation, 49:1, 1974.
18. —— Does thrombosis play a major role in the development of symptom-producing atherosclerotic plaques? Circulation, 48:1161, 1973.
19. —— Relationship between coronary thrombosis and myocardial infarction. Mod. Concepts Cardiovasc. Dis., 41:7, 1972.
20. —— Coronary arteries in fatal acute myocardial infarction. Circulation, 45:215, 1972.
21. —— The pathology of acute myocardial infarction. Hosp. Pract. 6:89, 1971.
22. —— Buja, L. M. The frequency and significance of coronary arterial thrombi and other observations in fatal acute myocardial infarction. A study of 107 necropsy patients. Am. J. Med., 52:425, 1972.
23. —— Buja, L. M., Bulkley, B. H., and Ferrans, V. J. Congestive heart failure and angina pectoris. Opposite ends of the spectrum of symptomatic ischemic heart disease. Am. J. Cardiol., 34:870, 1974.
24. —— Ferrans, V. J., Levy, R. I., and Fredrickson, D. S. Cardiovascular pathology in hyperlipoproteinemia. Anatomic observations in 42 necropsy patients with normal or abnormal serum lipoprotein patterns. Am. J. Cardiol., 31:557, 1973.
25. Spain, D. M. and Bradess, V. A. Sudden death from coronary heart disease. Survival time, frequency of thrombi, and cigarette smoking. Chest, 58:107, 1970.
26. —— Bradess, V. A.: The relationship of coronary thrombosis to coronary atherosclerosis and ischemic heart disease. (A necropsy study covering a period of 25 years.) Am. J. Med. Sci., 240:701, 1960.
27. Walston, A., Hackel, D. B., and Estes, E. H. Acute coronary occlusion and the "power failure" syndrome. Am. Heart J., 79:613, 1970.
28. Yarbrough, J. W., Roberts, W. C., Abel, R. M., and Reis, R. L. The cause of luminal narrowing in internal mammary arteries implanted into canine myocardium. Am. Heart J., 84:507, 1972.

Chapter 2 Prophylactic Antiarrhythmic Therapy in Acute Myocardial Infarction

EDWARD K. CHUNG, M.D.

General Considerations

Cardiac arrhythmias directly and indirectly influence the morbidity and mortality of patients with acute myocardial infarction. A reduction in the mortality rate of patients with acute myocardial infarction is directly achieved by improvements in the prevention and management of various arrhythmias. The mortality rate (about 80 percent) from the cardiogenic shock, however, seems to be unchanged, even though modern equipment and new drugs are being used.

Various arrhythmias may occur in nearly 95 percent of cases with acute myocardial infarction and may be divided into two major categories: bradyarrhythmias and tachyarrhythmias. Either an extremely slow (rate below 40 beats per minute) or an extremely rapid (rate above 160 beats per minute) rhythm may produce serious symptoms and even death.

It is well-documented that ectopic tachyarrhythmias, particularly ventricular ones, in acute myocardial infarction, often produce (a) reduction in cardiac output with hypotension (b) diminished perfusion of vital organs, particularly of the heart itself, (c) congestive heart failure, and (d) increased demand on the myocardium for oxygen at just the precise time when it can least afford it. On the other hand, marked bradyarrhythmias in acute myocardial infarction, regardless of the fundamental mechanism involved, frequently produce hypotension, shock, congestive heart failure, and the Adams–Stokes syndrome. In addition, it has been demonstrated that bradyarrhythmias usually enhance ventricular irritability and lower the threshold to ventricular fibrillation.

The purpose of this Chapter is twofold: (a) to assess the efficacy of the prophylactic use of antiarrhythmic drugs in acute myocardial infarction, particularly for life-threatening arrhythmias, and (b) to elucidate future challenges. The initial aim of the coronary care unit was the early recognition and management of various arrhythmias. However, the more important role of the coronary care unit, at present, is to prevent serious arrhythmias, particularly, ventricular fibrillation and ventricular standstill. Therefore, this presentation is primarily directed toward the prevention of ventricular fibrillation and ventricular standstill. The first thought should be directed as to whether the prophylactic management of arrhythmias in acute myocardial infarction would reduce the mortality rate and prevent sudden death.

When considering the prophylactic use of antiarrhythmic agents in acute myocardial infarction, the following three major questions should be asked:

1. Whom to treat
2. When to treat
3. How to treat

Obviously, these questions cannot be answered easily because such controversy exists among all physicians who treat patients with acute myocardial infarction.

Whom to Treat

The total incidence of arrhythmias has been reported to be between 75 and 95 percent in cases of acute myocardial infarction and every known type of cardiac arrhythmia may be observed (13, 18, 19, 21, 24, 31, 35, 40, 46). The incidence of individual arrhythmias in acute myocardial infarction varies markedly from study to study because of many factors. These included differing diagnostic criteria and classifications of individual arrhythmias, differing methods of timing and monitoring acute myocardial infarction, the transient nature of some arrhythmias, and difficulties in distinguishing supraventricular and ventricuiar tachyarrhythmias in certain cases. It is known that some arrhythmias are relatively benign, whereas others may be so serious that sudden death can result.

Tachyarrhythmias

Among the various arrhythmias complicating acute myocardial infarction, the most common and clinically significant are ventricular premature contractions, which occur in 70 to 80 percent of cases (8, 27, 30, 35). Ventricular fibrillation, which is believed to be the most common cause of sudden coronary death, is often preceded by ventricular premature contractions. Thus, it is generally agreed that prophylactic use of antiarrhythmic agents is justified in the following circumstances:

1. Frequent (six or more per minute) ventricular premature contractions (Figure 2-1).
2. Ventricular premature contractions with R-on-T phenomenon. (The ventricular premature contraction occurring during the vulnerable period which corresponds to the top of the T wave of the preceding beat, Figure 2-2) and which is prone to occur in the following conditions: long ventricular cycle lengths, prolongation of the Q-T interval, and increased amplitude of the T wave (16).
3. Grouped ventricular premature contractions (two or more, up to five consecutive ventricular premature contractions (Figure 2-3).
4. Multifocal ventricular premature contractions (Figure 2-3).
5. Ventricular premature contractions that occur after ventricular fibrillation, flutter, or tachycardia is terminated.
6. Ventricular tachycardia (Figure 2-2).

Although it has been said that the prophylactic use of antiarrhythmic agents is particularly desirable for high-risk coronary patients, the therapeutic efficacy of various of these drugs is far from ideal. High-risk coronary patients frequency suffer from massive or multiple acute myocardial infarction, often associated with severe congestive heart failure, cardiogenic shock, or serious arrhythmias. When ventricular fibrillation develops at the end-stage of progressive left ventricular deterioration (usually associated with cardiogenic shock and/or congestive heart failure), it is, as a rule, too late to treat and the clinical outcome, therefore, is often irreversible. In this situation, the term *secondary ventricular* fibrillation is used. Primary ventricular

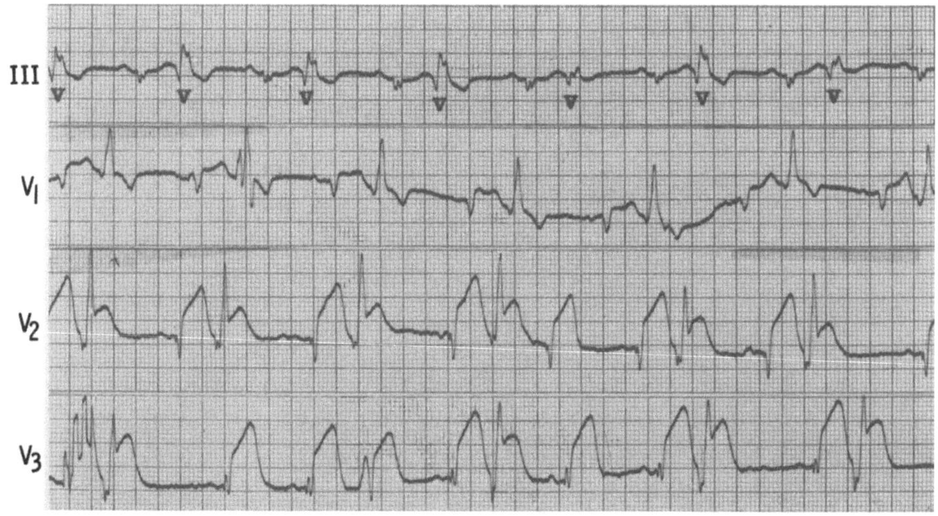

Fig. 2-1. Sinus rhythm with frequent ventricular premature contractions (marked V) producing ventricular bigeminy. Acute anteroseptal myocardial infarction manifested by marked S–T segment elevation, with Q or Q–S waves in Leads V_{1-3}. In addition, old diaphragmatic (inferior) myocardial infarction is a possibility.

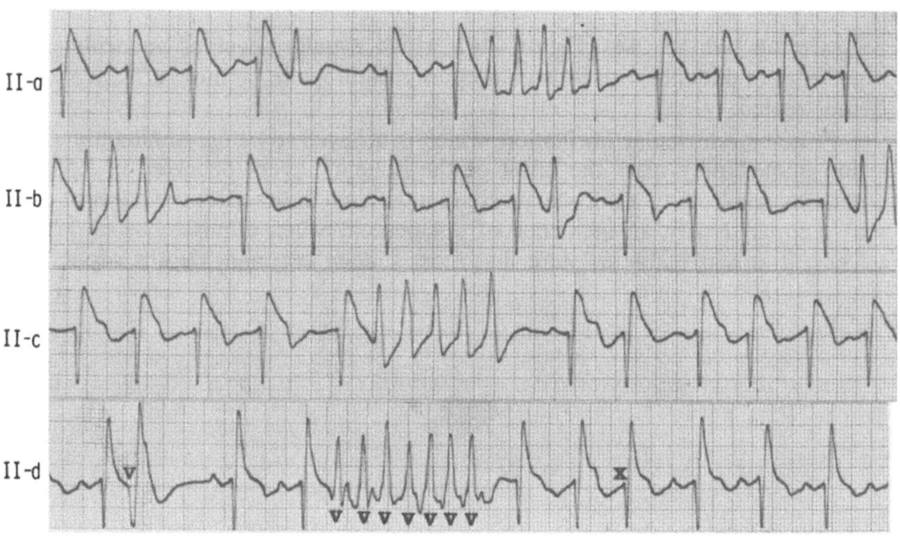

Fig. 2-2. This tracing and Figure 2-4 were obtained from a 57-year-old man with acute diaphragmatic myocardial infarction. Leads II—a, b, c, and d are continuous. The tracing shows sinus rhythm with paroxysmal ventricular tachycardia (marked V) initiated by a ventricular premature contraction (marked V). Since a coupling interval is so short, the ventricular premature beat is superimposed on the T wave of the preceding beat (R-on-T phenomenon). In addition, there are occasional atrial premature beats (marked X).

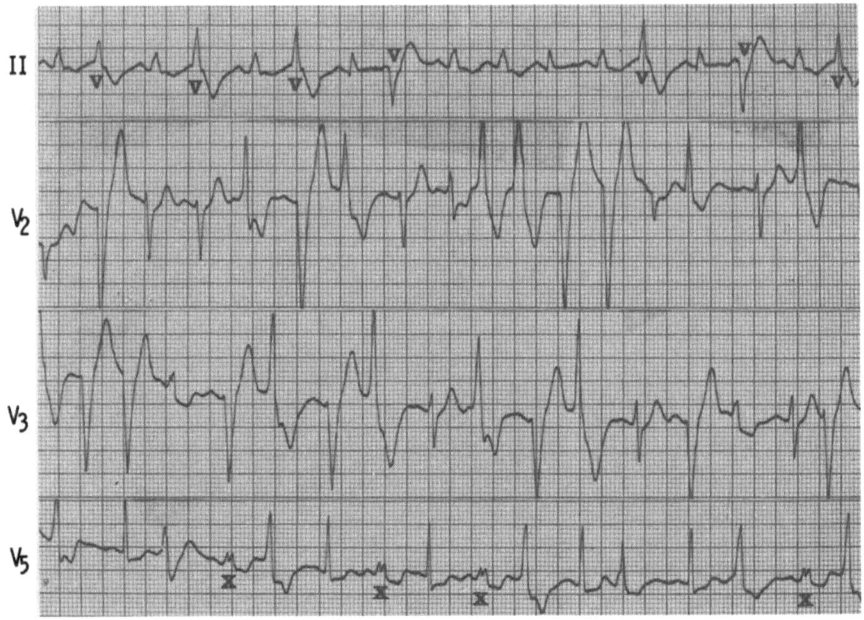

Fig. 2-3. This tracing was obtained from a 72-year-old man with acute anterior subendocardial infarction. The tracing shows sinus tachycardia (rate: 130 beats per minute) with frequent multifocal ventricular premature contractions and areas of group beats (marked V). In addition, left bundle branch block occurs intermittently (marked X).

fibrillation (28, 29, 48) (Figure 2-4), which usually develops suddenly, and unexpectedly in patients with little or no pump failure, can be most effectively prevented and treated.

Primary ventricular fibrillation, which is believed to be predominantly a complication immediately after the onset of the ischemic event occurred in 5.5 percent of patients admitted to a coronary care unit within 4 hours after the onset of chest pain, as compared with an incidence of 0.4 percent when admission was delayed (31). Thus, it is reasonable to state that most sudden coronary deaths occur before the

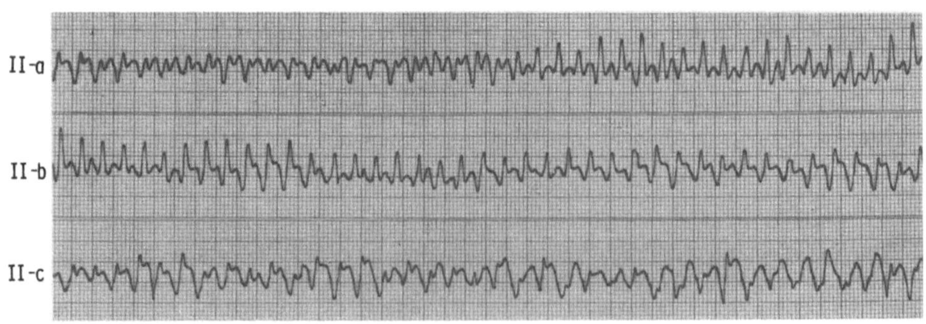

Fig. 2-4. Within several minutes following paroxysmal ventricular tachycardia (Figure 2-2), ventricular fibrillation is observed in this tracing. Leads II-a, b and c are continuous.

full-blown picture of acute myocardial infarction develops. Similarly, primary ventricular fibrillation was reported to be 25 times more frequent during the first 4 hours than the first 24 hours after the onset of symptoms (31). For the same reason, approximately 50 percent of sudden coronary death are estimated to occur during the first few hours after the onset of symptoms, and most of these deaths are considered to be caused by ventricular fibrillation (11, 25, 34). According to a study in which a mobile coronary care unit was used, the incidence of primary ventricular fibrillation was highest (9.9 percent) within the first hour and was reduced to 4.2 percent within the second hour in 284 patients seen within the first hour after the onset of symptoms (2, 31, 40).

It is important to note that the incidence of primary ventricular fibrillation was only 0.7 percent during the third and fourth hours in this study (2, 31, 40). Because of these observations, the prophylactic use of antiarrhythmic agents, even outside the hospital, has been proposed (2, 47, 49). However, the routine use of prophylactic antiarrhythmic therapy in all cases of suspected acute myocardial infarction, without knowing the actual rhythm disturbances, is still not accepted by most investigators. On the other hand, routine prophylactic drug therapy would seem reasonable when a coronary care unit is not available; or the unit is not well-equipped or staffed, provided that these drugs are used carefully in only selected patients. The blind use of prophylactic therapy in a well-equipped coronary care unit, with well-trained staffs, needless to say, is not justified.

Although frequent atrial or AV nodal (junctional) premature contractions may lead to atrial or AV nodal (junctional) tachyarrhythmias, respectively, the true value of prophylactic therapy for these arrhythmias is not well documented. When they develop, atrial or AV junctional tachyarrhythmias can be treated with very little difficulty in most instances. Furthermore, these supraventricular tachyarrhythmias are often transient in nature.

It should be noted that certain tachyarrhythmias associated with acute myocardial infarction, superficially, appear to be serious, but in actuality they are usually benign

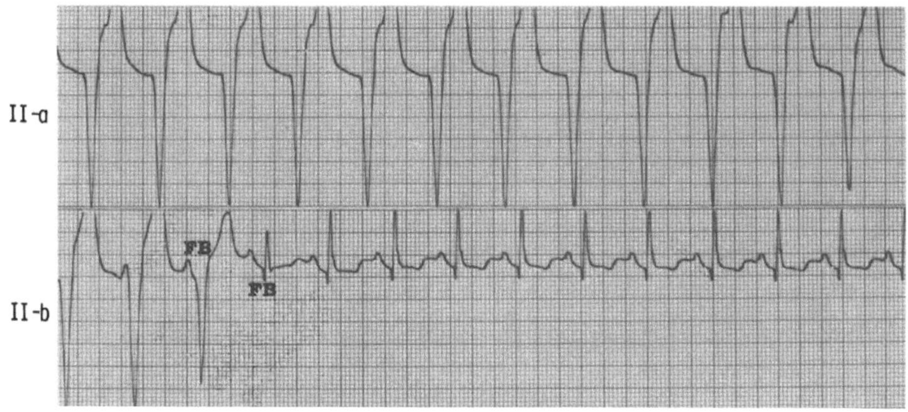

Fig. 2-5. This tracing was obtained from a 60-year-old woman with acute diaphragmatic myocardial infarction. Leads II-a and b are continuous. Nonparoxysmal (idioventricular) ventricular tachycardia (rate: 95 beats per minute) is abolished soon after intravenous injection of atropine sulfate, 0.6 mg. Note occasional ventricular fusion beats (marked FB).

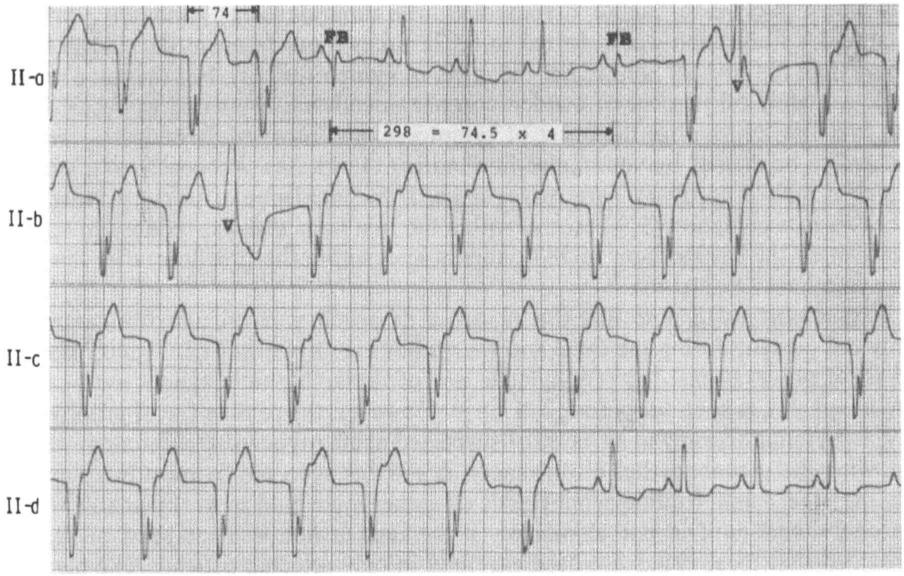

Fig. 2-6. These rhythm strips were obtained from another patient with acute anterior myocardial infarction. Leads II-a, b, c, and d are continuous. The tracing shows sinus rhythm (rate: 78 beats per minute) with intermittent parasystolic ventricular tachycardia (rate: 82 beats per minute). Note that a long interectopic interval is a multiple of the shortest interectopic interval. There are occasional ventricular fusion beats (marked FB) and ventricular premature contractions (marked V). (The numbers in this tracing represent hundredths of a second.)

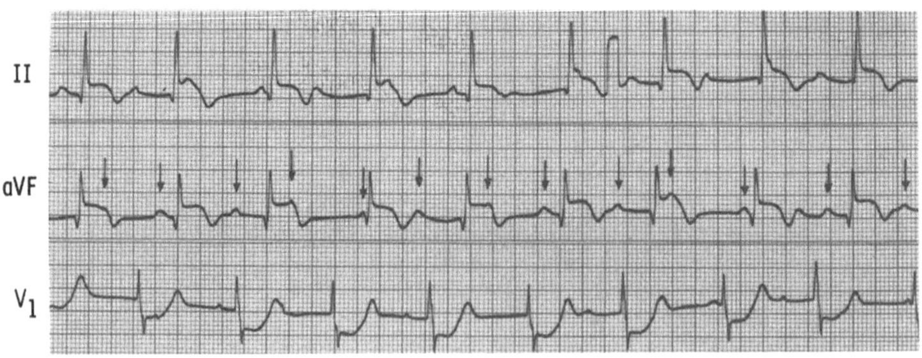

Fig. 2-7. This ECG tracing was recorded from a patient with acute diaphragmatic-posterior myocardial infarction. Arrows indicate sinus P waves. The rhythm is sinus arrhythmia (atrial rate: 85 to 110 beats per minute) with nonparoxysmal AV junctional tachycardia (rate: 70 beats per minute) and occasional ventricular captured beats (3rd and 7th QRS complexes in lead aVF) producing incomplete AV dissociation.

and self-limited. These arrhythmias include: nonparoxysmal ventricular tachycardia (idioventricular tachycardia, Figure 2-5), parasystolic ventricular tachycardia (Figure 2-6), and nonparoxysmal AV nodal (junctional) tachycardia (5, 8) (Figure 2-7). These arrhythmias as a rule do not produce significant hemodynamic alterations and often disappear spontaneously. They seldom last more than 72 hours. The usual ventricular rate in these arrhythmias is between 70 and 130 beats per minute (5). No therapy is indicated unless the rate is faster than usual or the patient is symptomatic.

Bradyarrhythmias

Bradyarrhythmias (ventricular rate slower than 60 beats per minute) are very common rhythm disorders associated with acute myocardial infarction (5, 42). Bradyarrhythmias alone may not only produce various untoward symptoms and even death, but also frequently predispose to ventricular arrhythmias, particularly ventricular fibrillation. Therefore, the prophylactic use of antiarrhythmic agents for bradyarrhythmias in acute myocardial infarction is justified in the following situations: (a) marked bradyarrhythmias alone (b) bradyarrhythmia with hypotension alone (c) bradyarrhythmias with congestive heart failure (d) bradyarrhythmias with ventricular tachyarrhythmias (brady-tachyarrhythmia syndrome; Figure 2-8).

Bradyarrhythmias usually occur as a very early complication of acute myocardial infarction, and are encountered much more frequently in patients with diaphragmatic (inferior) myocardial infarction than in those with anterior myocardial infarction (2, 31, 40). Among 284 patients with acute myocardial infarction seen by

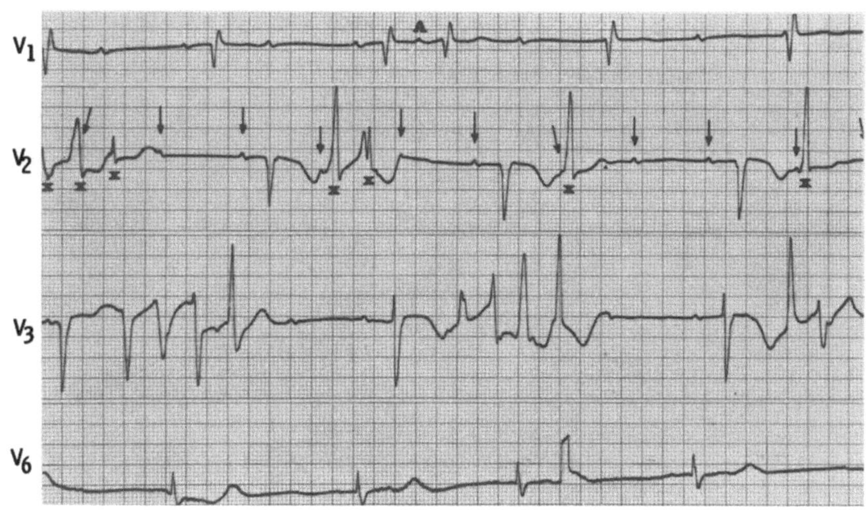

Fig. 2-8. This ECG tracing was obtained from a patient with acute anteroseptal myocardial infarction associated with right bundle branch block. Arrows indicate P waves. The tracing shows sinus rhythm (atrial rate: 83 beats per minute) with high-degree AV block and frequent ventricular premature contractions with group beats (marked X) producing bradytachyarrhythmia syndrome. Note an atrial premature contraction (marked A).

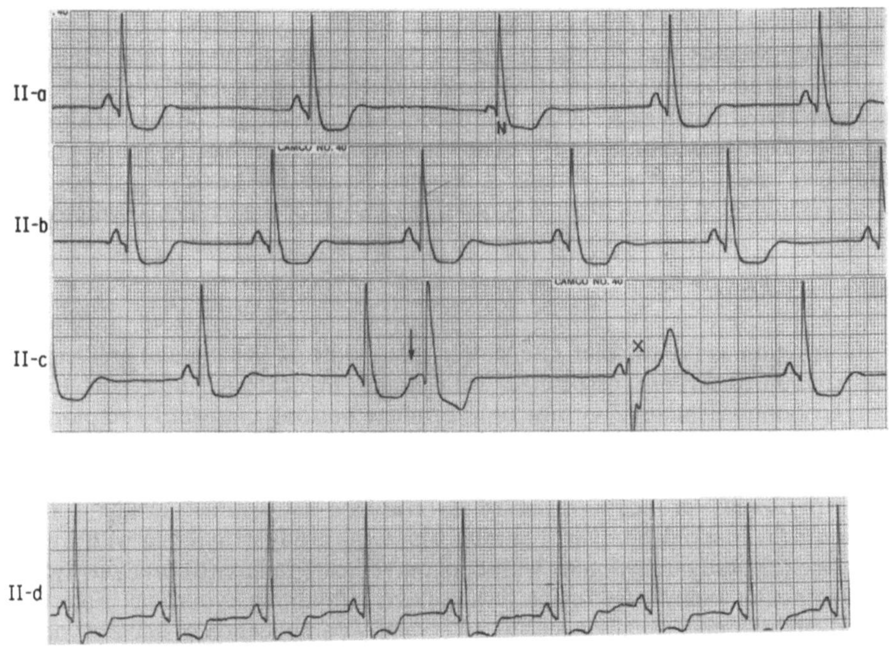

Fig. 2-9. These rhythm strips were obtained from a 74-year-old man with acute myocardial infarction. Leads II-a, b and c are continuous. The rhythm is marked sinus bradycardia (rate: 30 to 37 beats per minute) with occasional AV nodal and ventricular escape beats (marked N and X) and an atrial premature contraction (indicated by arrow). Lead II-d is taken following intravenous injection of atropine (0.4 mg) and the sinus rate is increased (rate: 57 beats per minute) considerably.

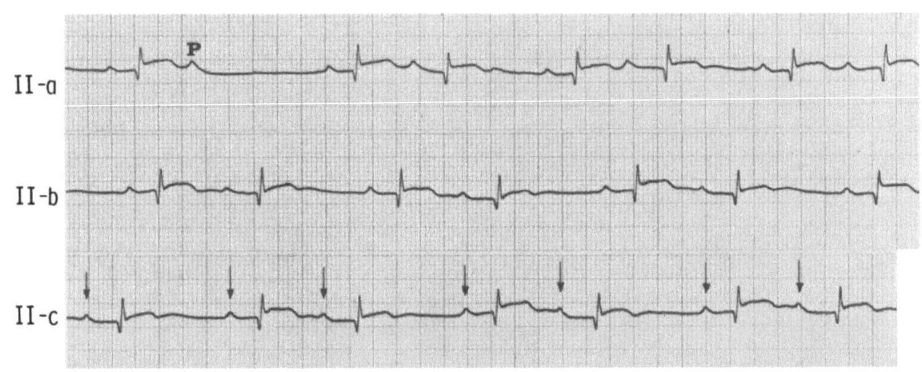

Fig. 2-10. These rhythm strips were obtained from a patient with acute diaphragmatic myocardial infarction. Leads II-a, b, and c are continuous. Arrows indicate sinus P waves. Long and short P–P cycles alternate throughout the tracing. The long P–P cycle is shorter than two short P–P cycles. This regular irregularity of the P–P cycles represents 3:2 Wenckebach sinoatrial block. In addition, there is Wenckebach AV conduction without actual blocked P waves throughout the tracing except for an early portion of lead II—a. A blocked P wave is indicated by P. It is extremely interesting to observe that a characteristic feature of Wenckebach AV block is altered by the 3:2 Wenckebach SA block.

a mobile coronary care unit within the first hour, 60 (45 percent) with diaphragmatic myocardial infarction had bradyarrhythmias within the first hour and 25 developed bradyarrhythmias later (2). In this study, therefore, 85 patients (64 percent) with diaphragmatic (inferior) myocardial infarction had bradyarrhythmias at some time (2).

Bradyarrhythmias may be due to various rhythm disturbances including: sinus arrhythmia, sinus bradycardia (Figure 2-9) with or without AV nodal (junctional) escape rhythm, sinus arrest, S-A block (Figure 2-10), second- or third-degree AV block (Figure 2-11), and ventricular standstill. Among these bradyarrhythmias, sinus

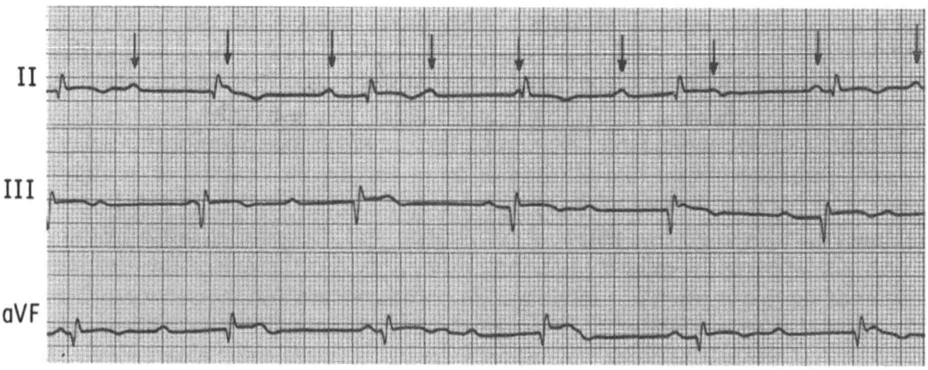

Fig. 2-11. This tracing was obtained from another patient with acute diaphragmatic myocardial infarction. Arrows indicate P waves. It shows sinus rhythm (atrial rate: 75 beats per minute) with AV nodal (junctional) escape rhythm (rate: 46 beats per minute) due to complete AV block.

bradycardia is the most common, and AV block of varying degree is the second most common rhythm disorder.

Experience with a mobile coronary care unit has shown that most patients who suffered cardiac arrest had ventricular fibrillation when efficient resuscitation was initiated within 4 minutes after the onset of symptoms (2, 31, 40). On the other hand, most patients with cardiac arrest demonstrated ventricular standstill when efficient resuscitation was not available within 4 minutes after the onset of symptoms (2, 31, 40). This observation suggests that a precursor of ventricular standstill is most likely ventricular fibrillation in most cases of acute myocardial infarction. Thus, ventricular standstill can be avoided by preventing or effectively treating ventricular fibrillation.

When to Treat

Prophylactic use of antiarrhythmic drugs in acute myocardial infarction may be valuable during (a) prehospital period (b) hospitalization and (c) posthospital period. Ideally, all potentially dangerous cardiac arrhythmias should be prevented and treated as soon as symptoms of acute myocardial infarction appear. Thus, the prophylactic use of antiarrhythmic drugs will be particularly beneficial before the patients reach the hospital (prehospital period) (2, 24, 37, 40, 41, 47, 49). For this reason a mobile coronary care unit has been used since 1966 primarily to prevent and treat life-threatening ventricular fibrillation and standstill (2, 4, 24, 31, 40, 41). Recently, a prehospital satellite industrial coronary care unit has been used for patients with suspected acute myocardial infarction in an industrial population to avoid hospitalization delay (12, 37). This unit shortened hospital arrival time when symptoms began at work, but had an adverse effect when symptoms occurred elsewhere (12, 37). Unfortunately, the sudden death mortality in patients with acute myocardial infarction was not reduced by this unit (12, 37).

In addition to prehospital and hospital care, posthospital care is equally important to prevent sudden death in patients with coronary heart disease (22). The long-term prophylactic use of antiarrhythmic drugs for high-risk ambulatory patients, such as survivors of myocardial infarction who have frequent or persistent ventricular arrhythmias, may be able to prevent sudden death from serious arrhythmias.

Although it has been emphasized repeatedly that the first line of treatment is to prevent life-threatening arrhythmias and sudden death, a delay in medical care, at present, is often unavoidable. Numerous factors are responsible for this delay in coronary care: the patient himself may delay in seeking medical aid or he may be unaware of the significance of his symptoms. In addition, the family physician may be unaware of the high-risk potential for sudden and preventable death in the patient with an apparently mild myocardial infarction. Furthermore, the ordinary ambulance service is often not familiar with coronary care and the service call may not be available immediately. It is extremely unfortunate that the longest delay frequently takes place between the patient's arrival at the hospital emergency room and his transfer to a coronary care unit. These various factors, which are responsible for delaying coronary care must be improved considerably before more favorable statistics can be expected.

How to Treat

The third question, how to treat, may be more difficult to answer even if the two previous questions (whom to treat and when to treat) can be answered. The main reason for this is that there is no universal antiarrhythmic agent. In addition, no antiarrhythmic drug is not potentially dangerous. It is well documented that various antiarrhythmic drugs are capable of producing serious side effects and toxicity. Serious toxicity may produce life-threatening arrhythmias, particularly ventricular fibrillation and even death (Figure 2-12). Side effects or toxicity may occur following a single (small) dose (either parenteral or oral) or during long-term oral therapy. Thus, no totally safe antiarrhythmic agent is available.

Nevertheless, *lidocaine* (*Xylocaine*) is considered to be the best and safest agent for the prevention and treatment of ventricular arrhythmias (3, 8, 18, 21, 27, 30). Lidocaine was reported to be effective in 95 percent of patients with ventricular arrhythmias in acute myocardial infarction (20). However, the efficacy of lidocaine was found to differ markedly, depending upon the time of treatment. For example, when lidocaine was given to 66 patients with ventricular arrhythmias in acute myocardial infarction, in a mobile coronary care unit, within the first 2 hours of the onset of symptoms, ventricular arrhythmias were abolished completely in only one-third (2). There was no effect of lidocaine in more than one-fourth of the patients in this study (2).

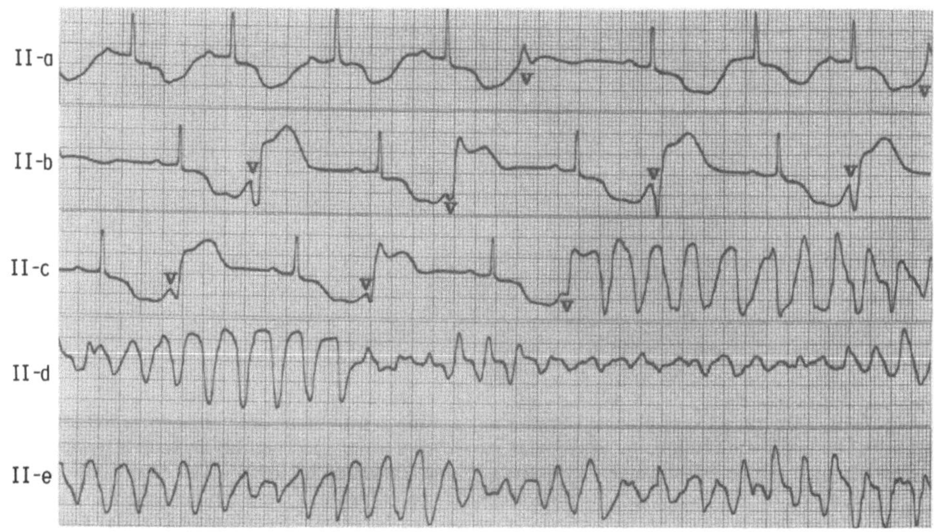

Fig. 2-12. This tracing was obtained from a 62-year-old woman with acute anterior myocardial infarction. Ventricular fibrillation is initiated by the ventricular premature contraction (marked V) because of the "R-on-T" phenomenon. Markedly prolonged Q–T interval, which is due to a combination of quinidine and propranolol, is responsible for the "R-on-T" phenomenon in spite of the fact that the coupling interval is relatively long.

Lidocaine is similar in structure to quinidine or procaine amide, but its electrophysiologic properties are quite different. Lidocaine depresses the diastolic depolarization and automaticity in the ventricles. It is of interest that lidocaine, in standard doses, has no effect on conduction velocity and in fact, generally shortens both the action potential and the refractory period (3, 10, 15, 20, 33). Approximately 90 percent of an administered dose of the drug is metabolized in the liver and the remaining 10 percent is excreted unchanged via the kidneys. The action of lidocaine is more transient than that of procaine amide and the former penetrates the cardiac tissues more rapidly than the latter (3, 10, 15, 20, 33).

Treatment of ventricular arrhythmias, as outlined previously begins with a direct intravenous injection of 75 to 100 mg of lidocaine (1–1.5 mg/kg) given slowly; the same dose may be repeated every 5 to 10 minutes until ventricular arrhythmias are suppressed (Figure 2-13). In general, the total dose should not exceed 750 mg, and it is advisable that no more than 300 mg be administered during a 1-hour period. When intravenous injection is not immediately feasible, alternatively, 200 to 250 mg of lidocaine may be given intramuscularly; the same dose may be repeated once or twice every 5 to 10 minutes. The ideal blood level of lidocaine has been shown to be 2 to 5 μg/ml, whereas more than 5 μg/ml often indicates toxicity (3, 10, 15, 20, 33). To maintain a better therapeutic blood level, simultaneous intravenous (75 to 100 mg) and intramuscular (200 to 250 mg) injections have been recommended by some investigators (31). In one study, different concentrations (6, 8, 9, and 10 percent) of lidocaine (200 mg) were injected intramuscularly at different sites in order to correlate with blood level (6). The results showed that the highest plasma level was obtained by administering a 6 percent solution, and an injection into the deltoid was

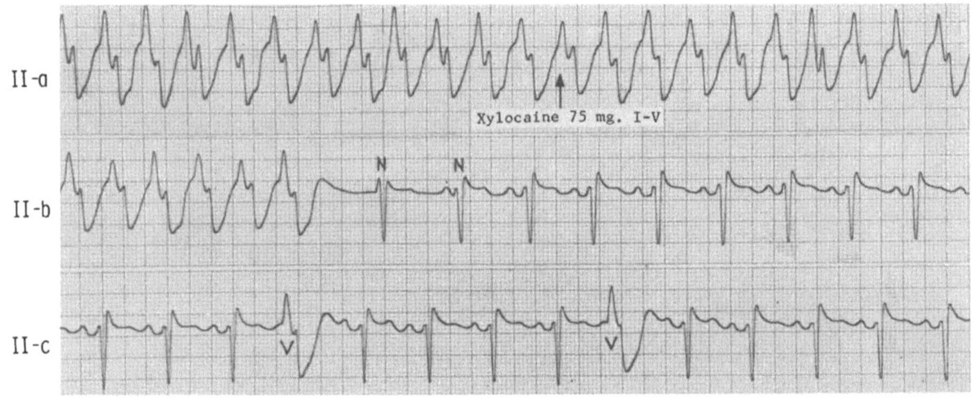

Fig. 2-13. This tracing was obtained from another patient with acute anterior myocardial infarction. Leads II-a and b are continuous. Ventricular tachycardia (rate: 155 beats per minute) is terminated by intravenous injection of lidocaine (Xylocaine), 75 mg (indicated by arrow). The configuration of the QRS complex of the ventricular premature contraction (Marked V) and the tachycardia is identical. This finding proves that the tachycardia is ventricular in origin. Note two AV nodal (junctional) premature beats (marked N).

superior to one in the lateral thigh or buttock (6). Following the suppression of ventricular arrhythmias, the continuous intravenous infusion of lidocaine at a rate of 1 to 5 mg/kg is needed for 24 to 72 hours in most cases to prevent the arrhythmias from recurring. The second drug of choice (parenteral use) for ventricular arrhythmias is *procainamide* (*Pronestyl*). Oral administration of lidocaine was found to be ineffective for ventricular arrhythmias (9).

Long-term prophylactic use of antiarrhythmic drugs in high-risk patients is probably equally important. Presently, the most commonly used agents for long-term prophylaxis are procainamide (250–500 mg every 3 hours) and quinidine (300–400 mg q.i.d.) (17, 23). However, these agents are poorly tolerated by many patients because of side effects and toxicity during long-term therapy. *Diphenylhydantoin* (*Dilantin*) *or propranolol* (*Inderal*) are less reliable for the prevention and management of ventricular arrhythmias in coronary heart disease. *Bretylium tosylate*, which was found to be effective in the treatment of refractory ventricular arrhythmias, is still an investigational agent (7, 45). In addition, new beta-receptor blocking agents such as *oxprenolol* or *alprenolol*, have been used for various arrhythmias in acute myocardial infarction, but these agents need further investigation (38, 43).

For bradyarrhythmias, the most commonly used agent is *atropine*, and the second most commonly used drug is *isoproterenol* (*Isuprel*) (2, 42, 49).

Indications for these agents were described previously. Needless to say, an artificial pacemaker is indicated in drug-resistant bradyarrhythmias or Adams–Stokes syndrome due to complete AV block, especially when they result from bilateral bundle branch block in acute anterior myocardial infarction.

Atropine is used primarily to accelerate the sinus rate by vagal inhibition. Thus, this is the drug of choice for marked sinus bradycardia (Figure 2-9). Atropine often suppresses ventricular arrhythmias by accelerating the atrial rate (Figure 2-5).

Atropine is also effective in the treatment of sinus arrest, SA block, and first or second-degree AV block. In addition, atropine may be useful in complete AV block associated with diaphragmatic myocardial infarction when the ventricles are controlled by the AV junctional pacemaker.

Atropine is best administered intravenously in a dose between 0.3 and 1 mg (up to 2.0 mg), and a similar dose may be repeated every 4 to 6 hours as needed. The total dose of atropine should not exceed 4 mg. The drug may be given subcutaneously or intramuscularly if the intravenous route is not feasible immediately. The onset of action is usually prompt. Oral use of atropine is not reliable.

Intravenous administration of atropine to all patients with a rate below 60 beats per minute, and lidocaine to all patients with a rate faster than 60 beats per minute, for prophylactic purposes has been proposed by some investigators (1, 14, 49). However, the routine use of prophylactic antiarrhythmic agents is still not accepted. Several authors have recommended intravenous *isoproterenol* (1 to 2 μg/min) in patients unresponsive to atropine (32, 44). Furthermore, routine prophylaxis, administered by the patient himself, a family member, various health personnel, or a family physician have been proposed by some but rejected by others. It should be pointed out that the routine prophylactic use of antiarrhythmic agents may not only be without benefit, but even deleterious in some patients with acute myocardial infarction.

Future Challenges and Conclusion

Obviously, there is no uniform agreement as to whom to treat, when to treat, or how to treat. However, most physicians agree that treatment should be initiated soon after symptoms begin. Thus, the prehospital coronary care unit, such as a mobile coronary care unit, should hopefully be available in every community in the near future so that proper prophylactic therapy can be applied according to the type and nature of each arrhythmia. When prehospital coronary care units are available widely, the mortality rate in acute myocardial infarction may be reduced to 10 to 13 percent (2, 31, 40). At present, the lowest mortality rate in acute myocardial infarction, utilizing the usual coronary care unit, was reported to be 17.5 percent (26). Even if a mobile coronary care unit is not available, the unnecessary delay in transporting coronary patients to the hospital coronary care unit should be avoided. Public education, with emphasis on early warning symptoms and signs of acute myocardial infarction is another important factor that hopefully will minimize transportation delay. In addition, professional education should be improved and continued for better coronary care.

Although lidocaine and atropine are the most commonly used agents, the routine use of these drugs for all patients with acute myocardial infarction is not justified.

In addition to coronary care during the prehospital and hospital periods, long-term antiarrhythmic therapy during posthospital care is also extremely important for high-risk patients, such as survivors of myocardial infarction with persistent ventricular arrhythmias. Identification of individuals prone to sudden death is essential.

At present, no antiarrhythmic agent has been sufficiently accepted by the medical community to be used routinely. Implantation of the transvenous automatic defibrillator (a device that automatically recognizes and treats ventricular fibrillation) in patients with previous myocardial infarction or those recovered from previous ventricular fibrillation may prevent sudden death (36).

In conclusion, there is much to be done to prevent unnecessary coronary death. The early administration of proper antiarrhythmic agents will reduce the mortality rate in acute myocardial infarction, and better antiarrhythmic agents are urgently needed.

References

1. Adgey, A. A. J., Geodes, J. S., Mulholland, H. C., Keegan, D. A. J., and Pantridge, J. F. Incidence, significance and management of early bradyarrhythmias complicating acute myocardial infarction. Lancet, 2:1097, 1968.
2. Adgey, A. A. J. and Pantridge, J. F. The prehospital phase of treatment for myocardial infarction. Geriatrics, 27:102, 1972.
3. Bonanno, J. A., Amsterdam, E. A., Massumi, R. A., Zelis, R. and Mason, D. T. Principles of antiarrhythmic therapy. Drug. Ther., 24–35, July, 1971.
4. Chamberlain, D. A., White, N. M., Binning, R. *et al.* Mobile coronary care provided by ambulance personnel. Br. Heart J., 35:550, 1973.
5. Chung, E. K. Electrocardiography: Practical Applications with Vectorial Principles. Hagerstown, Harper and Row, 1974.
6. Cohen, L. S., Rosenthal, J. E., Horner, D. W., Jr., Atkins, J. M., Matthews, O. A., and Sarnoff, S. J. Plasma levels of lidocaine after intramuscular administration. Am. J. Cardiol., 29:520, 1972.
7. Day, H. W. and Bacaner, M. Use of bretylium tosylate in the management of acute myocardial infarction. Am. J. Cardiol., 27:177, 1971.
8. DeSanctis, R. W., Block, P., and Hutter, A. M. Jr. Tachyarrhythmias in myocardial infarction. Circulation, 45:681, 1972.
9. Fehmers, M. C. O. and Dunning, A. J. Intramuscularly and orally administered lidocaine in the treatment of ventricular arrhythmias in acute myocardial infarction. Am. J. Cardiol., 29:514, 1972.
10. Gianelly, R., von der Groeben, J. O., Spivack, A. P., and Harrison, D. C. Effect of lidocaine on ventricular arrhythmias in patients with coronary heart disease. N. Engl. J. Med., 277:1215, 1967.
11. Goble, A. J., Sloman, G., and Robinson, J. S. Mortality reduction in a coronary care unit. Br. Med. J., 1:1005, 1966.
12. Goldstein, S., Moss, A. J., and Greene, W. Sudden death in acute myocardial infarction. Arch. Intern. Med., 129:720, 1972.
13. Grace, W. J. Intermediate coronary care unit. In Chung, E. K. ed. Cardiac Emergency Care, Philadelphia, Lea and Febiger, 1975.
14. Gregory, J. J. and Grace, W. J. The management of bradycardia, nodal rhythm, and heart block for the prevention of cardiac arrest in acute myocardial infarction. Prog. Cardiovasc. Dis., 10:505 1968.
15. Grossman, J. I., Lubow, L. A., Frieden, J., and Rubin, I. R. Lidocaine in cardiac arrhythmias. Arch. Intern. Med., 121:396, 1968.
16. Han, J. and Goel, B. G. Electrophysiologic precursors of ventricular tachyarrhythmias. Arch. Intern. Med., 129:749, 1972.
17. Jelinek, M. V., Lohrbauer, L., and Lown, B. Antiarrhythmic drug therapy for sporadic ventricular ectopic arrhythmias. Circulation, 49:659, 1974.
18. Jewitt, D. E., Balcon, R., Raferty, E. B., and Oram, S. Incidence and management of supraventricular arrhythmias after acute myocardial infarction. Lancet, 2:734, 1967.
19. Julian, D. G., Valentine, P. A., and Miller, G. G. Disturbances of rate, rhythm and conduction in acute myocardial infarction. A prospective study of 100 consecutive unselected patients with the aid of electrocardiographic monitoring. Am. J. Med., 37:915, 1964.
20. Killip, T. Acute myocardial infarction. In Julian, D. G. and Oliver, M. F. eds. University of Edinburgh Symposium. Edinburgh, E. and A. Livingstone, 1968, p. 111.
21. Kimball, T. J. and Killip, T. Aggressive treatment of arrhythmias in acute myocardial infarction. Prog. Cardiovasc. Dis., 10:483, 1968.

22. Koch-Weser, J. Antiarrhythmic prophylaxis in ambulatory patients with coronary heart disease. Arch. Intern. Med., 129:763, 1972.
23. Kosowski, B. D., Taylor, J., Lown, B., and Ritchie, R. F. Long term use of procaine amide following acute myocardial infarction. Circulation, 47:1204, 1973.
24. Kubik, M. M., Bhowmick, B. K., Stokes, T., and Joshi, M. Mobile cardiac unit. Experience from a west midland town. Br. Heart J., 36:238, 1974.
25. Kuller, L. Sudden death in arteriosclerotic heart disease. Am. J. Cardiol., 24:617, 1969.
26. Lawrie, D. M., Greenwood, T. W., Goddard, M., *et al.* A coronary care unit in the routine management of acute myocardial infarction. Lancet, 2:109, 1967.
27. Lawrie, D. M., Higgins, M. R., Godman, M. J., Oliver, M. F., Julian, D. G., and Donald, K. W. Ventricular fibrillation complicating acute myocardial infarction. Lancet, 2:523, 1968.
28. Liberthson, R. R., Nagel, E. L., Hirschman, J. C., and Nussenfeld, S. R. Prehospital ventricular defrillation: Prognosis and follow-up course. N. Engl. J. Med., 291:317, 1974.
29. Liberthson, R. R., Nagel, E. L., Hirschman, J. C. *et al.* Pathophysiologic observations in prehospital ventricular fibrillation and sudden cardiac death. Circulation, 49:790, 1974.
32. Lown, B., Fakhro, A. M., Hood, W. B., and Thorn, G. W. The coronary care unit: new perspectives and directions. J.A.M.A., 199:188, 1967.
30. Lown, B., Klein, M. D., and Hershberg, P. Coronary and Pre-coronary care. Am. J. Med., 46:705, 1969.
31. Lown, B. and Wolf, M. Approaches to sudden death from coronary heart disease. Circulation, 44:130, 1971.
33. Malach, M., Kostis, J. B., and Fischetti, J. L. Lidocaine for ventricular arrhythmias in acute myocardial infarction. Am. J. Med. Sci., 257:52, 1969.
34. McNeilly, R. H. and Pemberton, J. Duration of the last attack in 988 fatal cases of coronary artery disease and its relation to possible cardiac resuscitation. Br. Med. J., 3:139, 1968.
35. Meltzer, L. E. and Kitchell, J. B. The incidence of arrhythmias associated with acute myocardial infarction. Prog. Cardiovasc. Dis., 9:50, 1966.
36. Mirowski, M., Mower, M. M., Staewen, W. S., Denniston, R. H., and Mendeloff, A. I. The development of the transvenous automatic defrillator. Arch. Intern. Med., 129:773, 1972.
37. Moss, A. J., Goldstein, S., Greene, W., and DeCamilla, J. Prehospital precursors of ventricular arrhythmias in acute myocardial infarction. Arch. Intern. Med., 129:750, 1972.
38. Norris, R. M. Alprenolol in acute myocardial infarction: double-blind trial. N.Z. Med. J., 71:135, 1970.
39. Pantridge, J. F. Pre-hospital coronary care. Br. Heart J., 36:233, 1974.
40. Pantridge, J. F. and Adgey, A. A. J. Rational approach to the prehospital management of acute myocardial infarction. In Chung, E. K. ed. Cardiac Emergency Care. Philadelphia, Lea and Febiger, 1975.
41. Paul, O. Prehospital management of acute myocardial infarction. Med. Clin. North Am., 57:119, 1973.
42. Rotman, M., Wagner, G. S., and Wallace, A. G. Bradyarrhythmias in acute myocardial infarction. Circulation, 45:703, 1972.
43. Sandler, G. and Pistevos, A. C. Use of oxprenolol in cardiac arrhythmias associated with acute myocardial infarction. Br. Med. J., 1:254, 1971.
44. Shillingford, J. and Thomas, M. Treatment of bradycardia and hypotension syndrome with acute myocardial infarction. Am. Heart J., 75:843, 1968.
45. Taylor, S. H., Saxton, C., Davis, P. S., and Stoker, J. B. Bretylium tosylate in prevention of cardiac dysrhythmias after myocardial infarction. Br. Heart J., 32:326, 1970.
46. Weiner, L. Coronary care unit. In Chung, E. K. Cardiac Emergency Care. Philadelphia, Lea and Febiger, 1975.
47. Wyman, M. G. Prevention of primary ventricular fibrillation in acute myocardial infarction. Am. J. Cardiol., 29:298, 1972 (Abstr).
48. Wyman, M. G. and Hammersmith, L. Comprehensive treatment plan for the prevention of primary ventricular fibrillation in acute myocardial infarction. Am. J. Cardiol., 33:661, 1974.
49. Yu, P.N. Prehospital care of acute myocardial infarction. Circulation, 45:189, 1972.

Chapter 3 Mobile Intensive Care Units—Are They Really Needed?

MICHAEL LUXTON, M.B., THOMAS PETER, M.D., and GRAEME SLOMAN, M.B.

General Considerations

The treatment of acute myocardial infarction in coronary care units has provided a substantial reduction in hospital mortality. Any further reduction using present techniques is unlikely without major advances in the present form of therapy. Today cardiogenic shock and congestive heart failure account for most of the deaths in the coronary care unit. Some centers have emphasized use of the aortic balloon to assist in the management of these conditions and will proceed to select patients for coronary artery surgery. The number of patients who may be benefited by these heroic procedures will probably continue to be small. Interest has moved sharply to the prehospital phase of acute ischemic heart disease in the belief that the lessons learned from experience in the coronary care unit can be applied much earlier in the history of acute ischemic heart disease and additional lives saved. This has led to the concept of prehospital care for all patients with suspected acute ischemic heart disease, and the development of various types of mobile intensive care units. In this chapter we discuss the place of these units, their benefits, organization, and administration and the results obtained in some centers as examples of their success as well as some of the problems encountered in developing an efficient system.

Historic Considerations

Acute ischemic heart disease is the most common lethal cardiovascular emergency in many countries. A World Health Organization project was established to register definite and suspected acute episodes in the natural history of acute ischemic heart disease in the community from 19 geographic areas. A standardized protocol was followed in all countries and information was collected concerning 9,692 subjects in the calendar year 1971. The average annual attack rate was calculated from the pooled data and was found to be (in the group aged 20 to 64 years) 3.4 per 1,000 population for males and 0.9 per 1,000 for females (WHO 1974). Several studies of coronary heart disease have shown that fatalities are concentrated within the first hour of the acute attack (3, 7, 12, 18). Nearly three-fourths of those who die during an acute attack do so outside the hospital (7). Death is often sudden, with little or no immediate warning. In a study of 998 fatal cases McNeilly (18) found that 596 (59.7 percent) had died before admission to a hospital. Of these 229 (23 percent) of the 998 patients were known to have survived for more than half an hour after the onset of the fatal attack; 182 (18 percent) survived for more than 1 hour and 143 (14 percent) survived for more than 2 hours.

A World Health Organization working group (31) studied the role of mobile coronary care and concluded that 40 percent of deaths from acute myocardial ischemia occurred during the first hour, more than 50 percent had occurred within 2 hours, and 65 percent within 12 hours after the onset of the first major symptoms. Immediately after the onset of symptoms, the incidence of bradycardia is high (2), as is the incidence of ventricular fibrillation (22, 24). When death occurs at this time, it is suggested that it is due to dysrhythmia. It has been generally assumed that the majority of early deaths are due to ventricular fibrillation and this is being increasingly substantiated by experience on mobile coronary care units (21). Lawrie, in 1968 (13), reported from Edinburgh that 60 percent of the episodes of ventricular fibrillation in coronary care units occurred within 4 hours after the onset of symptoms and 80 percent within 12 hours. It is probable that the highest incidence of ventricular fibrillation occurs immediately after the onset of myocardial infarction; thereafter the incidence declines rapidly.

Direct current counter shock (15) has made it possible to treat patients who develop ventricular fibrillation, and a number of follow-up reports show a good prognosis after successful defibrillation (14). McNamee, in 1970 (17) reported that of 160 patients who survived ventricular fibrillation, 80 had a clinically mild coronary episode and long-term prognosis was similar to those whose course was not complicated by this dysrhythmia.

In summary, these observations indicated that ventricular fibrillation is a major cause of death immediately after acute myocardial infarction, and if prompt electrical defibrillation is available, the prognosis of these patients is related to the size of the infarct, which may be small. This is a strong argument for the availability of portable defibrillating devices wherever there are clusters of people who are known to be subject to episodes of acute ischemic heart disease, with or without acute myocardial infarction.

In some communities there is a great delay in the delivery of emergency medical services capable of defibrillation and resuscitation. It has been shown that without a mobile intensive care unit, the delay between the onset of symptoms and admission to a coronary care unit is considerable (8, 9, 19). The Belfast study of fatal ischemic heart disease showed a mean delay of 8 hours of which the major part followed a call for medical help. The median time from the onset of symptoms until a doctor was called was 1 hour and 17 minutes. The subsequent delay was made up of time taken by the doctor to reach the patient, delay in diagnosis, delay in conventional ambulances arriving and transferring him to hospital and of great importance, delay in the hospital casualty rooms.

Benefits of Mobile Intensive Care Units

Although we are discussing the role of prehospital coronary care, the concept of the mobile intensive care unit embraces all medical and surgical emergencies, such as road accidents, poisonings, and so on. In acute ischemic heart disease, apart from prompt diagnosis and reversion of malignant dysrhythmias, the mobile intensive care unit provides a number of secondary benefits.

Prevention of Malignant Ventricular Dysrhythmias

Multifocal or frequent ventricular ectopic activity or both has been considered a precursor of so-called malignant or lethal ventricular tachycardia and fibrillation (14, 16, 26). This ectopic activity can be treated promptly in a mobile intensive care unit and may decrease the incidence of life-threatening dysrhythmias.

Prophylactic intramuscular lidocaine (300 mg, 10 percent solution) has been shown to reduce mortality in the first 2 hours after acute myocardial infarction (28). The most impressive reduction in mortality was seen in male patients 55 years of age. A possible explanation for this result, is provided in the work of Lie *et al.* (14) who found that primary ventricular fibrillation was frequent in younger males, especially those with an inferior infarction. Wyman (33) reported only one episode of ventricular fibrillation in 732 patients with acute myocardial infarction treated in a coronary care unit, and who received prophylactic lidocaine. However, further community studies are needed before the routine use of prophylactic lidocaine can be advised in all subjects with suspected acute myocardial infarction.

Sinus Bradycardia

Although there has been some difference of opinion with regard to the treatment of sinus bradycardia without hypertension (10, 16, 20), there is little doubt about the prompt administration of atropine sulfate in patients with acute myocardial infarction and obvious hemodynamic disturbances. Care should be taken that the rate is not increased to an inappropriate level, as this might cause the area of infarction to extend (6). We found the automatic Atropen tissue spray injection of 2 mg atropine citrate free of this detrimental rise in heart rate (24).

Cardiac Failure in Acute Myocardial Infarction

Cardiac failure in acute myocardial infarction is observed in 20 and 60 percent depending on the clinical and hemodynamic or radiologic criteria employed. A study reported from our coronary care unit (25) showed left ventricular failure in 48 percent of patients admitted to the coronary care unit. This finding is of considerable importance if the postulate, prompt treatment of cardiac failure will improve myocardial perfusion and limit the extension of infarcted tissue, proves correct (23). For similar reasons, early administration of diuretics in the mobile intensive care unit may decrease the incidence of cardiogenic shock.

Pantridge (23) demonstrated a reduction in mortality in patients transported by a mobile coronary care unit within 2 hours after the onset of chest pain compared to patients transported by other means even if those transported in the mobile intensive care unit did not require defibrillation. This finding, although based on a small group of patients, supports the concept that early treatment, provided by special mobile units, is of benefit in aspects of care other than the reversion of malignant arrhythmias. In road trauma, drowning, asphyxiation, acute pulmonary embolism, and so forth, there can be no doubt that early, on site, treatment is beneficial and potentially life-saving.

Organization

During the early planning stage, if a prehospital emergency care service is to be instituted, a decision must be made as to whether a very specialized transport system, such as a mobile coronary care unit, is to be established and its use restricted to patients "calling for help" for definite or suspected symptoms of acute infarction or whether a less specialized service should be set up suitable for all definite or suspected cardiovascular emergency cases. As all cardiovascular emergencies have many characteristics in common, particularly with respect to their management, there is much that can be said in favor of a very broadly based mobile intensive care unit capable of dealing with all cardiovascular emergencies.

The organization of mobile coronary care units in various cities varies considerably with local requirements and existing emergency facilities. They may be divided into units based at hospitals and those based at emergency vehicle depots outside hospitals; for example, fire departments or ambulance centers. In the former situation the units are usually staffed by a physician and other medical personnel, including trained coronary care nurses and paramedical personnel. Nonhospital based emergency care vehicles are staffed by ancillary workers and a physician who may be picked up at a local hospital, or medical advice may be obtained by radio communication. Three different mobile intensive care units can be illustrated in detail.

Hospital Based Unit

In the Belfast unit both a physician and a nurse are on the ambulance, which is based at a depot on the grounds of the hospital (22). When this service was being established, the medical profession of Belfast was informed about the theoretic basis of mobile coronary care and were instructed in the procedures they were to carry out when attending a patient suspected of having a myocardial infarction. In this system a doctor and, more recently, the patient themselves or a relative, telephone a widely publicized emergency number, which immediately connects them to the coronary care unit of a general hospital. On receiving the call, a resident doctor and a nurse are paged and instructed to join the ambulance. This arrangement provides the benefit that calls from the general public are screened by medical personnel before the ambulance is mobilized, thereby minimizing the number of false alarms. Another advantage is that medical personnel are at the site of the incident quickly and are able to give skilled advice. However, a major disadvantage is the delay inherent in mobilizing the team. As the program developed, more calls were received directly from the public. This minimized the delay in the system when the family doctor attended the patient. With this system 50 percent of patients are now reached within 10 minutes after the call is received at the coronary care unit. The ambulance itself is a standard, virtually unmodified, vehicle carrying a battery operated defibrillator, monitoring apparatus, selected drugs, and intravenous solutions. A facility for cardiac pacing from transvenous wires is also provided. All equipment is portable. Care in the ambulance during transport is similar to that received by the patient in the coronary care unit, i.e., relief of pain, prophylaxis against dysrhythmias, and treatment of ventricular dysrhythmias should they occur.

Fire Department Based Mobile Intensive Care Units

In contrast to the Belfast unit, the unit in Seattle, Washington, is based at the local fire department (4). Local citizens of Seattle telephoned the fire department in any type of emergency situation. The fire department had been providing an "out of hospital" emergency service for many years prior to the inception of a mobile coronary care unit. It was therefore very appropriate to upgrade the existing service. This service is not only used for cardiac problems but for other medical emergencies as well.

Seattle has a population of 600,000 with 13 hospital coronary care units. The mobile intensive care unit enables a patient to be reached by a coronary care unit within 2 to 5 minutes after the call received by the fire department. The public has been given a widespread educational program in which they were encouraged to telephone the fire department the moment an emergency arises rather than first waste time telephoning a hospital or doctor. As soon as the fire department receives such a call, it dispatches the closest of 10 strategically placed "aide cars." These cars carry paramedical personnel capable of cardiopulmonary resuscitation. If a dispatcher feels that emergency represents a cardiac problem, he would also dispatch the mobile intensive care unit with its specialized paramedical personnel. These more sophisticated units have radio communication to the duty physician at the coronary care unit and are also able to transmit the patient's electrocardiogram. They are also authorized to carry out definitive emergency therapy (following standard written orders) in situation where a physician is not present. If the patient has possible acute ischemic heart disease he is transported to a prearranged hospital coronary care unit selected by the fire department dispatcher and is admitted directly, avoiding delays in emergency rooms. This system provides for a very rapid response and maximum use of facilities but relies heavily on the knowledge and cooperation of the general public to call for help and on medical practitioners to use the system. It is essentially a community service in improved health care.

Combined Hospital and Paramedical Mobile Intensive Care Units

The system in Melbourne, Australia combines local ambulance service facilities staffed solely by ambulance officers who have been trained in a coronary care program and medical control and guidance from the staff of a hospital coronary care unit. The details of this service are discussed later in the chapter to illustrate problems encountered in establishing mobile intensive care units.

Results of Mobile Intensive Care Units

The potential of mobile intensive care units can be gauged from results of centers that operate units especially for the prehospital care of acute ischemic heart disease.

Belfast

The Belfast unit received 2,753 calls between 1966 and 1969. Of these patients, myocardial infarctions were subsequently diagnosed in 43 percent and coronary insufficiency in 33 percent. During the 3 years, there were no deaths during transport due primarily to dysrhythmias. This contrasts favorably with experiences before the mobile coronary care unit when up to 10 percent of the deaths occurred in the ambulance.

In patients with proven infarction, 25 percent were under intensive care within 1 hour, 52 percent within 2 hours, and 76 percent within 4 hours. These figures improved over the 4-year period, reflected by the reduction in median delay from 8 hours in 1965 to 1 hour and 4 minutes in 1969.

Cardiac arrest occurred outside the hospital in 193 patients and 12 of these occurred in the ambulance. Resuscitation was not attempted in 38 cases because cardiac arrest had been prolonged before cardiopulmonary resuscitation was applied. Of the remaining 155 patients in whom resuscitation was attempted, there were 55 initial survivors and 38 left the hospital alive. In the group of patients who received prehospital coronary care in the Belfast unit, the overall hospital mortality was 17.3 percent, which compares favorably with the collective mortality of 23.5 percent from four different coronary care units (23). Pantridge attributes part of this improvement to a reduced incidence of shock and pump failure in patients who were treated early after the onset of chest pain.

Seattle

In Seattle during the first 3 years of operation, 202 patients were resuscitated by the unit. Of these, 70 percent in ventricular fibrillation were defibrillated and subsequently discharged (4). However, this would be the bare minimum of lives saved, as it is likely that treatment of other dysrhythmias and hemodynamic disturbances would have indirectly prevented death. Of the patients who had ventricular fibrillation and survived, half had no evidence of myocardial infarction after they were admitted to the hospital. Some of these patients subsequently had coronary angiograms and most showed severe coronary artery disease (5).

It is important to note that the percentage of patients who had ventricular fibrillation and ultimately survived increased greatly from the first to the third year during which this service operated (increasing from 11 percent during the first 2 years to over 20 percent during the third year). This improvement was attributed to dispatching the unit more rapidly, firemen were being given better training, and an intensive public education system had been established.

The importance of this education is reflected by the fact that at the time of the review 20 percent of resuscitations were initiated by a member of the community already at the scene, in contrast to the 5 percent before cardiopulmonary resuscitation education had been started. This was achieved by educating 40,000 people during this 3-year period.

Does Mobile Intensive Care Contribute to Improved Patient Care?

In any attempt to judge the value of mobile intensive care a number of questions must be asked:

1. Is mobile intensive care valuable from a medical point of view?
2. Is it economically sound?
3. Is it practical in a large city beset by problems of communication and traffic congestion?

With regard to the first question, the data from the Belfast and the Seattle units show that many lives have been saved and patients subsequently returned to gainful employment. Similar experience has been reported by the Melbourne unit.

Economic evaluation is very difficult. However, it may be based in a very approximate way on an envisaged cost per life saved. In the American setting, Dr. Jan Paul Acton has estimated that the cost per life saved would range from US$2,200 to US$4,600 (1). The mobile unit he envisaged, was staffed by a physician. Although these figures may be quite different in other communities, they do give some idea of the magnitude of the cost. Against this debit must be balanced the loss of community earnings due to premature deaths and also the costs of other high-grade medical care currently being undertaken in hospitals. It would be reasonable to say that mobile intensive care is economically a sound proposition in those communities that can afford sophisticated medical care at all levels. It would be unreasonable to suggest the system be implemented in a community where medicine is less developed and money, if available, could be spent more wisely in basic fields of health care.

The third point to consider is implementation of a system. To be effective, care must reach a potential coronary patient in a very short time, ideally a few minutes. This is becoming increasingly difficult in modern cities, with traffic congestion and communication problems. These problems can be overcome, as has been demonstrated by the Seattle program, by intelligent use of existing community facilities, such as less specialized units backed up by one or two vehicles containing a monitor and a defibrillator.

Other problems that may limit the value of prehospital coronary care lie in the field of community medicine. A major delay is that between the onset of the patient's symptoms and his first call for any form of medical help (8). This may be overcome by very intensive educational programs, such as those attempted in Seattle, Belfast, and a number of other cities. This may be coupled with instruction in cardiopulmonary resuscitation. One criticism leveled against these programs is that they will increase public anxiety regarding coronary artery disease. This is an inherent problem in any community health education program such as the fight against cancer, tuberculosis, or, indeed, any current program attempting to reduce the risk of coronary artery disease. A further concern about public education is an excessive number of false alarms if the patient is not seen initially by a local medical practitioner. However, the Seattle and Belfast experience shows that after a short period of time, the number of false alarms is remarkably small.

Prediction of Patients Admitted with Acute Coronary Heart Disease

Another important aspect of prehospital coronary care is the potential for recognizing people at risk of acute myocardial infarction or sudden death from coronary artery disease so that prophylactic treatment can be instituted. Kinlen (11), in a study of acute ischemic heart disease, in Oxford interviewed relatives of 140 patients who died suddenly and found that 49 percent of the patients had had preceding chest or epigastric pain a month prior to infarction and 25 percent saw their general practitioner within a week before the event and 50 percent within a month. If these patients could be identified, they may form a group in which advice regarding the availability of prehospital coronary care could be given. In addition, it has been suggested that when effective antiarrhythmic agents have been developed, these may be given to such patients to be used prophylactically while they are waiting for the mobile intensive care unit. We mention this aspect of coronary artery disease because it may well prove to be an important adjunct to prehospital mobile coronary care. The World Health Organization established a study (30, 31) to evaluate the significance of symptoms and signs that precede sudden coronary deaths.

General Purpose of Mobile Intensive Care Units (With Particular Reference to Cardiovascular Emergencies)

The Melbourne Mobile Intensive Care Unit Program, demonstrates one method of developing such a service and also highlights some of the problems that might be encountered in other centers intending to start a similar community program. The system has been developed in the metropolitan and city areas of Melbourne (population approximately 2 million). In 1969 a pilot mobile intensive care unit was established, based at a university teaching hospital, and was staffed at that time by specially trained senior ambulance officers and medical graduates. However, professional acceptance was poor and dividends were low with respect to lives saved. A special committee was established to advise on such special emergency care in the state and coordinate guidelines for staff training, equipment, and communications of such a unit. A general policy was established, and two university teaching hospitals with active nurse training programs associated with their coronary care units, were requested to undertake training of ambulance officers to fit them for the special mobile intensive care unit. After a number of trial courses, the ambulance officers' course training was integrated with the technical training given to coronary care nurses at the start of their standard 30-week in-service training course. The detailed syllabus made use of all forms of audiovisual training and practical experience in the coronary care unit and on the emergency ambulance. When they completed the course, the ambulance officers underwent a further 3 months of practical training in the mobile intensive care unit and attended the coronary care unit, one half-day each week for additional training, lectures, and case presentations. When this 3 months' service was completed, the ambulance officer's suitability for certification as a trained special mobile intensive unit medical assistant was assessed by a special board.

The number of officers qualified was gradually increased, and by January 1974 enough staff were trained to man four special mobile intensive care units, which were then distributed in the Melbourne metropolitan area. Each vehicle was sponsored by a major hospital and at all times, one medical officer was immediately available for radio-telephone consultation. In addition, facilities were available in each vehicle for the transmission of electrocardiograms over the radiotelephone, either to the coronary care unit or to the cardiologist (Figure 3-1). Calls for the mobile intensive care

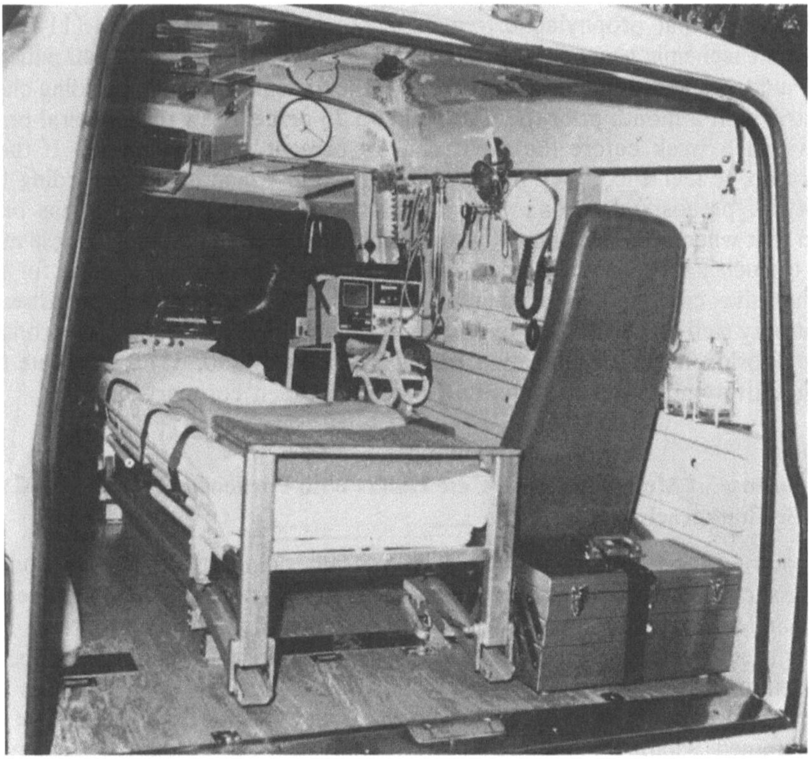

Fig. 3-1. Interior of Melbourne Mobile Intensive Care Units showing portable monitor, defibrillator, and drug box.

unit originated either from the general public or from doctors directly to the ambulance central common room. As soon as a call is received, the mobile intensive care unit closest to the patient was dispatched by ambulance control. There were two mobile intensive care units serving the metropolitan area of Melbourne until December 1973, and since this was grossly inadequate, two more were commissioned in January 1974. This, in itself, is one lesson learned from this project: the area covered by a unit should be carefully limited to keep delays to a minimum. In the calendar year 1973, there were 3,516 calls for the two mobile intensive care units. Of these calls 1,835 were for patients whose history suggested acute ischemic heart disease, 662 were general medical cases, 144 were a miscellaneous group termed collapses, 378 were various forms of accidents, in 260 cases the ambulance was not required on arrival, and 236 calls were cancelled. (Table 3-1). Of the 1,835 patients who were presumed to have acute ischemic heart disease, 29 were resuscitated successfully from either ventricular fibrillation or standstill (Table 3-2). Nine of these patients subsequently died in hospital. There was no follow-up information on 3. Of 17 patients discharged from the hospital after resuscitation, 1 died a month after discharge, 6 were alive and well after 1 year, and in 10 the follow-up period was less than 1 year. These figures may be compared with the first full calendar year during which the ambulance was used in 1972 in which 19 patients were resuscitated from ventricular fibrillation or ventricular standstill, and of these 10 left the hospital alive.

Table 3-1. Data From Melbourne Mobile Intensive Care Unit—1973

	No. of patients
History suggestive of acute ischemic heart disease	1,835
General medical	662
Motor car accidents	188
Other accidents	190
Noncardiac syncope	144
Total patients transported	3,019
Mobile intensive care unit attended but not required	260
Calls cancelled	236
Total calls	3,515

In the first 3 months of 1974, when four units began to operate (each totally manned by ambulance personnel), 14 patients were resuscitated from ventricular fibrillation or standstill. This experience demonstrates the important point that the number of lives saved in the initial phase of any service is relatively small while the program is being developed and the response time is being reduced. This should be anticipated by any community setting up a similar program and should not lead to excessive pessimism.

The cost of keeping one mobile intensive care unit on the road for 1 year, 24 hours a day, is A$140,000, which includes salaries of ambulance officers. The cost of a new vehicle in our service is approximately A$12,000. These figures must be assessed in light of the fact that our ambulance also services trauma and other medical emergencies.

There are various aspects of our mobile intensive care unit program that deserve attention. The concept of paramedical care is relatively new in Australia. There was a problem getting the medical profession and, to a lesser extent, the general public, to accept the unit. Paramedical care has now been accepted in many areas of the United States, as demonstrated by the Seattle unit. The concept has been developed in the United Kingdom, as shown in the Brighton program described by White *et al.* (29). Using ambulance officers has certain very clear advantages: (a) these men have already selected themselves in the sense that they have a particular interest in health

Table 3-2. Status of 1,835 Patients with Suggested Ischemic Heart Disease Treated in Mobile Intensive Care Unit

		No. of patients
1973	Alive at 1 yr	6
	Alive more than 1 yr	10
	Died in hospital	9
	Late deaths	1
	Lost to follow-up	3
	No. of successfully resuscitated (ventricular fibrillation or standstill)	29
1974	First 3 mo. No. successfully resuscitated	14

care, (b) they have been trained by their service and have experienced the fundamentals of medical care, and (c) the ambulance service is a recognized emergency care service in our community and to this extent is accepted by the general public. The ambulance officers selected for training have shown a considerably high pass rate, both in written and practical aspects. Further, it has led to an increased interest throughout the ambulance service. We hope that this training will eventually lead to a higher status for ambulance officers as medical coworkers in the Australian community.

Despite these optimistic aspects, difficulties have arisen due to the over-confidence shown by ambulance officers and a tendency for them to overuse forms of therapy, such as intravenous infusion, with a consequent and unnecessary time delay in transport. This problem has been overcome by forcing them to adhere to detailed orders and emphasizing the importance of transporting patients to hospital care as soon as possible. The use of intramuscular therapy for emergency dysrhythmias (atropine, Atropen tissue spray, and lidocaine 10 percent) has been taught as an alternative procedure to immediate intravenous therapy.

The need for a refresher course has also become apparent, and this must be an important aspect of any training programme. The degree of practical experience in any one aspect of mobile intensive care may be insufficient. To overcome this problem, ambulance officers are encouraged to become involved in the functions of coronary care and other emergency areas of the hospital while awaiting calls.

Another major aspect of the prehospital care of acute ischemic heart disease has been the education of patients, relatives, and the lay public in general, in cardiopulmonary resuscitation. Early in our program, it became apparent that medical practitioners were not aware of recently documented features of the natural history of acute ischemic heart disease. The ambulance service was often called for patients who were in pulmonary edema or cardiogenic shock, yet not for patients who had chest pain but were otherwise well. A cardiopulmonary resuscitation program for the lay public was started in June 1973 at the Royal Melbourne Hospital. The teaching team consisted of a course supervisor, who was a trained coronary care nurse. Cine film and, more recently, video tape are used by the staff of the mobile intensive care unit. Detailed cardiopulmonary resuscitation brochures have been produced with the help of the National Heart Foundation. To date, 4,000 people have been instructed.

It can be concluded that mobile intensive care units are a valuable extension of health care in any community that can afford an adequate coronary care unit service. To obtain maximum benefit, widespread public and medical education programs are required. These projects are relatively inexpensive once they are established and will repay the community not only in lives saved but also from the economic point of view in terms of working hours otherwise lost due to premature death. In addition, the community will directly benefit by upgrading their emergency services in many other areas. We consider the mobile intensive care unit for prehospital care of a patient with acute ischemic heart disease a step relatively easy to take to reduce mortality from coronary artery disease.

Summary

Considerable evidence indicates that the high early mortality from acute ischemic episodes is due mainly to ventricular fibrillation. Furthermore, if such patients can be defibrillated promptly, their prognosis is good and depends mainly on the size of the infarction. This has led to the concept of prehospital care and the development of mobile coronary care units staffed by personnel trained to deal with cardiovascular emergencies. Such training includes the ability to recognize ventricular fibrillation and defibrillate patients, monitoring arrhythmias, and administering intravenous medication, endotracheal intubation, and performing cardiopulmonary resuscitation when necessary.

The organization of such units can be based on that of the hospital in Belfast or on emergency services such as those provided by the fire department in Seattle, or it can be based on combined hospital and ambulance facilities, as in Melbourne.

The mobile intensive care unit in Melbourne is staffed by trained paramedical personnel capable of performing emergency procedures. They are in voice communication with designated physicians or trained coronary care nurses at a nearby hospital. Where indicated, they are able to transmit the electrocardiogram to the hospital staff for interpretation. In Melbourne the ambulance officers staffing the units receive the same basic training as do coronary care nurses and have similar pass rates.

The value of a mobile intensive care unit can be assessed in terms of the numbers of lives saved and the cost per life saved. Experience over the past 3 years has shown that:

1. These units can be run at a reasonable cost to the community.
2. The area covered by one unit should be carefully limited to keep delays at a minimum.
3. Well-trained ambulance officers are capable of handling emergency situations.
4. A program of public education, stressing the necessity for early calls for medical help will considerably increase the number of lives saved.
5. A cardiopulmonary resuscitation teaching program for the lay public is a valuable adjunct to a mobile intensive care program.

Acknowledgments

We wish to thank the Victorian Hospitals and Charities Commission, the Victorian Civil Ambulance, the Executive Committee of the Royal Melbourne Hospital, the staff of the Royal Melbourne Hospital and the National Heart Foundation of Australia.

Videotape on CPR is available in three-quarter inch Sony cassette from the National Heart Association of Australia, Victorian Division, 3050, Australia.

References

1. Acton, J. P. Evaluating public programmes to save lives: The case of Heart Attacks. The Rand Corporation, Santa Monica, California, January 1973.
2. Adgey, A. A. J., Geddes, J. S., Webb, S. W., Allen, J. D., James, R. G. G., Zaidi, S. A., and Pantridge, J. F. Acute phase of myocardial infarction. Lancet, 2:501, 1971.
3. Bainton, C. R. and Peterson, D. R. Deaths from coronary heart disease in persons fifty years of age and younger. N. Engl. J. Med., 268:569, 1963.
4. Cobb, L. A. and Alvarez, H. Three years' experience with a system for prehospital emergency care. National Heart Foundation of Australia. Notes on Cardiovasc. Dis., 9:36, 1973.

5. Dodge, H. T. Personal communication.
6. Epstein, S. E., Goldstein, R. E., Redwood, D. R., Kent, K. M., and Smith, E. R. The early phase of acute myocardial infarction: Pharmacologic aspects of therapy. Ann. Intern. Med., 78:918, 1973.
7. Fulton, M., Julian, D., and Oliver, M. Sudden death and myocardial infarction. Circulation, 40:Suppl. 4:182, 1969.
8. Gilchrist, I. C. Patient delay before treatment of myocardial infarction. Br. Med. J., 1:535, 1973.
9. Hacket, T. P. and Cassem, N. H. Factors contributing to delay in responding to the signs and symptoms of acute myocardial infarction. Am. J. Cardiol., 24:651, 1969.
10. Meltzer, L. E. and Kitchell, J. R. Cardiac pacing and cardioversion. Philadelphia, The Charles Press Publishers Inc., 1967.
11. Kinlen, L. J. Incidence and presentation of myocardial infarction in an English community. Br. Heart J., 35:616, 1973.
12. Kuller, L., Lilienfeld, A., and Fisher, R. Epidermiological study of sudden and unexpected deaths due to arteriosclerotic heart disease. Circulation, 34:1056, 1966.
13. Lawrie, D. M., Higgins, M. R., Goodman, M. J., Oliver, M. F., Julian, D. L., and Donald, K. W. Ventricular fibrillation complicating myocardial infarction. Lancet, 2:524, 1968.
14. Lie, K. I., Wellens, H. J., and Durrer, D. Characteristics and predictability of primary ventricular fibrillation. Eur. J. Cardiol. 1:379, 1974.
15. Lown, B., Amarasingham, R., and Norma, J. New methods for terminating cardiac arrhythmias. Use of synchronized capacitator discharge. J.A.M.A., 182:548, 1962.
16. Meltzer, L. E. and Kitchell, J. R. The current state of intensive coronary care. Philadelphia, The Charles Press Publishers Inc., 1966.
17. McNamee, B. T., Robinson, T. J., Adgey, A. A., Scott, M. E., Geddes, J. S., and Pantridge, J. F. Longterm prognosis following ventricular fibrillation in acute ischaemic heart disease. Br. Med. J., 4:204, 1970.
18. McNeilly, R. H. and Pemberton, J. Duration of last attack in 998 fatal cases of coronary artery disease and its relation to possible cardiac resuscitation. Br. Med. J., 3:139, 1968.
19. Moss, A. J., Wynar, B., and Goldstein, S. Delay in hospitalization during the acute coronary period. Am. J. Cardiol., 24:659, 1969.
20. Norris, R. M., Mercer, C. J., and Yeates, S. E. Sinus rate in acute myocardial infarction. Br. Heart J., 34:901, 1972.
21. Pantridge, J. F. and Geddes, J. S. Cardiac arrest after myocardial infarction. Lancet, 1:807, 1966.
22. ——, ——. A Mobile Intensive Care in the management of myocardial infarction. Lancet, 2:271, 1967.
23. —— Adgey, A. A. J. The prehospital phase of acute myocardial infarction. In Meltzer, L. E. and Dunning, A. J., eds. Textbook of Coronary Care. Amsterdam, Excerpta Medica, 1972.
24. —— Geddes, J. S. Primary ventricular fibrillation. Eur. J. Cardiol., 1:335, 1974.
25. Sloman, J. G. and Brown, R. W. Hospital registration in patients with acute myocardial infarction. Am. Heart J. 79:761, 1970.
26. Smirk, F. H. and Palmer, D. G. A myocardial syndrome with particular reference to the occurrence of sudden death and premature systoles interrupting antecedent "T" waves. Am. J. Cardiol., 6:620, 1960.
27. Stuckey, J., Pitt, M., and Sloman, G. Atropine solution administered with an automatic device in the coronary care unit. Am. J. Cardiol., 32:988, 1973.
28. Valentine, P. A., Frew, J. L., Mashford, M. L., and Sloman, J. G. Lidocaine in the prevention of sudden death in the prehospital phase of acute infarction. A double blind study. N. Engl. J. Med. 291: 1327, 1974.
29. White, N. M., Parker, W. S., Binning, R. A., Kimber, E. R., Ead, H. W., Chamberlain, D. A., Mobile coronary care provided by ambulance personnel. Br. Med. J., 3: 618, 1973.
30. WHO. The role of mobile coronary care units. Report of a working group. Moscow, February 3–6, 1970.
31. WHO. The prodromal symptoms of myocardial infarction and sudden death. Report of a working group. Copenhagen, March 1–3, 1970.
32. WHO. Study on symptoms and signs predicting acute myocardial infarction and sudden death. Report of a working group. Copenhagen, February 21–25, 1972.
33. WHO. Committee report on cardiovascular emergencies. Geneva, May 1974.

Chapter 4 The Use of Artificial Pacemakers in Acute Myocardial Infarction

DORIS J. W. ESCHER

General Considerations

Artificial pacing to control bradyarrhythmias and Adams–Stokes syndrome dates back to the introduction of external cardiac pacing by Zoll (135). The pain, morbidity, and limited dependability of this method (18, 71, 91, 92, 96, 100, 109), however, limited its usefulness and artificial pacing to control bradyarrhythmias associated with acute myocardial infarction did not achieve popularity until after the transvenous endocardial approach was introduced (40, 41). The earliest hopeful specific reports on the use of transvenous endocardial pacing in acute myocardial infarction date from 1963 (23, 109). A decade later, during which period hundreds of cases have been reported, we still appear hopeful and still uncertain of its overall value.

A major problem is the baseline against which improvement in mortality and morbidity as effected by pacing is measured. A sampling of the references quoted as controls by early users of pacing in myocardial infarction (9, 19, 23, 27, 32, 88, 109, 118, 136) shows that most were written before the onset of coronary care monitoring, used retrospective material or further referenced still earlier similar studies (3, 6, 15, 20, 25, 29, 39, 52, 53, 55, 57, 58, 61, 81, 89, 95, 102, 106, 112, 116, 131, 132). Several were designed primarily as studies of AV block rather than of myocardial infarction (39, 57, 89, 106, 132). Detailed data that could be used to correlate the incidence and mortality of AV block with age, sex, site of infarction or complications of syncope, shock, or congestive failure, were rarely available. Definitions of bradyarrhythmias, degree of AV block, or bundle branch blocks (if they were considered at all) often were unclear.

Clinical Data

Table 4-1 reviews what little data are available in 11 of these references on the percent incidence and percent mortality (in parentheses) in acute myocardial infarction, of the bradyarrhythmias, and conduction disturbances. The studies of Rosenbaum, Woods, Rathe, Mintz, Smith, Johnson, Imperial and Hurwitz total 2,942 cases with an overall incidence of some degree of AV block of 4.9 (3.1 to 9.6) percent (not necessarily bradycardic) and of third-degree AV block of 1.7 (0.9 to 3.8) percent. Although AV blocks, in general, had mortalities ranging from 25 to 50 percent and third-degree AV block from 29 to 100 percent mortality, only the "advanced" blocks (second- and third-degree) were considered prognostically serious

Table 4-1. Reported Incidence and Mortality of Bradycardias in Acute Myocardial Infarction: Prepacing

Study	Rosenbaum and Levine (102)	Woods *et al.* (131)	Rathe (95)	Mintz and Katz (81)	Smith *et al.* (16)	Cohen *et al.* (15)
Published	1941	1942	1942	1947	1951	1957
No. of patients	208 (38)	128 (47)	274 (20)	572 (22)	920 (23)	68 (47)
Duration of follow-up	1 month	6 weeks	1 month	Hosp	6 weeks	2 months
Sex M	69 (31)	84 (42)	71 (19)	68 (19)	81 (22)	63 (–)
F	31 (35)	16 (75)	29 (24)	32 (29)	19 (30)	37 (–)
Myocardial Infarction						
Ant	52 (30)	48 (42)	32 (26)	55 (20)	59 (26)	24 (75)
Post	31 (36)	41 (42)	35 (19)	36 (23)	40 (18)	75 (37)
Both		2.5 (100)		4.2 (25)		1.5 (100)
Unclassified	5.8 (8.3)	8.5 (82)	17 (26)	4.6 (31)	1.5 (21)	
Percent Arrhythmias	38 (42)			16 (44)	16 (–)	
SA Block						
Sin. Brady				0.5 (0)		
Block Uncl.[a]	3.4 (43)	4.7 (50)	5.1 (36)	6.9 (44)		100 (47)
1°				4.0 (23)		
2° I		3.1 (25)		1.9 (55)		49 (33)
2° II						32 (50)
3°	2.4 (60)	1.6 (100)		0.9 (100)	1.2 (55)	19 (77)
BBB Uncl.						
Cond. Abn.	4.3 (78)	12 (67)	19 (15)	13 (38)		13 (78)
RBBB						
LBBB						

[a]Inclusive of values for 1°, 2°, or 3° block as listed below.

and demonstrated an increased mortality as they progressed in degree (52, 53, 58, 81, 95, 102, 116, 131).

Three of the studies, totaling 124 cases, selectively deal with AV block in myocardial infarction (15, 20, 106). The male to female ratio and ages in this group are similar to those of the general incidence in myocardial infarction. However, the prevalence of diaphragmatic (inferior) wall infarction is 71 to 100 percent, while in the general group it is 37 to 52 percent. This association between AV block and diaphragmatic (inferior) wall infarction is consistent with the fact that in 90 percent of hearts, the blood supply to the AV node is from the right coronary artery. In the remaining 10 percent (in a ratio of 3 males to 1 female), it usually is from the left circumflex artery (54). The higher incidence of death with AV block in anterior wall infarction reflects either a prior diaphragmatic wall infarction or involvement of the His conduction system, the bundle branches, or both, by septal infarction (15, 51, 54, 55, 70).

Rowe and White (106)	Johnson and Miner (58)	Imperial *et al.* (53)	Courter *et al.* (20)	Hurwitz and Eliot (52)	Totals in studies of acute MI	Totals in studies of heart block
1958	1958	1960	1963	1964		
38 (42)	187 (24)	153 (35)	18 (39)	500 (24)	2942 (26)	124 (44)
1 month	Hosp	Hosp	Hosp	Hosp		
68 (46)	76 (20)		89 (47)	67 (–)	70 (23)	69 (48)
32 (33)	24 (33)		11 (0)	33 (–)	30 (34)	31 (10)
16 (–)	48 (29)	53 (36)		45	49 (66)	18 (75)
39 (–)	52 (18)	39 (30)	100 (39)	28 (30–45)	37 (27)	68 (38)
45 (–)		7.8 (50)		8		
				19		
	17 (29)	73 (46)		80 (27)		
	0.5 (100)	15 (17)		9 (11)		
100 (32)	5.9 (–)	6.6 (50)	100 (39)	9.6 (–)	10 (44)	100 (39)
				5.8 (–)		
	2.1 (–)	3.3 (20)		2.0 (60)	5.6 (31)	
			17 (33)			
100 (32)	3.8 (29)	3.8 (80)	88 (37)	1.8 (22)	2.2 (55)	100 (45)
		7.8 (50)				

With these figures in mind, the mixed enthusiasm of the early investigators is understandable. Samet (109) had a 50 percent mortality among his 4 cases (probably all anterior wall infarctions), with one survivor requiring permanent pacing. Bruce *et al.* (9), with 7 cases (6 confirmed as inferior wall infarcts), had only one death (14 percent) and one patient was permanently paced; a good record in view of the severity of illness in his patients. Paulk *et al.* (88), with 43 patients, 75 percent with inferoposterior wall, 7 percent anterior wall, and 18 percent with combined infarction, had a disappointing 40, 67, and 50 percent mortality rate, respectively, despite pacing. This is an overall mortality of 44 percent, with a 77 percent mortality where there was a history of previous infarction and persistence in AV block by 79 percent of those who died.

Despite modern monitoring methods and treatment, the incidence of shock, congestive failure, and mortality were no different from those reported by prepacing groups (15, 89, 106). Epstein *et al.* (32) with 9 patients, 56 percent with anterior or combined infarctions and all severely ill clinically, reported 7 deaths (78 percent). Both survivors, one requiring permanent pacing, were female, with inferior wall lesions. Seven had third-degree AV block, but 2 with 2:1 AV block nevertheless succumbed to shock or congestive failure. Importantly, the records of these cases show that sudden death supervened in 3 patients after sinus rhythm had returned, and days after pacing had been discontinued. Also, when death did not occur immediately, pacing seemed to accelerate improvement of the clinical state. Cosby (19), studying patients with AV block and myocardial infarction (site unknown), reported an 85-percent incidence of death in 13 unpaced patients but only a 60-percent incidence in 10 paced patients and felt that it improved prognosis in the absence of serious complications. Except for the results reported by Bruce, these results are in the ranges of the controls.

For the past 8 to 10 years, circumstances changed in that most study groups have the benefit of continuous rhythm monitoring, which was introduced at the same time as was pacing, for rhythm changes in myocardial infarction (7, 8, 14, 22, 36, 48, 60, 61, 66, 76, 80, 82, 84, 96–98, 115, 120, 121).

Table 4-2 lists eight representative studies, giving the percent incidence and, when available, the percent mortality (in parentheses) in unpaced patients. Little had changed in the incidence of sex ratio or site of infarction, but the tendency to better define the location of the infarction in terms of presumed anatomic disruption is evident, as is the increasing awareness of the diagnostic and prognostic association of bundle branch block. Of interest, is the clearly increased appreciation of the incidence of cardiac arrhythmias in general. Arrhythmias of some sort will be seen in 75 to 95 percent of continuously monitored patients, whereas arrhythmias of diagnostic, prognostic, or therapeutic value will be present in perhaps 50 ± 10 percent. In the bradyarrhythmias, continuous monitoring demonstrates that their incidence is two to three times that found on intermittent observation and is actually in the order of 10 to 20 percent for SA block or sinus bradycardia, 1.7 (1.2 to 3.9) percent for unclassified block, 6 (4 to 8) percent for third-degree AV block, and 15 percent for bundle branch block. Mortality continues to be higher in females than males by about 9 ± 2 percent, attributable, by most, to the fact that females are older than males by 5 to 10 years at the time of their first infarction. While the incidence of anterior versus inferior myocardial infarction varied from study to study, complete AV block was seen two to five times more frequently with posteroinferior than with anterior infarction. The mortality in AV block was lowest if the block was posteroinferior and the QRS narrow and highest if the lesion was anterior with a broad QRS complex. Pump failure was the major cause of death in anterior wall infarction with complete AV block (particularly if there was bundle branch block), with shock, congestive failure, or both occurring within hours to less than 1 week after onset. In inferior wall lesions, shock, failure, or both occurred less precipitously, starting in 1 or 2 days and lasting for up to 2 weeks in survivors (7, 14, 36, 48, 66, 84, 115, 121).

Studies on the effect of pacing, primarily in third-degree and second- to third-degree AV block, abound (4, 10, 12, 38, 46, 62, 64, 68, 72, 83, 87, 90, 108, 113, 114, 119, 122, 127). Tabulations of overall mortality of several groups are listed by Parsonnet *et al.* (87), Friedberg *et al.* (38), Schluger *et al.* (113), and Narvas *et al.* (83) as well as in Table 4-3. Many of the individual studies listed are not statistically valid because of small numbers, and it is from these papers that biased reports of zero percent, 100 percent, and similar widely different figures are derived. All of the summaries duplicate many listings. Nevertheless, they arrive at dissimilar figures of death. Parsonnet compares an unpaced mortality of 47 percent from a group of 276 patients with 43 percent of 80 paced patients (87). Friedberg (38) compares an unpaced group of 131 cases (primarily, but not purely, third-degree AV block) with a 52 percent mortality, with a paced series of almost 600 cases in which the overall mortality is only 40 percent but that for third-degree AV block is 58 percent and for second-degree AV block, 34 percent. Sutton *et al.* (122) reinforce the difference between second- and third-degree AV block in his comparison of a mortality of 11 percent for second-degree AV block with that of 48 percent with third-degree AV block.

In comparing Tables 4-1, 4-2, and 4-3 in this report, it is easy to see where problems arise, even when an effort has been made to adjust figures to a common method of presentation and only studies with large case loads included. Unclassified block in Table 4-2 reveals the higher incidence of blocks observed (especially first-degree), which may dilute mortality figures. This appears to have occurred in both total unclassified block and third-degree AV block. In the paced series (Table 4-3) it would appear that there is a small but clearcut improvement in survival in third-degree AV block and probably for second-degree AV block as well.

If pacing, with its dramatic impact and ability to improve cardiac output by stabilizing cardiac rhythm and increasing ventricular rate in AV block and other bradycardias does not yield a better salvage, what then is the problem? There is no question that it is pump failure giving rise to shock and congestive failure. Syncope, also a serious problem, may be a combination of electrical failure or failure of mechanical response, one reinforcing the other. Wiggers (129) discussion of the problem, 30 years ago, is still precisely to the point. Noncontractile muscle will not pump, ischemic muscle is poorly contractile, and nonperfused muscle not only will not pump but acts as a sump, absorbing in flaccid dilatation variably significant amounts of contractile force generated by whatever functional muscle remains postinfarction. As a compensatory response depends on the condition of the remaining myocardium, mortality rises swiftly with histories of previous infarction. Severe shock or congestive failure will double or triple the mortality of the uncomplicated course from a similar but possibly less massively affected site (12, 67, 69, 76, 87, 88, 93, 130). Cardiogenic shock is discussed in detail in Chapter 5.

Pacing in these patients frequently offers an early, remarkable, improvement in clinical appearance due, primarily, to an increase in cardiac output from the increase in ventricular rate and often an accompanying increase in systolic blood pressure. Unlike chronic AV block, where the myocardium often is minimally affected, the infarcted heart has a limited ability to increase cardiac output by increasing stroke volume. The rates of maximal improvement appear to be about 100 beats per minute or even a little higher. When there has been excessive damage, however, no amount of increase in ventricular rate can improve cardiac output or elevate blood pressure. When the remaining vascular supply is also compromised, too great an increase in ventricular rate has a deleterious effect, as the inadequate perfusion results in an ischemic state with anaerobic metabolism (17, 37, 67, 69, 133). Even the survivor of an acute episode, with or without the use of temporary or even permanent pacing, in the event of persistent AV block, still encounters the late effect of myocardial damage. Many remain in heart failure and their life expectancy, in contradistinction

Table 4-2. Reports on the Incidence and Mortality of Bradycardias in Acute Myocardial Infarction: Continuous Monitoring

Study	Julian *et al.* (61)	Meltzer and Kitchell (80)	Restieaux *et al.* (97)	Lown *et al.* (76)	Stock and Macken (121)	Day (22)	Brown *et al.* (7)	Simon *et al.* (115)	Total in studies of acute MI
Published	1964	1966	1967	1967	1968	1968	1969	1972	
Duration followed	4–5 wk	—	3 wk	1–2 wk	2 wk	Hosp	Hosp	Hosp	
No. of patients	100 (31)	141 (–)	150 (14)	300 (18)	364 (–)	273 (27)	446 (25)	757 (20)	2531 (–) 2026 (17)
Sex M	76 (30)		83 (–)	64 (14)				67 (–)	69 (19)
F	24 (33)		17 (–)	36 (25)				33 (–)	32 (26)
MI Ant	46 (–)		67 (–)	29 (26)	39 (–)		52 (–) 4 (56)[f]		38 (–)
Post	44 (–)		33 (–)	27 (24)	43 (–)		42 (–) 18 (17)[f]		38 (–)
Both	4 (100)			6 (39)	0.8 (–)		3 (–) 54 (100)[f]		3 (–)
Unclassified	6 (–)			38 (10)	18 (–)		3 (–) 21 (0)[f]		11 (–)
Percent Arrhythmias	95 (–) 56 (36)[b]	75 (–)	19 (64)[b]	90 (–)		78 (–) (50 (–)[b]			84 42 (45)[b]
SA Block	14 (21)	11 (–)		26 (–)					20 (–)
Sin. Brady				15 (4.4)[b]					
Block[a]	39 (–)	21 (–)			16 (–)	16 (24)	12 (33)	18 (39)	17 (29)
1°	13 (46)	8.5 (–)		11 (–)[e]	5.0 (–)	4.4 (0)	6.1 (–) 2.2 (10)[e]	11.8 (–) 7.9 (18)[e]	8.5 (–)
2°	10 (30)	3.5 (–)		6.0 (–)	4.4 (–)	5.9 (13)	4.7 (–) 3.0 (27)[e]	4.8 (50) 3.8 (41)[e]	5.1 (–)
I					1.4 (–)				
II					3.0 (–)				
3°	8 (37)	4.2 (–)	6 (33)	7 (38)[d,e]	6.6 (–)	6.2 (53)	6.5 (45)	5.9 (64)	6.3 (47)
Narrow									
Broad									
IVCD					11 (–) 1.7 (–)[f]				

Study	Julian *et al.* (61)	Meltzer and Kitchell (80)	Restieaux *et al.* (97)	Lown *et al.* (76)	Stock and Macken (121)	Day (22)	Brown *et al.* (7)	Simon *et al.* (115)	Total in studies of acute MI
BBB[c]	13 (62)	18 (–)	15 (–)		15 ( ) 5.5 (–)[f]	14 (76)			15 (73)
RBBB	6 (–)		11 (–)		9.9 (–) 3.6 (–)[f]	5.5 (80)			8.3 (–)
LBBB	7 (–)		4 (–)		5.2 (–) 1.4 (–)[f]	8.1 (73)			6.1 (–)
BBBB					0.6 (–) 0.6 (–)[f]				

[a] Total unclassified block.
[b] Serious arrhythmia.
[c] Total unclassified bundle branch block.
[d] Despite pacing.
[e] Figure is for number of patients with this degree of block the highest reached.
[f] Percent associated with heart block.

Mortalities calculated from those studies providing the necessary data.

Table 4-3. Selected Reports on the Incidence and Mortality of Paced Patients and Second- and Third-degree Heart Block and Myocardial Infarction

Study	Paulk *et al.* (88)	Parsonnet *et al.* (87)	Sutton *et al.* (122)	Chatterjee *et al.* (12)	Watson and Goldberg (127)	Totals in study
Study limit	3° Block	3° Block	2°, 3° Block	2°, 3° Block	2°, 3° Block	
Published	1966	1967	1968	1969	1971	
Duration followed	Hosp	Hosp	Hosp	Hosp	Hosp	
No. of patients	43 (44)[a] (63)[c]	19 (37)[a] (–)	55 (46)[a] (40)	82 (33)[a] (–)	58 (28)[a] (–)	257 (37)
Sex M	63 (44)	63 (42)	78 (–)			70 (43)
F	37 (44)	37 (29)	22 (–)			30 (39)
MI Ant	7 (67)	21 (100)	20 (100)	20 (76)	16 (67)	33 (43)
Post	75 (41)	47 (11)	78 (30)	80 (23)	84 (20)	77 (26)
Both	18 (50)		2 (100)			
Unclass.		32 (33)				
Block 2°			13 (12)		22 (23)	18 (20)
I						
II						
3°	100 (44)		84 (48)		78 (29)	86 (40)
Persisted 3°	49 (71)	53 (86)	33 (89)	27 (82)		46 (60)
RSR	53 (17)	47 (11)	67 (24)	60 (16)		65 (19)
Narrow QRS			60 (24)	69 (16)		65 (20)
Broad QRS			36 (75)	31 (73)		34 (74)
RBBB					10 (83)	
LBBB					6.9 (50)	
Syncope	30 (–)	47 (62)		42 (52)	17 (60)	41 (57)
Arrest	44 (63)					
Shock	58 (40)[b] (80)[d]	37 (14) (86)			74 (43)	
CHF	77 (55)[b] (84)[d]	63 (67)[e]				
Survived Perm. Paced	56 (8)	63 (33)				

[a] Overall.
[b] Clinically moderate.
[c] Within first 1–3 days.
[d] Clinically severe.
[e] Clinically moderate plus clinically severe.

to chronic AV block, is sharply curtailed (5, 33, 59, 69). It has been suggested that AV sequential pacing in these patients would be helpful as it would restore the push of the atrial contribution to ventricular function and raise cardiac output somewhat above that of simple ventricular pacing (11). It could make some difference, as it would in the management of any paced patient at the limits of function, but cannot restore myocardium. Two of 10 percent of patients are permanently paced postinfarction (5, 33, 69).

Given what appears to be a salvage situation with perhaps a 10 percent gain in overall mortality with pacing despite initial clinical improvement, who then should be paced, when, and how? Some clue seems offered by a study of bundle branch blocks, as together with the site of infarction the blocks are an index to the severity of muscle and conduction tissue damage, before, during, and after the acute event. Rosenbaum and Lepeschkin (104) discussed the effect of bilateral bundle branch in the nonacute patient, as long as 30 years ago. Sambhi and Zimmerman (107), with an almost 50-percent incidence of anterior wall infarction in a series of 234 cases reported an almost 20-percent incidence of bundle branch blocks but a normal 5 percent incidence of third-degree AV block. As might be expected, all of their postmortem studies (31 percent of deaths) revealed infarctions of the left ventricle and septum. Sutton and Davies (123), correlating the electrocardiogram with autopsy findings in 19 patients found seven of eight anterior wall (anteroseptal) infarctions to have bundle branch block on the electrocardiogram. The one exception, a patient with a narrow QRS complex, was found to have a posteroseptal lesion at postmortem. On the other hand, only three of nine diaphragmatic myocardial infarctions by electrocardiography, had bundle branch block. The mortality in the bundle branch blocks was 77 percent, with 4 of 5 survivors left with residual third-degree or bilateral bundle branch block. Mortality with a narrow QRS complex was 24 percent (123). Many other publications reinforce this pattern (2, 24, 28, 30, 35, 40–45, 50, 65, 73, 74, 78, 79, 86, 99, 101, 103, 110, 111, 126, 128). In summary, they accept mortalities from 40 to 90 percent, but more in the order of 65 $\pm$ 10 percent in bilateral bundle branch block, almost all of which are associated with septal damage. Isolated left anterior hemiblock (see Chapter 15) is relatively benign, often transient, associated half the time with single vessel disease, and does not affect mortality (45, 65). Right bundle branch block is a serious involvement, often associated with 60 to 70 percent mortality, when associated with left anterior hemiblock. Right bundle branch block with left posterior hemiblock implies a more extensive septal damage (44). Atkins *et al.* (2) raise the question of elective permanent pacing in recovered patients with right bundle branch block and left anterior hemiblock as they have had sudden late deaths in 5 of 6 patients in this category (with anterior myocardial infarcts and/or syncope. Third-degree AV block in anterior myocardial infarction is in the same category, as it again results from septal damage. Second- and third-degree AV blocks associated with posterior-inferior infarctions are much more benign and result from ischemia or closure of the AV nodal artery (90 percent from the right coronary artery). They are often transient and shift through various stages of AV block, giving warning that they are progressing in depth and allowing time to pace electively. Unless septal collaterals are jeopardized by anterior myocardial damage, they remain in the 15 to 25 percent morbidity range. Interestingly, Lie *et al.* (74) take exception to the thesis that broadening of the QRS complex is always an ominous sign. In inferior myocardial infarctions with third-degree AV block, its presence did not affect mortality (74).

Anterior lesions are abrupt in onset, often present on admission and rarely advertising their advent by lesser grades of AV block. Despite these depressing figures and facts, it is difficult to accept the almost nihilistic approach of Scheinman and Brenman who virtually state that statistics will be unchanged with or without pacing and they withhold it except in first-degree AV block in categories likely to progress abruptly to high-grade AV block, anterior infarctions or first-degree AV block with bundle branch blocks (trifascicular block) (111).

Indications for Pacing

It would seem preferable to pace where intellect or even when emotion dictates. This should include anterior wall infarctions with bundle branch block, particularly when newly present and particularly with right bundle branch block, bifascicular, or trifascicular block. First-degree AV block in anterior infarction can be viewed with suspicion but should be "ignored" in inferior infarction. Mobitz type I (Wenckebach) AV block does not require pacing unless it progresses to Mobitz type II AV block with a slow ventricular rate and clinical distress. In *good* hands temporary pacing is a relatively atraumatic procedure. It eliminates surprise and crisis and, at least for a while, particularly in those with a potential for survival, gives them the appearance and feeling of well-being earlier and more securely. If the difference is no more than an ephemeral 10 percent, it would seem worth it, as it is not always possible to pick the survivor in advance (126). When pacing, attention should be given to rate. Higher pacing rates may result in a better output, but they are energy consumers and can precipitate higher degrees of block (21, 30).

The role of sinus bradycardia and sick sinus syndrome in acute, usually inferior wall, myocardial infarction is generally understated. It is considered benign and not likely to affect mortality unless there is sinus arrest or profound bradycardia. Mild, vagal bradycardias, or blocked extrasystoles, are rarely of clinical importance (31, 75, 105, 134). Slower rates are hemodynamically deleterious and also open the cardiac cycle to a greater risk of ectopic activity such as bigeminal beats (which further depress effective output) or ventricular tachycardias (bradytachycardia syndrome). While atropine or Isuprel are a logical recourse, in many of these patients, pacing is a valuable backup (134). This is especially true in the patient with recurrent sinus arrest who should be paced rather than depend on Isuprel or atropine.

Pacing is increasingly used to treat tachyarrhythmias in myocardial infarction (1, 16, 31, 47, 49, 56, 77, 85, 94, 117). Their incidence is much higher than that of the bradyarrhythmias, about 20 to 30 percent with an approximate 50 percent mortality. They are commonly associated with cardiogenic shock or heart failure. Normally, the upper physiologic rates function as a compensatory response to increase cardiac output by increasing beats per minute instead of increasing stroke volume, but excessive rates reduce output and potentiate hypotension and heart failure. An infarcted heart is at least temporarily, in this category (26). The tachyarrhythmia may, as in ventricular lesions, be in response to the irritation of pericarditis, secondary to ischemia and responsive to catecholamines. Rapid rhythms can be approached by using over-riding rates (10 to 20 beats over the spontaneous rate) to capture and suppress the underlying irritable mechanism and gradually bring the paced rate down to a normal physiologic level. Very rapid pacing rates can be used as a brief blocking drive. Antiarrhythmic drugs (see Chapter 2) can be used in high doses, backed by pacing at a normal rate to prevent over suppression (26, 117). Overdrive, not in excess of 140 to 180 per minute, can also be used to capture ventricular rhythms. Here, overdrive is used with greater caution as, depending upon the failing state of the heart, fibrillation can be induced at lower rates of overdrive. It is frequently used in demand mode at physiologic rates in the ventricle as a back stop, again, for drug use (13, 34, 124, 125).

A cookbook prescription for pacing (63) the heart in myocardial infarction is difficult to expect. Pacing in myocardial infarction usually is by the temporary approach. If the three modalities for the use of a pacemaker are kept in mind, good usefulness can result. For the bradyarrhythmias, the ventricle, in the absence of AV conduction, or the atria (via the coronary sinus electrode) with intact AV conduction, can be stimulated to contract and maintain a rate in physiologic ranges. In tachyarrhythmias, the pacer can be overdriven to suppress underlying irritable ectopic foci and "bring down" the tachyarrhythmias as its rate is reduced. Alternatively, it can be kept at a normal rate as drugs are used to reduce irritability with the pacemaker as an overshoot safeguard against bradyarrhythmia.

Summary

In the bradyarrhythmias, a good working plan is to pace on standby in anterior wall myocardial infarctions if the patient arrives at the hospital in second- or third-degree AV block, or if bilateral bundle branch block develops later. In diaphragmatic (inferior) myocardial infarctions, it seems reasonable to prophylactically pace on standby for a Mobitz type II or third-degree AV block, but not plan to put in an electrode for the first-degree or Mobitz type I (Wenckebach) AV block. The pacing has not proved to be of prophylactic value in hemiblocks associated with acute myocardial infarction. (Hemiblocks are discussed in detail in Chapter 15.) Mortality may not improve dramatically, as pacing will not reverse deaths by cardiogenic shock or congestive heart failure due to massive muscle damage. It should prevent asystole and be useful in damping ventricular tachycardia or fibrillation by suppressing frequent or multifocal extrasystoles much of the time. It will surely allow slight relaxation from some of the sense of crisis an unstable case may bring to the coronary care unit.

In the following situations, artificial pacing is recommended:

1. Symptomatic bradyarrhythmias of any origin or mechanism (particularly complete AV block in anterior myocardial infarction)
2. Bradytachyarrhythmia syndrome
3. Drug-resistant tachyarrhythmias
4. Bilateral bundle branch block, right or left bundle branch block with acute onset in anterior myocardial infarction
5. Mobitz type II or complete AV block (even asymptomatic).

References

1. Askey, J. M. Aurecular paroxysmal tachycardia in association with myocardial infarction. Am. Heart J., 37:425, 1949.
2. Atkins, J. M., Leshin, S. J., Blomquist, G., and Mullins, C. B. Ventricular conduction blocks and sudden death in acute myocardial infarction: potential indications for pacing. N. Engl. J. Med., 288:281, 1970.

3. Ball, C. O., Billings, F. T., Jr., Furman, R. H., Brothers, G. B., Thomas, J., and Meneely, G. R. The functional circulatory consequences of myocardial infarction. Circulation, 11:749, 1955.
4. Beregovich, J., Fenig, S., Lasser, J., and Allen, D. Management of acute myocardial infarction complicated by advanced atrioventricular block. Am. J. Cardiol., 23:54, 1969.
5. Bernard, R., Van Durme, J. P., Beaujean, M., Colay, G., Collignon, P., Cornel, A., Daenen, W., Derom, Fr., D'Heer, H., Dodinot, B., Helmer, J., Laurent, Cl., Ponlot, R., Primo, G., Tremouroux, J., Vandroux, A., and Vermeire, P. Le Pacemaker definitif post-infarctus. Ann. Cardiol., Angeiol., 20:435, 1971.
6. Blondeau, M., Rizzon, P., and Lenègre, J. Les troubles de la conduction auriculoventriculaire dans l'infarctus myocardique récent. Arch. Mal Coeur, 54:1104, 1961.
7. Brown, R. W., Hunt, D. and Sloman, J. G. The natural history of atrioventricular conduction defects in acute myocardial infarction. Am. Heart J., 78:460, 1969.
8. Brown, K. W. G., MacMillan, R. L., Forbath, N., Med'grano, F. and Scott, J. W. Coronary Unit: an intensive care center for acute myocardial infarction. Lancet, 2:349, 1963.
9. Bruce, R. A., Blackmon, J. R., Cobb, L. A., and Dodge, H. T. Treatment of asystole or heart block during acute myocardial infarction with electrode catheter pacing. Am. Heart J., 69:460, 1965.
10. Chamberlain, D. and Leinbach, R. Electrical pacing in heart block complicating acute myocardial infarction. Br. Heart J., 32:2, 1970.
11. —— —— Vassaux, C. E., Kastor, J. A. DeSanctis, R. W, and Sanders, C. A. Sequential atrioventricular pacing in heart block complicating acute myocardial infarction. N. Engl. J. Med., 282:577, 1970.
12. Chatterjee, K., Harris, A. and Leatham, A. The risk of pacing after infarction and current recommendations. Lancet, 2:1061, 1969.
13. Chodda, K. D., Banka, V. S., and Helfant, R. H. Rate dependent ventricular ectopia following acute coronary occlusion. Circulation, 49:654, 1974.
14. Christiansen, I., Haghfelt, T., and Amtorp, O. Complete heart block in acute myocardial infarction: drug therapy. Am. Heart J., 85:162, 1973.
15. Cohen, D. B., Doctor, L., and Pick, A. The significance of atrioventricular block complicating acute myocardial infarction. Am. Heart J., 55:215, 1957.
16. Cohen, H. E., Kahn, M., and Donoso, E. Treatment of supraventricular tachycardias with catheter and permanent pacemakers. Am. J. Cardiol., 20:735, 1967.
17. Conti, C. R., Pitt, B., Gundel, W. D., Friesinger, G. C., and Ross, R. Myocardial blood flow in pacing induced angina. Circulation, 42:815, 1970.
18. Corday, E., Irving, D. W., Gold, H., Bernstein, H., and Jaffe, H. L. Recent advances in the treatment of arrhythmias and conduction defects. Am. Heart J., 64:126, 1961.
19. Cosby, R. S., Lau, F., Rhode, R., Cafferky, E., and Mayo, M. Complete heart block: Prognostic volume of electrocardiographic features and clinical complications. Am. J. Cardiol., 17:190, 1966.
20. Courter, S. R., Moffat, J., and Fowler, N. O. Advanced atrioventricular block in acute myocardial infarction. Circulation, 27:1034, 1963.
21. Danzig, R., Alpern, H., and Swan, H. J. C. The significance of atrial rate in patients with atrioventricular conduction abnormalities complicating acute myocardial infarction. Am. J. Cardiol., 24:707, 1969.
22. Day, H. W. Acute coronary care—a five year report. Am. J. Cardiol., 21:252, 1968.
23. Delman, A. J., Schwedel, J. B., and Escher, D. J. W. An intracardiac pacemaker in Adams–Stokes attacks in acute myocardial infarction. J.A.M.A., 184:1040, 1963.
24. DePasquale, N. P., and Bruno, M. S. Natural history of combined bundle branch block and left anterior hemiblock (bilateral bundle branch block). Am. J. Med., 54:297, 1973.
25. DeSaint Pierre, G., Toscani, A., and Massi, A. Il blocco atrioventricolare completo conseguente ad infarto del miocardio. descrizione di due casi trattati con successo mediante alupent. Settimana Med., 51:1243, 1963.
26. DeSanctis, R. W., Block, P., and Hutter, A. M., Jr. Tachyarrhythmias in myocardial infarction. Circulation, 45:681, 1972.
27. —— Short term use of intravenous electrode in heart block, J.A.M.A., 184:544, 1963.
28. Dhingra, R. C., Denes, P., Wu, D., Chuguimia, R., and Rosen, K. M. The significance of second degree atrioventricular block and bundle branch block. Circulation, 49:638, 1973.
29. Dimond, E. G., Dunn, M., and Brosius, F. Management of arrhythmias in acute myocardial infarction. Prog. Cardiovasc. Dis., 3:1, 1960.
30. El-Sherif, N. Intermittent trifascicular block. Am. J. Cardiol., 31:71, 1973.

31. —— Tachycardia and bradycardia dependent bundle branch block after acute myocardial ischemia. Br. Heart J., 36:291, 1974.
32. Epstein, E. J., Coulshed, N., McKendrick, C. S., Clarke, J., Kearns, W. E. Artificial pacing by electrode catheter for heart block or asystole complicating acute myocardial infarction. Br. Heart J., 28:546, 1966.
33. Escher, D. J. W., Furman, S., and Solomon, N. Transvenous emergency cardiac pacing. Ann. N.Y. Acad. Sci., 167:582, 1969.
34. Feldman, A. E., Hellersteen, H. K., Driscol, T. E., and Botti, R. E. Repetitive ventricular fibrillation in myocardial infarction refractory to Bretylium Tosylate subsequently controlled by ventricular pacing. Am. J. Cardiol., 27:227, 1971.
35. Fenig, S., and Lichstein, E. Incomplete bilateral bundle branch block and AV block complicating acute anterior wall myocardial infarction. Am. Heart J., 84:38, 1972.
36. —— —— Incomplete bilateral bundle branch block and AV block complicating acute anterior wall myocardial infarction. Am. Heart J., 84:38, 1972.
37. Forrester, J. S., Helfant, R. H., Pasternac, A., Amsterdam, E. A., Most, A. S., Kemp, H. G., and Gorlin, R. Atrial pacing in coronary heart disease. Am. J. Cardiol., 27:237, 1971.
38. Friedberg, C. K., Cohen, H., and Donoso, E. Advanced heart block as a complication of acute myocardial infarction, role of pacemaker therapy. Prog. Cardiovasc. Dis., 10:466, 1968.
39. —— Donoso, F., and Stein, W. G. Nonsurgical acquired heart block. Ann. N.Y. Acad. Sci., 111:835, 1964.
40. Furman, S., and Robinson, G. The use of intracardiac pacemaker in correction of total heart block. Surg. Forum., 9:245, 1958.
41. —— Schwedel, J. B. An intracardiac pacemaker for Stokes–Adams seizures. N. Engl. J. Med., 261:943, 1959.
42. Godman, M. J., Lassers, B. W., and Julian, D. G. Complete bundle branch block complicating acute myocardial infarction. N. Engl. J. Med., 282:237, 1970.
43. —— Alpert, B. A., and Julian, D. G. Bilateral bundle branch block complicating acute myocardial infarction. Lancet, 2:345, 1971.
44. Gould, L., Venkataraman, K., Mohammad, N. and Gomprecht, R. F. Prognosis of right bundle branch block in acute myocardial infarction, J.A.M.A., 219:502, 1972.
45. Hamby, R. J., Tabrah, F., and Gupta, M. Intraventricular conduction disturbances and coronary artery disease. Am. J. Cardiol., 32:758, 1973.
46. Harris, A. and Bluestone, R. Treatment of slow heart rates following acute myocardial infarction. Br. Heart J., 28:631, 1966.
47. Hass, J. Mechanisms of ventricular arrhythmias associated with myocardial infarction. Am. J. Cardiol., 24:800, 1969.
48. Hatee, L. and Rokseth, R. Conservative treatment of AV block in acute myocardial infarction. Br. Heart J., 33:595, 1971.
49. Heiman, D. F. and Helwig, J., Jr. Suppression of ventricular arrhythmias by transvenous pacing. J.A.M.A., 195:172, 1966.
50. Hunt, D., and Sloman, G. Bundle branch block in acute myocardial infarction. Br. Med. J., 1:85, 1969.
51. —— Lie, J. T., Vohra, J., and Sloman, G. Histopathology of heart block complicating acute myocardial infarction. Circulation, 48:1252, 1973.
52. Hurwitz, M., and Eliot, R. S. Arrhythmias in acute myocardial infarction. Dis. Chest, 45:616, 1964.
53. Imperial, E. S., Carballo, R., and Zimmerman, H. A. Disturbances of rate, rhythm and conduction in acute myocardial infarction. Am. J. Cardiol., 5:24, 1960.
54. James, T. N. Pathogenesis of arrhythmias in acute myocardial infarction. Am. J. Cardiol., 24:791, 1969.
55. —— Arrhythmias and conduction disturbances in acute myocardial infarction. Am. Heart J., 64:416, 1962.
56. Jewett, D. E., Dalcon, R., Raferty, E. B., and Oram, S. Incidence and management of supraventricular arrhythmias after acute myocardial infarction. Lancet, 2:734, 1967.
57. Johannsson, B. Complete heart block. Acta. Med. Scand. 180 (Suppl. 451): 1, 1966.
58. Johnson, C. C. and Miner, P. F. The occurrence of arrhythmias in acute myocardial infarction. Dis. Chest, 33:414, 1958.
59. Julian, D. G., Lassers, B. W., and Godman, M. J. Pacing for heart block in acute myocardial infarction. Ann. N.Y. Acad. Sci., 167:911, 1969.

60. —— Valentine, P. A., and Miller, G. G. Routine electrocardiographic monitoring in acute myocardial infarction. Med. J. Austr., 1:433, 1964.
61. —— —— —— Disturbances in rate, rhythm and conduction in acute myocardial infarction. Am. J. Med., 37:915, 1964.
62. Julian, D. G. and Oliver, M. F. eds. Acute Myocardial Infarction. Edinburgh and London, E. and S. Livingston, Ltd., 1968.
63. Kaltman, A. J. Indications for temporary pacemaker insertion in acute myocardial infarction. Am. Heart J., 81:837, 1971.
64. Kimball, J. T., Klein, S. W., and Killip, T. Cardiac pacing in acute myocardial infarction. Am. J. Cardiol., 19:136, 1967.
65. Kinkaid, D. T., and Botti, R. E. Significance of isolated left anterior hemiblock and left axis deviation during acute myocardial infarction. Am. J. Cardiol., 30:797, 1972.
66. Kostuk, W. J. and Beanlands, D. S. Complete heart block associated with acute myocardial infarction. Am. J. Cardiol., 26:380, 1970.
67. Lassers, B. W., Anderton, J. L., George, M., Muir, A. L., and Julian, D. G. Hemodynamic effects of artificial pacing in complete heart block complicating myocardial infarction. Circulation, 38:308, 1963.
68. —— Julian, D. G. Artificial pacing in management of complete heart block complicating acute myocardial infarction. Br. Med. J., 2:142, 1968.
69. —— First year follow-up after recovery from acute myocardial infarction with complete heart block. Lancet, 1:1172, 1969.
70. Lev, M., Suman, G. K., and Pick, A. The pathogenesis of atrioventricular block in coronary disease. Circulation, 42:409, 1970.
71. Levowitz, B. S., Ford, W. B., and Smith, J. W. Jr. The use of direct stimulating myocardial electrodes in complete atrioventricular block. J. Thorac. Cardiovasc. Surg., 40:283, 1960.
72. Lewinson, R. B., Cornil, A., and Thys, J. P. L'entrainement electrosystolique da s l'infarctus due myocarde. Aeta Cardive, 27:665, 1972.
73. Lichstein, P. R., Gupta, P. K., Chudda, K., Liu, H., and Sayeed, M. Findings of prognostic valve in patients with incomplete bilateral bundle branch block complicating acute myocardial infarction. Am. J. Cardiol., 32:913, 1973.
74. Lie, K. I., Wellens, H. J., Schuiilenburg, R. M., and Durrer, D. Mechanisms and significance of widened QRS complexes during complete atrioventricular block in acute inferior myocardial infarction. Am. J. Cardiol., 33:833, 1974.
75. Lightfoot, P. R. Sinoatrial block with Wenckebach phenomenon and ventricular parasystole after myocardial infarction. Chest, 65:664, 1974.
76. Lown, B., Hood, W. B., Fakhro, A. M., Kaplinsky, E., and Roberge, G. Unresolved problems in coronary care. Am. J. Cardiol., 20:494, 1967.
77. —— Kosowsky, B. D. Artificial pacemakers. N. Engl. J. Med., 283:971, 1970.
78. Luy, G., Bahl, O. P., and Massie, E. Intermittent left bundle branch block. Am. Heart J., 85:332, 1973.
79. McNally, E. M., and Benchimol, A. Medical and physiologic considerations in the use of artificial cardiac pacing. Am. Heart J., 75:380, 1968.
80. Meltzer, L. E., and Kitchell, J. B. The incidence of arrhythmias associated with acute myocardial infarction. Prog. Cardiovasc. Dis., 9:50, 1966.
81. Mintz, S. S., and Katz, L. N. Recent myocardial infarction. Arch. Intern. Med., 80:205, 1947.
82. Nachlas, M. M., Miller, D. I., and Siedband, M. P. Continuous monitoring of patients with acute myocardial infarction. J.A.MA., 198:1, 1966.
83. Narvas, R. M., Kilgour, J. M., and Basu, S. K. Heart block in acute myocardial infarction: prognostic factors and role of transvenous catheter pacemaker. Can. Med. Assoc. J., 102:55, 1970.
84. Norris, R. M. Heart block in posterior and anterior infarction. Br. Heart J., 31:352, 1969.
85. —— Mercer, C. J., and Yeates, S. E. Idioventricular rhythm complicating acute myocardial infarction. Br. Heart J., 32:617, 1970.
86. —— —— Croxon, M. S. Conduction disturbances due to anteroseptal myocardial infarction and their treatment by endocardial pacing. Am. Heart J., 84:560, 1970.
87. Parsonnet, V., Zucker, I. R., Gilbert, L., Rothfeld, E. L., Brief, D. K. and Alpert, J. An evaluation of transvenous pacing of the heart in complete heart block following acute myocardial infarction. Israel, J. Med. Sci., 3:306, 1967.
88. Paulk, E. A., and Hurst, J. W. Complete heart block in acute myocardial infarction: A clinical evaluation of the intracardiac bipolar catheter pacemaker. Am. J. Cardiol. 17:695, 1966.

89. Penton, G. B., Miller, H., and Levine, S. Some clinical features of complete heart block. Circulation, 13:801, 1956.
90. Peretz, D. I. Advanced heart block during acute myocardial infarction treated with an electrode pacing catheter. Can. Med. Assoc. J., 96:451, 1967.
91. Portal, R. W., Davies, J. G., Leatham, A., and Siddons, A. H. M. Artificial pacing for heart block, Lancet, 2:1369, 1962.
92. —— Robinson, B. F., and Leatham, A. G. Notes on cardiac resuscitation including external cardiac message. Br. Med. J., 1:636, 1963.
93. Rackley, C. E., and Russell, R. O. Left ventricular function in acute myocardial infarction and its clinical significance. Circulation, 45:231, 1972.
94. Raferty, E. B., Rehman, M. F., Banks, D. C., and Oram, S. Incidence and management of ventricular arrhythmias after acute myocardial infarction. Br. Heart J., 31:273, 1969.
95. Rathe, H. W. Myocardial infarction: Clinical features and prognosis. J.A.M.A., 120:99, 1942.
96. Reiff, T. R., Oppenheimer, J., and Ferguson, G. Cardiac injury presumably due to use of the external electric cardiac pacemaker in Stokes–Adams disease. Am. Heart J., 54:437, 1957.
97. Restieaux, N., Bray, C., Bullard, H., Murray, M., Robinson, J., Brigden, W., and McDonald, L. 150 patients with cardiac infarction treated in a coronary unit. Lancet, 1:1285, 1967.
98. Robinson, J. S., Sloman, G., and McRae, C. Continuous electrocardiographic monitoring in the early stages after acute myocardial infarction. Med. J. Aust., 1:427, 1964.
99. Roos, J. C., and Dunning, A. J. Right bundle branch block and left axis deviation in acute myocardial infarction. Br. Heart J., 32:847, 1970.
100. Rose, L. B. and Wartonick, W. Treatment of a case of Stokes–Adams Disease by external electric stimulation. J.A.M.A., 159:1015, 1955.
101. Rosen, K. M., Loeb, H. S., Chuguima, R., Sinno, M. Z., Rahimtoola, S. H., and Gunnar, R. M. Site of heart block in acute myocardial infarction. Circulation, 42:925, 1970.
102. Rosenbaum, F. F., and Levine, S. Prognostic value of various clinical and electrocardiographic features of acute myocardial infarction: I: immediate prognosis. Arch. Intern. Med., 68:913, 1941.
103. Rosenbaum, M. B. The hemi-blocks: Diagnostic criteria and clinical significance. Mod. Concepts Cardiovasc. Dis., 39:141, 1970.
104. —— Lepeschkin, E. Bilateral bundle branch block. Am. Heart J., 50:38, 1955.
105. Rotman, M., Wagner, G. S., and Wallace, A. G. Bradyarrhythmias in acute myocardial infarction. Circulation, 45:703, 1972.
106. Rowe, J. C., and White, P. D. Complete heart block: A follow-up study. Ann. Int. Med., 49:260, 1958.
107. Sambhi, M. P., and Zimmerman, H. Acute myocardial infarction: an analysis of 234 cases. Ohio State Med. J., 52:718, 1956.
108. Samet, P. Indications for cardiac pacing in acute myocardial infarction. J. Florida Med. Assoc., 55:1079, 1968.
109. —— Jacobs, W., and Bernstein, W. H. Electrode catheter pacemaker in the treatment of complete heart block in the presence of acute myocardial infarction. Am. J. Cardiol. 11:379, 1963.
110. Scheidt, S., and Killip, T. Bundle branch block complicating acute myocardial infarction, J.A.M.A., 222:919, 1972.
111. Scheinman, M., and Brenman, B. Clinical and anatomic implications of intraventricular blocks in acute myocardial infarction. Circulation, 46:753, 1970.
112. Scherf, D. Therapy of arrhythmias in myocardial infarction. Am. J. Cardiol., 1:242, 1958.
113. Schluger, J., Iraj, I., and Edson, J. N. Cardiac pacing in acute myocardial infarction complicated by complete heart block. Am. Heart J., 80:116, 1970.
114. Scott, M. E., Geddes, J. S., Patterson, G. C., Adgey, A. A. J., and Pantridge, J. F. Management of complete heart block complicating acute myocardial infarction. Lancet, 2:1382, 1967.
115. Simon, A. B., Steinke, W. E., and Curry, J. J. Atrioventricular block in acute myocardial infarction. Chest, 62:156, 1972.
116. Smith, F. J., Keyes, J. W., and Denham, R. M. Myocardial infarction: A study of the acute phase in 920 patients. Am. J. Med. Sci., 221:508, 1951.
117. Sowton, E. Overdriving of dysrhythmias following acute myocardial infarction. In Julian, D. G. and Oliver, M. F. eds. Acute Myocardial Infarctions. Edinburgh and London, E. and S. Livingstone, Ltd., 1968.
118. —— The use of artificial pacemaking in cardiac resuscitation. Proc. R. Soc. Med., 57:368, 1964.

119. —— Cardiac Pacemakers and pacing. Mod. Concept. Cardiovasc. Dis., 36:31, 1967.
120. Spann, J. F., Moellering, R. C., Haber, E., and Wheeler, E. O. Arrhythmias in acute myocardial infarction. N. Engl. J. Med., 271:427, 1964.
121. Stock, R. J., and Macken, D. L. Observations on heart block during continuous electrocardiographic monitoring in myocardial infarction. Circulation, 38:993, 1968.
122. Sutton, R., Chatterjee, K., and Leatham, A. Heart block following acute myocardial infarction. Lancet, 2:645, 1968.
123. —— Davies, M. The conduction system in acute myocardial infarction complicated by heart block. Circulation, 38:987, 1968.
124. Talano, J. V., and Ronan, J. A., Jr. The effect of sinus tachycardia on the phases of left ventricular systole during acute myocardial infarction in man. Am. Heart J., 87:428, 1974.
125. Van Durme, J. P., Vermeire, P., and Pannier, R. Atrial and ventricular pacing in the treatment of tachyarrhythmias following acute myocardial infarction. Acta. Cardiol., 27:749, 1972.
126. Waters, D. D., and Mizgala, H. F. Long term prognosis of patients with incomplete bilateral bundle branch block complicating acute myocardial infarction: Role of cardiac pacing. Am. J. Cardiol., 34:1, 1974.
127. Watson, C. C., and Goldberg, M. J. Evaluation of pacing for heart block in myocardial infarction. Br. Heart J., 33:120, 1971.
128. Waugh, R. A., Wagner, G. S., Haney, T. L., Rosati, R. A., and Morris, J. A., Jr. Immediate and remote prognostic significance of fascicular block during acute myocardial infarction. Circulation, 47:765, 1973.
129. Wiggers, C. J. The functional consequence of coronary occlusion. Ann. Int. Med. 23:158, 1945.
130. Wolk, M. J., Scheidt, S., and Killips, T. Heart failure complicating acute myocardial infarction. Circulation, 45:1125, 1972.
131. Woods, R. M., and Barnes, A. R. Factors influencing immediate mortality after acute coronary occlusion. Am. Heart J., 24:4, 1942.
132. Wright, J. C., Hejtmancik, M. R., Herrmann, G. R., and Shields, A. H. A clinical study of complete heart block. Am. Heart J., 52:369, 1956.
133. Yoshida, S., Gang, W., Donoso, R., Marcus, H. S., and Swan, H. J. C. Coronary hemodynamics during successive elevation of heart rate by pacing subjects with angina pectoris. Am. J. Cardiol., 27:1062, 1971.
134. Zipes, D. The clinical significance of bradycardic rhythms in acute myocardial infarction. Am. J. Cardiol., 24:814, 1969.
135. Zoll, P. M. Resuscitation of the heart in ventricular standstill by external electric stimulation. N. Engl. J. Med., 247:768, 1952.
136. Zucker, I. R., Parsonnet, V., Gilbert, L., and Asa, M. Bipolar electrode in heart block. J.A.M.A., 184:549, 1963.

Chapter 5 Treatment of Cardiogenic Shock

Calvin L. Weisberger, M.D., Nicholas Ruggiero, M.D., and
Eward K. Chung, M.D.

General Considerations

In this era of the coronary care unit and electrocardiographic monitoring of patients with acute myocardial infarction, a major problem is that of cardiogenic shock. Some 10 to 20 percent of hospitalized patients with acute myocardial infarction experience "pump failure" or cardiogenic shock (2). Of these patients, 80 to 100 percent die as a direct result of the shock state (27). Various approaches to the management of this entity have been used by different investigators (11, 21, 29), and yet, a significant controversy exists as to the ideal therapeutic approach with a proper selection of various pharmacologic agents in cardiogenic shock.

Cardiogenic shock is defined as a clinical state in which the heart is no longer intrinsically capable of maintaining sufficient cardiac output to meet the requirement of body functions. This condition is characterized by (31):

1. Systolic blood pressure less than 90 mm Hg in normotensive individuals or a reduction of more than 30 mm Hg in systolic blood pressure in known hypertensive patients.
2. Urine output less than 20 ml/hr associated with various symptoms, including diaphoresis, pallor, cyanosis, mottling, and altered mentation.

Many etiologic factors may produce cardiogenic shock. It may occur when the heart is unable to fill adequately, as seen in acute cardiac tamponade or ball-valve obstruction (e.g., thrombus or myxoma) of the atrioventricular valves. Pump failure is more commonly observed when the heart is incapable of emptying adequately. This may be due to aortic valvar stenosis or insufficiency, mitral insufficiency, or cardiac rhythm disturbances. In the case of acute myocardial infarction it is usually caused either by an insufficient volume of normally functioning ventricular myocardium or wasted contractile force by systolic expansion of the infarcted myocardium. Cardiogenic shock is more likely encountered when myocardial infarction is complicated by mitral insufficiency (due to papillary muscle dysfunction or chordea tendinae rupture), ventricular septal defect, or rupture of the ventricular wall. The fundamental controversy exists as to the best therapeutic approach to cardiogenic shock of the acute functional muscle decrement type in acute myocardial infarction.

In the course of myocardial infarction, cardiogenic shock is observed more frequently in patients with anterolateral than with diaphragmatic (inferior) myocardial infarction. Patients with multiple myocardial infarctions (old or new), long-standing hypertension, diabetes mellitus, and those over 60 years of age seem to be an increased risk for development of cardiogenic shock (22, 35). It has been shown that 30 to 51 percent of the left ventricular myocardium is usually infarcted in patients who die of cardiogenic shock (14, 28). Frequently this is due to subendocardial extension of infarction from a narrow based transmural focus rather than being a widespread transmural infarction (28). When the myocardial damage approaches the critical extent, the left ventricle is relatively unable to eject blood against systemic resistance. This is the reason cardiac output is reduced relative to tissue demand, leading to a reduction of blood pressure with increased end-systolic and diastolic left ventricular volumes.

The decrease in cardiac output initiates reflex catecholamine output, with positive chronotropic, inotropic, and after load effects. These effects may cause the required increase in cardiac output; they may also produce a positive feedback mechanism. They increase the demand for oxygen by the myocardium, which, in the presence of falling coronary blood flow, increases the metabolic derangement of myocardial cells and can cause extension of ischemic or infarcted tissue. This extension would cause a further reduction in cardiac output and failing pulsatile blood flow, perpetuating the positive feedback circuit, while the microcirculation undergoes changes characteristic of the shock syndrome.

Therapeutic approaches to this positive feedback mechanism have taken several forms, including pharmacologic and physiologic techniques, mechanical circulatory assistance, and surgical correction of coronary flow and myocardial infarctectomy. The initial medical management of cardiogenic shock in the coronary care unit is to identify the high-risk patient, as previously described, including also those who develop a ventricular diastolic gallop with poor heart tones and hypotension. Ideally, a pulmonary artery catheter and peripheral or central arterial catheter are inserted to monitor the patient's hemodynamic status precisely, including pulmonary artery wedge and diastolic pressure, cardiac output, and systemic blood pressure. The optimal average wedge pressure during acute myocardial infarction (representing left ventricular filling pressure), appears to be 14 to 25 mm Hg (9, 30), but this can be titrated with cardiac output for the individual patient. In patients with cardiogenic shock syndrome or just with falling cardiac output and blood pressure but whose filling pressure are less than the optimal range, blood volume can be expanded rapidly with appropriate solutions (colloid) and cardiac output sampled immediately when higher filling pressures are reached. This determines whether volume loading has a beneficial effect. If left ventricular filling pressures are raised progressively to the 20 to 25 mm Hg range without a beneficial effect on cardiac output, it must be assumed that something more is needed. Traditionally, agents that augment myocardial contractility, peripheral vascular resistance, or both, have been used. These agents include digitalis, isoproterenol, epinephrine, norepinephrine, dopamine, glucagon, and other agents, such as steroids.

Various Therapeutic Approaches

Digitalis

Digitalis augments contractility in both the normal and failing myocardium (6). If the glycoside caused a reduction in end-diastolic volume with an increase in cardiac output and blood pressure, it could reduce myocardial oxygen demand. Nevertheless, there is no clear evidence that digitalis produces the above-mentioned effects in cardiogenic shock associated with myocardial infarction (6, 20). Therefore, it is

Table 5-1. Drugs and Dosages in Cardiogenic Shock

Drug	IV dosage	Method
Norepinephrine	4–8 mg in 1 liter of D5W or D5/S	Microdrip to titrate mean arterial pressure (MAP) to 90 mm Hg or systolic BP to 100 mm Hg
Isoroterenol	1 mm in 500 ml of D5W (2 μg/ml)	Microdrip to MAP 90 mm Hg or systolic BP 100 mm Hg; arrhythmias frequent at doses greater than 6 μg/min
Dopamine	200 mg in 500 ml D5W (400 μg/ml)	2 to 5 mg/kg-min up to 50 mg/kg-min to maintain MAP at 90 mm Hg or systolic BP at 100 mm Hg; average dose rate less than 20 mm/kg-min
Glucagon	10 mg in 50 ml D5W	Average rate 4 mg/hr; glucagon not stable for long periods and fresh infusion must frequently be prepared (approximately every hour)
Methyl prednisolone	30 mg/kg	IV bolus every 4 to 6 hr

generally agreed that cardiac glycosides have little or no direct beneficial effect in cardiogenic shock despite the probability that they do augment the contractility of the functional myocardial remnant (6, 20, 29).

Glucagon

Glucagon is a pancreatic hormone that increases myocardial contractility. This effect is mediated by activating cyclic AMP. It does not appear to be affected by beta-adrenergic blocking agents. In man, glucagon results in increased cardiac output, heart rate, and mean arterial blood pressure, with a slight reduction in systemic vascular resistance. The increments in the above parameters, however, are not great with glucagon. Therefore, its use in cardiogenic shock would seem questionable (29, 38), except for patients with myocardial depression due to beta-blocking drugs.

Catecholamines

Catecholamine drugs such as isoproterenol, norepinephrine, and dopamine are widely used pressor agents. Their pharmacologic properties are fairly similar to each other with respect to the heart. They all possess beta-adrenergic stimulating effects to various degrees. Stimulation of beta-receptors accelerates heart rate, increases the force of myocardial contraction, and dilates some muscle arteriolar beds (3). The increased myocardial contractility and accelerated heart rate concomitantly increase myocardial oxygen consumption (19, 25).

Isoproterenol essentially stimulates only beta-receptors. In studies of patients with cardiogenic shock, it has generally caused an increase in cardiac output with or without a rise in systemic mean arterial pressure (21, 24, 37). This drug uniformly increases heart rate, and ventricular irritability is a frequent untoward effect of its use. Isoproterenol has been advocated for use especially when bradycardia-associated hypotension is present. The decrease in total peripheral resistance seen with this drug may also be of benefit in selected cases.

Norepinephrine has mixed alpha- and beta-adrenergic effects. Besides causing increases in heart rate and contractility, it also causes an increase in peripheral vascular resistance. In most studies of patients in shock, it raised mean arterial blood pressure at least temporarily (5, 24). Its use must be monitored closely through an intra-arterial cannula and through controlled administration. Excess norepinephrine can easily raise peripheral resistance to levels that would present an intolerable after load to the failing myocardium and exacerbate the positive feedback mechanism of shock (1).

Dopamine is a precursor of norepinephrine and possesses both alpha- and beta-adrenergic effects. It has been claimed that one effect of dopamine is to dilate both the renal and mesenteric systems. Dilation of renal arterioles obviously would be of great advantage in the patient with oliguria secondary to shock. Its use might also be beneficial, in general, in the hypotensive patient with increased systemic vascular resistance but who requires additional inotropic support (13, 18, 29, 37).

Steroids

Other pharmacologic agents that have been used are the steroids. These agents have been shown to exert the following effects when used in pharmacologic doses (approximately 100 times physiologic levels):

1. They decrease peripheral vascular resistance.
2. They decrease coronary vascular resistance.
3. They increase cardiac output.
4. They increase coronary blood flow.

In addition to several other effects, the steroids counteract myocardial depressant factors (16). Their use has been shown to reduce the size of experimental myocardial infarction and they may, through a related effect, increase myocardial compliance (19).

Afterload Reduction

One of the newest pharmacologic concepts of treating cardiogenic shock, is afterload reduction. The rationale for afterload reduction is that some patients may be in pump failure, which is exacerbated when the left ventricle is required to pump against very high systemic vascular resistance. In patients with cardiogenic shock, when left ventricular end-diastolic pressure is elevated, the cardiac index low, and mean blood pressure elevated, normal, or just slightly low (80 to 90 mm Hg) peripheral vasodilating agents have been used (14, 16). It is hoped that by decreasing systemic vascular resistance, the ventricles will be able to empty more efficiently and blood pressure will be maintained by increased cardiac output. Presumably the net effect would be to break the positive feedback circuit of the shock syndrome and allow the left ventricle to stabilize at a functional level. The principle drugs used to reduce the afterload were regitine and sodium nitroprusside (16, 29). Their use is

Table 5-2. Physical Signs of Low Cardiac Output

Physical signs	Pathophysiology
Small femoral or carotid pulse volume	Decreased stroke volume
Decreasing intensity of heart sounds	Decreased stroke volume, low cardiac output
Cold, clammy extremities	Sympathetic mediated vasoconstriction and stimulation of sweat glands
Sinus tachycardia	Possible compensation for low stroke volume
Confusion, lethargy, somnolence	Decreased cerebral blood flow
Concentrated urine less than 30 ml/hr volume	Compensation for decreased renal blood flow
Tachypnea	Compensation for decreased Po_2 or for acidosis
Mean arterial blood pressure less than 80 to 90 mm Hg $\left(\text{Mean arterial BP} = \frac{\text{systolic} + 2(\text{diastolic})}{3}\right)$	Low cardiac output

still in the research stage and requires invasive monitoring of both left ventricular end-diastolic pressure, systemic pressure, and cardiac output. Similarly, the delivery system for a drug, such as nitroprusside, must be able to prevent a too rapid and fatal massive reduction in systemic resistance.

Combined Drug Therapy

The literature is filled with studies of various agents in the treatment of cardiogenic shock. Each agent has therapeutic advantages as well as inherent dangers in a given situation. If the medical treatment method reverses the shock syndrome and the patient is able to perfuse without assistance, then a specific method has been successful. From a statistical viewpoint, no drug regimen has shown to improve the overall survival rate in cardiogenic shock. Recent reports have, in fact, demonstrated relative increases in the area of myocardial infarction with the use of pressor agents (19).

Mechanical Circulatory Assistance

Several types of mechanical devices to assist circulation have been tried in an attempt to augment circulatory hemodynamics while decreasing the work load on the heart. Basically, these devices are of two types: pulsatile and nonpulsatile. The basic example of a nonpulsatile pump is the heart-lung bypass, which employs a roller device to deliver a constant flow of blood to the arterial system, augmenting both systolic and diastolic pressure. Since this system is asynchronous, i.e., it pumps through all phases of the cardiac cycle, it presents the myocardium with an increased afterload, thus increasing myocardial oxygen consumption.

The pulsatile system is synchronized to the cardiac cycle. The most widely used example is the intra-aortic balloon (11), which consists of a flexible balloon catheter that is introduced into the aorta through the femoral veins. This is connected to a console, which senses the patient's electrocardiogram and triggers a pulse of carbon dioxide or helium to inflate the balloon in diastole. Another sensing function ensures the balloon deflates at or before the beginning of left ventricular systole. The effect of this balloon is to augment mean blood pressure by increasing diastolic blood pressure (25). This also increases coronary blood flow in diastole. The device produces little or no afterload increase because the balloon deflates before or at the beginning of systole. The net effect is to increase systemic perfusion pressure while increasing coronary blood flow and decreasing myocardial oxygen consumption. The complications associated with intra-aortic balloon pumping include rupture of the balloon, systemic embolization, and myocardial rupture (11, 32). The rupture probably occurs because patients who otherwise would have succumbed to massive myocardial infarction survive longer. There has been extensive experience with the balloon pump (11, 24, 32); the overall complication rate has been low and its use is initiated easily. Almost all patients show beneficial effects hemodynamically while on the pump. However, the overall mortality in patients with myocardial infarction associated with cardiogenic shock remains at 80 percent (32).

Several other methods of mechanical circulatory assistance have been used, but no study has shown that any particular method is superior to others from a hemodynamic viewpoint.

Surgical Approach

The other main line of treating cardiogenic shock has been coronary aortography and emergency coronary bypass surgery (34). The goal of this approach is to identify the anatomic lesions and to surgically improve coronary circulation in the hope that the size of the myocardial infarction will be minimized and, by augmenting flow, enable the heart muscle to function more efficiently. The surgical approach is, of course, extremely valuable when a ventricular aneurysm is thought to impair ventricular dynamics (26). On the other hand, surgical treatment for cardiogenic shock may produce various surgical and postoperative complications. The large series of patients treated surgically show that this form of therapy is feasible but that the basic mortality statistics have not been altered (12, 26). The question of quality of life of surgical survivors as compared with medically treated survivors has not yet been answered.

Comments and Conclusion

The controversy over the best therapeutic approach for cardiogenic shock has been fueled for years by reports of successful results with one approach or another. Surgeons claimed that only by revascularizing the myocardium can survival be improved. Various medical investigators have made and are still making claims for improved statistics with one therapeutic regimen or another. However, a review of the literature on this subject clearly indicates that at present one point is not controversial—no current therapeutic approach to cardiogenic shock of the muscle decrement type has significantly altered the basic statistics on mortality.

Therefore, what can be done about the problem is of concern. As in every other area of medicine, the primary goal should be to prevent cardiogenic shock. If our inability to prevent myocardial infarction is accepted, then we can attempt to discover whether or not cardiogenic shock can be prevented once myocardial infarction has occurred. During the acute stage of the infarction, there is a zone of ischemic muscle surrounding the infarcted area, which is potentially salvageable (8). However, cardiogenic shock is frequently produced when the ischemic muscle is not salvaged.

Let us consider ways in which this ischemic tissue can be saved. There are two major therapeutic approaches to the problem. The first is to decrease the oxygen demand of the myocardium and thereby reduce the requirements of the threatened cardiac muscle by preload and afterload reduction, as with nitrates. Myocardial oxygen consumption may also be reduced with propanolol (23). The treatment would be similar to that of angina pectoris. Some patients who are dependent upon increased peripheral resistance or beta stimulation can be expected to suffer from this type of regimen. These patients would, in general, be those who suffer from chronic congestive heart failure. Therefore, propanolol would be contraindicated in these patients. Severe bradycardia would be another contraindication to the use of beta blockers in patients suffering from acute myocardial infarction (23), unless an artificial pacemaker were inserted.

The use of agents to improve delivery of oxygen to the ischemic area could also be considered. If the concept of inflammatory cell infiltration of the infarcted and peri-infarcted area is accepted, then the use of corticosteroids would be a reasonable attempt at muscle salvage. The effectiveness of this approach in the experimental animal has already been demonstrated (3). Presumably the steroids would need to be given only for the first few days of myocardial infarction, until the acute process stabilizes. It has been suggested that long-term steroid therapy in acute myocardial infarction may predispose to poor ventricular healing and myocardial rupture. No clinical study has yet demonstrated that the use of steroids in the early stage of myocardial infarction decreases the incidence of cardiogenic shock.

Other agents have also been shown to minimize the size of infarction in experimental animals. These agents include hyaluronidase, glucose, glucose-insulin-potassium solution, and mannitol (3). They may affect sludging of the microcirculation and lead to improved circulation to the endangered peri-infarction tissue.

There is a possibility that earlier surgical intervention for myocardial revascularization may be an answer. If the metabolism of the myocardium is studied by sampling the effluent from the coronary sinus, some indications of the state of the myocardial circulation can be gained. In the patient with acute myocardial infarction, the concentration of creatine phosphokinase (CPK) in coronary sinus blood usually is higher than that in the systemic circulation. By sampling lactate in the coronary sinus effluent, the extent of myocardial ischemia present can be inferred. That is, aerobically metabolizing myocardium uses lactate as a substrate, and consequently the concentration of lactate in normal coronary sinus effluent blood is lower than that in systemic arterial blood. When the myocardium is ischemic, hypoxic, or otherwise impaired metabolically, it may shift to the anaerobic type metabolism and begin to produce lactate (12). The extent to which lactate is produced correlates with the volume of ischemic myocardium (12). By measuring the above parameters in high-risk patients with extensive lactate production, large areas of ischemic myocardium could possibly be salvaged by reparative surgery following coronary arteriography. A study of this nature is in progress at the Thomas Jefferson University Hospital (34).

In conclusion, there is no single regimen or combination regimen, including drugs, or surgery, or both, which alters mortality from cardiogenic shock. However, new methods, as suggested previously in this Chapter, may be shown to alter the incidence of this syndrome and thus the mortality rate from it.

In the absence of proof for any specific prophylactic approach, we suggest, for the present, the following regimen: (a) Pulse, blood pressure, and urine output should be monitored very frequently (preferably continuously) every hour initially in any patient with acute myocardial infarction who belongs in a high-risk group for cardiogenic shock. Any patient whose systolic blood pressure is less than 110 mm Hg or whose respiratory rate is greater than 28 per minute belongs to this category. (b) Chest pain should be alleviated with intravenous morphine, administered in small doses (5 mg) as needed; oxygen may be given. (c) In any patient who shows signs of falling cardiac output, such as an increased sinus heart rate, a decreased femoral pulse volume, a drop in blood pressure heart sounds of decreased intensity, altered mental status, or a urine colume less than 30 ml/hr, a pulmonary artery catheter should be inserted and wedge pressures recorded if possible (9, 33). Wedge pressure or pulmonary artery diastolic pressure should be maintained at approximately 20 mm Hg or at an optimal level determined by serial cardiac output studies, as wedge pressure is raised using albumin dextran or saline. The cardiac index should be greater than or equal to 2.2 liters/min-M^2. When the cardiac index and mean and arterial blood pressure (80 to 90 mm Hg) can be maintained with these methods, no further steps are needed. If cardiac index, blood pressure, or both continue to fall after adequate ventricular filling pressures are assured, vasopressors would then be recommended. Isoproterenol or dopamine, to titrate mean arterial blood pressure to 90 mm Hg would be our choice (5). When a patient does not respond to these measures, others, such as myocardial revascularization, should strongly be considered (35). In treating the patient in cardiogenic shock, precious time must not be lost. If the left ventricle is operating under an inadequate filling pressure (wedge), rapid elevation of wedge pressure to more adequate levels, by administering a colloid solution (albumin, dextran) will probably result in positive hemodynamic improvement (increased blood pressure and cardiac output). Similarly, the effect of pressor agents should be rapid (14). It cannot be emphasized too strongly that the best hope of successful therapy lies in detecting cardiogenic or impending shock early and correcting hemodynamic abnormalities immediately, before the syndrome is well established.

References

1. Abrams, E., Forrester, J. S., Chatterjee, K., Danzig, R., Swan, H. J. C. Variability in response to norepinephrine in acute myocardial infarction. Am. J. Cardiol., 32:919, 1973.
2. Binder, M. J., Ryan, J. A., Jr., Marcus, S., Mugler, F. Jr., Strange, D., and Agress, C. M. Evaluation of therapy in shock following acute myocardial infarction. Am. J. Med., 18:622, 1955.
3. Braunwald, E. and Maroko, P. R. Protection of ischemic myocardium. In The Myocardium Failure and infarction. New York, H.P. Publications, 1974.
4. Chatterjee, K., Parmley, W., Ganz, W., Forrester, J., Walinsky, P., Crexells, C., and Swan, H. J. C. Hemodynamic and metabolic responses to vasodilator therapy in acute myocardial infarction. Circulation, 48:1183, 1973.

5. Cohn, J. N. and Luria, M. H. Studies in clinical shock and hypotension. II. Hemodynamic effects of norepinephrine and angiotensin. J. Clin. Invest., 44:1494, 1965.
6. —— Tristani, F. E., and Khatri, I. M. Cardiac and peripheral vascular effects of digitalis in clinical cardiogenic shock. Am. Heart J., 78:318, 1969.
7. Corday, E. and Swan, H. J. C. Myocardial Infarction. Baltimore, Williams and Wilkins, 1973.
8. Cox, J. L., McLaughlin, K. W., Flowers, N. C., and Horan, L. G. The ischemic zone surrounding acute myocardial infarction: its morphology as detected by dehydrogenase staining. Am. Heart J., 76:650, 1968.
9. Crexells, C., Chatterjee, K., Forrester, J. S., Dikshit, K., and Swan, H. J. C. Optimal level of filling pressure in the left side of the heart in acute myocardial infarction. N. Engl. J. Med., 289:1263, 1973.
10. Dietzman, R. H. and Lillehei, R. C. The treatment of cardiogenic shock. V. The use of cortico steroids in the treatment of cardiogenic shock. Am. Heart J., 75:274, 1968.
11. Dunkman, W. B., Leinbach, R. C., Buckley, M. J., Mundth, E. D., Kantrowitz, A. R., Austen, W. G., and Sanders, C. A. Clinical and hemodynamic results of intra aortic balloon pumping and surgery for cardiogenic shock. Circulation, 41:469, 1972.
12. Gorlin, R. Evaluation of myocardial metabolism in ischemic heart disease. Circulation Suppl. to Vol. XXXIX and XL, p. 155–163, 1969.
13. Gunnar, R. M. and Loeb, H. S. Use of drugs in cardiogenic shock due to acute myocardial infarction. Circulation, 45:1111, 1972.
14. Hanarceyan, C., Bennet, M. A., Pentecost, B. L., and Brewer, D. B. Quantitative study of infarcted myocardium in cardiogenic shock. Br. Heart J., 32:728, 1970.
15. Huddy, F. J. Pathophysiology and therapy of the shock of myocardial infarction. Ann. Intern. Med. 73:809, 1970.
16. Lefer, A. M., Cowgill, R., Marshall, F. F., Hall, L. M., and Brand, E. D. Characterization of a myocardial depressant factor present in hemorrhagic shock. Am. J. Physiol., 213:492, 1967.
17. Loeb, H. S., Rahimtoola, S. H., Rosen, K., Sunno, M. Z., Chyquimia, and Gunnar, R. Assessment of ventricular function after myocardial infarction by plasma volume expansion. Circulation, 47:720, 1973.
18. —— Winslow, E., Rahimtoola, S. H., Rosen, K., and Gunnar, R. Acute hemodynamic effects of dopamine in patients with shock. Circulation, 44:163, 1971.
19. Maroko, P. R., Kjekshus, J. K., Sobel, B. E., Watanabe, T., Covell, J. W., Ross, J. Jr., and Braunwald, E. Factors influencing infarct size following experimental coronary artery occlusion. Circulation, 43:67, 1971.
20. Mason, D. T. Digitalis pharmacology and therapeutics: Recent advances. Ann. Intern. Med., 80:520, 1974.
21. Misra, S. N. and Kezdi, P. Hemodynamic effects of adrenergic stimulating and blocking agents on cardiogenic shock and low output state after myocardial infarction. Am. J. Cardiol., 31:724, 1973.
22. Morris, R. M., Brandt, P. W. T., Caughey, D. F., Lee, A. J., and Scott, P. J. A new coronary prognostic index. Lancet, 1:274, 1969.
23. Mueller, H. S., Ayres, S. M., Religa, A., and Evans, R. G. Acute myocardial infarction: effect on myocardial oxygenation and hemodynamics. Circulation, 49:1078, 1974.
24. —— —— Gianelli, S., Conklen, E. F., Mazzara, J. T., and Grace, W. J. Effect of isoproterenol, L-norepinephrine, and intra aortic counterpulsation on hemodynamics and myocardial infarction. Circulation, 45:335, 1972.
25. —— —— Gianelli, S. Jr., Conklin, E. F., Mazzara, J. T., and Grace, W. J. Effects of isoproterenol, L-norepinephrine and intra-aortic balloon counterpulsation on hemodynamics and myocardial metabolism in shock following acute myocardial infarction. Circulation, 45:335, 1972.
26. Mundth, E. D., Buckley, M. J., Leinbach, R. C., DeSanctis, R. W., Sanders, C. A., Kantrowitz, A., and Austen, W. G. Myocardial revascularization for the treatment of cardiogenic shock complicating acute myocardial infarction. Surgery, 70:78, 1971.
27. Nyquist, O. Shock complicating acute myocardial infarction. Acta Med. Scand. Suppl. 536, p. 54–63, 1972.
28. Page, D. L., Caulfied, J. B., Kastor, J. A., DeSanctis, R. W., and Sanders, C. A. Myocardial changes associated with cardiogenic shock. N. Engl. J. Med., 285:133, 1971.
29. Perlroth, M. G. and Harrison, D. C. Cardiogenic shock: A review. Clin. Pharmacol. Ther. 10:449, 1969.
30. Rackley, C. E. and Russel, R. O. Jr. Left ventricular function in acute myocardial infarction and its clinical significance. Circulation, 45:231, 1972.

31. Ratshin, R. A., Rackley, C. E., and Russel, R. O. Jr. Hemodynamic evaluation of left ventricular function in shock complicating myocardial infarction. Circulation, 45:127, 1972.
32. Scheidt, S., Wilner, G., Mueller, H., Summers, D., Lesch, M., Wolff, G., Krakauer, J., Ruberfire, M., Fleming, P., Noon, G., Aldham, N., Killip, T., and Kantrowitz, A. Intra-aortic balloon counterpulsation in cardiogenic shock. N. Engl. J. Med., 288:979, 1973.
33. Scheinman, M., Evans, G. T., Weiss, A., and Rapaport, E. Relationship between pulmonary artery end-diastolic pressure and left ventricular filling pressure in patients in shock. Circulation, 42:317, 1973.
34. Smullens, S. N., Wiener, L., Kasparian, H., Brest, A. N., Bacharach, B., Noble, P. H., and Templeton, J. Y. III. Evaluation and surgical management of acute evolving myocardial infarction. J. Thorac. Cardiovasc. Surg., 64:495, 1972.
35. Stock, E. Prognosis of myocardial infarction in a coronary care unit. Med. J. Austr. 2:377, 1969.
36. Swan, H. J. C., Forrester, J. S., Diamond, G., Chatterjee, K., and Parmley, W. Hemodynamic spectrum of myocardial infarction and cardiogenic shock. Circulation, 45:1097, 1972.
37. Talley, R. C., Goldberg, L. I., Johnson, C. E., and McNay, J. L. A hemodynamic comparison of dopamine and isoproterenol in patients with shock. Circulation. 39:361, 1969.
38. Vander Ark, C. R. and Reynolds, E. W. Clinical evaluation of glucagon by continuous infusion in the treatment of new cardiac output states. Am. Heart J., 79:481, 1970.
39. Walinsky, P., Chatterjee, K., Forrester, J., Parmely, W., and Swan, H. J. C. Enhanced left ventricular performance with phentolamine in acute myocardial infarction. Am. J. Cardiol., 33:37, 1974.
40. Wiener, L. Personal communication.

Chapter 6 Serum Digitalis Level—Practical Value

JAMES E. DOHERTY, M.D.

General Considerations

Although digitalis serum levels were reported for [^{14}C] digitoxin by Okita *et al.* (15) and later for [^{3}H] digoxin by Doherty, Perkins, and Mitchell (4), it was not until Lowenstein (12) reported glycoside inhibition of rubidium uptake by the red cell that a reasonably practical method for determining digitalis in serum and excreta became available. The development of antibodies to digoxin reported by Butler and Chen (2) lead directly to the accurate and practical radioimmunoassay of digoxin developed by Smith, Butler, and Haber (18) and its counterpart for digitoxin reported by Oliver, *et al.* (16). In this chapter we shall attempt to briefly examine the value, pro and con, of serum assays for digitalis.

A number of questions will be asked to bring out important points about serum levels of digitalis. They will be answered in both a positive and negative sense. Finally a critique will be given and some guidelines provided for the rational and appropriate use of this new tool in cardiology—the digitalis serum level.

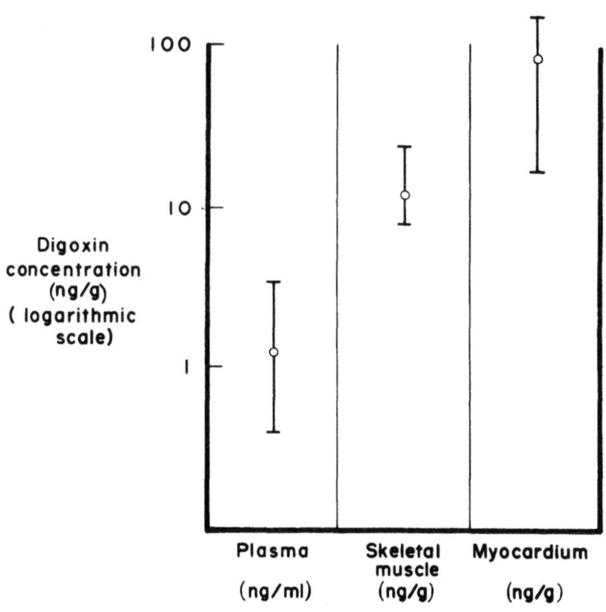

Fig. 6-1. Mean and range of plasma, skeletal and myocardial muscle digoxin concentrations. Note the wide range of myocardial: plasma concentrations (39:1 to 155:1). Reproduced with permission from Coltart *et al.* Br. Med. J. 2:318, 1972.

Controversial Opinions

Question 1: Does the digitalis serum level reflect the level of digitalis at the tissue or myocardial level where digitalis is expected to exert its major therapeutic action?

No. Reports published by Coltart *et al.* (3) indicate a rather striking lack of correlation between serum digoxin and tissue levels from human papillary muscle obtained at the time of valvular surgery. This would seem to indicate that there is no consistent relationship between serum and myocardial levels; thus, serum levels are valueless for clinical assessment (see Figure 6-1).

Yes. Doherty, Perkins, and Flanigan (5) reported a rather rough, yet still close, grouping of left ventricular serum ratios in postmortem examinations performed on patients who received tritium-labeled digoxin. Subsequent studies by Murphy and Doherty (14) in rabbits indicate an even more direct relationship between myocardial and serum levels under carefully controlled experimental conditions. Further, in tissue turnover studies in 34 dogs, Doherty *et al.* (6) demonstrated that the half-times of heart tissue digoxin closely parallel those observed in serum.

It may be conclusively stated, from analysis of these data, that *accurate* serum levels of digitalis should reflect the left ventricular tissue level of digoxin. Whether or not serum levels would prove useful in the management of patients depends on correlation with toxicity to the glycoside, inotropic effects, and underdigitalized patients.

Question 2: Does the serum level of digitalis reflect the toxic effects of the drug as suggested by other clinical parameters, such as the electrocardiogram; visual, gastrointestinal, neurologic, and other general noncardiac symptoms?

No. Fogelman *et al.* (11) report no correlation between the toxic effects of digitalis and serum levels obtained in their study of 104 patients at Los Angeles County Hospital. Wotman *et al.* (22) report there is not a reliable relationship between serum digoxin level and toxic effect, but indicate that salivary electrolytes will unmask digitalis intoxication not detected by serum levels. Thus, one may conclude that serum levels of digitalis have no relationship to toxicity.

Yes. Smith and Haber (20) report a high degree of correlation between the usual clinical manifestations of digitalis intoxication (cardiac and noncardiac). Over 90 percent of digitalis toxic patients had serum levels of 2.0 ng/ml and greater degrees of correlation have been demonstrated by other investigators (19). A high degree of correlation exists between elevated digitalis serum levels and digitalis intoxication, thus establishing this relationship as a valuable clinical measurement in the presence of digitalis excess. Duhme, Greenblatt, and Koch-Weser (10) noted a reduction in digitalis toxicity when serum levels are available, indicating that use of the assay will reduce adverse reactions or toxicity to digoxin.

Question 3: Does the serum digoxin level measure the lack of effect of digoxin as shown by low digitalis levels in the underdigitalized patient who will benefit from increased doses of the drug?

No. Fogelman *et al.* (11) and Wotman (22) failed to relate underdigitalization to the patient's clinical status. Digitalis serum levels were of no value in assessing the patient who required additional digitalis.

Yes. Smith and Haber (19) demonstrated low digitalis serum levels with lack of digitalis effect. This area, however, is more difficult to analyze, as so many symptoms of digitalis intoxication are also manifestations of serious heart disease; i.e., arrhythmia, heart block, or heart failure. An accurate history is of more value than a digitalis serum level in this instance. Clinical judgment of any problem in digitalis dosage is of greatest importance (7), but it is useful to monitor judgment with digitalis serum levels.

Question 4: Does the digitalis serum level show optimal control of digitalized patients.

No. Fogelman *et al.* (11) find no difference in toxic, nontoxic, and optimally digitalized serum levels in patients. Digitalis serum levels are of no value in the management of cardiac patients.

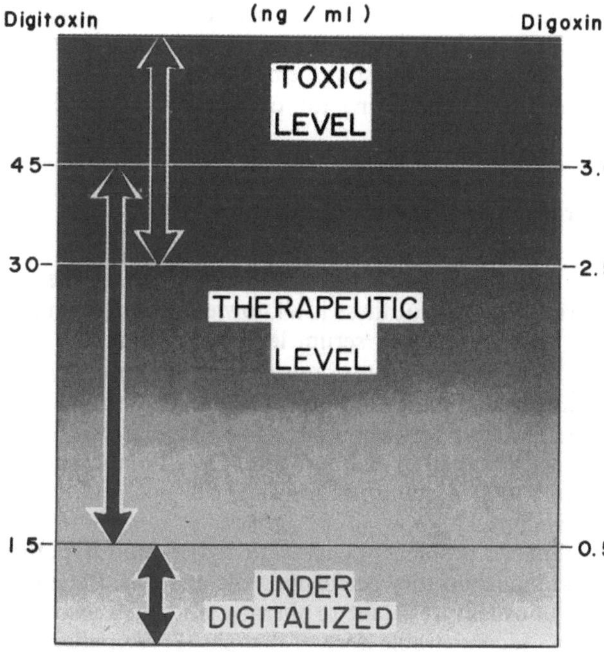

Fig. 6-2. Serum digitalis levels. Note that the scale for digitoxin is shown on left vertical axis, digoxin on the right in nanograms per milliliter. A considerable degree of overlap is present and one must apply clinical judgment for appropriate evaluation.

Yes. Doherty (7) and Smith and Haber (19) and Shapiro, Narahara and Taubert (17) demonstrated the value of the serum digitalis levels in the management of the cardiac patient. A serum level of 0.5 ng/ml to 2.0 to 2.5 ng/ml *usually* is associated with good control of cardiac problems for which digoxin is indicated. Figure 6-2 shows optimal, underdigitalized, and toxic levels of digitalis serum levels. The overlap should be noted and may vary slightly from one laboratory to another.

Question 5: Does every cardiac patient on digitalis need a digitalis serum level?

No. Fogelman *et al.* (11) and Wotman *et al.* (22) indicate no relationship between serum level and clinical effect, so there is no help here! It is also costly and unnecessary if there are no problems with management of a patient.

Yes. It will reassure the patient and the physician regarding status of medication (7) and will assist in evaluation should problems develop in the future.

Question 6: Does the digitalis serum level cost more than it is worth?

No. The rubidium assay and the radioimmunoassay are no more expensive than an electrocardiogram and are a great deal more help to the physician in a clinical situation in which the patient's exact digitalis status must be known.

Yes. Since it has been shown to be of little or no value, money is wasted and the best interest of the patient is not served.

Question 7: Does one need to know the level of serum immediately if the data are to be of value?

No. Although it is and would be of great value to know the serum level immediately in digitalis intoxication, no further digitalis should be used, regardless of the serum level, if clinical judgment favors digitalis toxicity.

Yes. Immediate help is often needed to assess life-saving measures. An *accurate* serum level would be very helpful in this situation. Mortality and morbidity of digitalis toxicity is so bad an immediate 1-hour answer is needed.

These simple questions emphasize the problems faced by the physician and cardiologists in managing the cardiac patient on digitalis (usually digoxin).

Critique and Summary

A few simple guidelines are in order for the best interpretation of serum digoxin levels. The first of these is a knowledge of digoxin blood levels and pharmacokinetics to help know *when* serum levels are required.

Figure 6-3 indicates comparative serum digoxin levels after intravenous (IV), intramuscular (IM), and oral (O) administration. Note that plateau levels (indicating equilibration between serum and tissue) occur 2 to 4 hours after IV, 5 to 6 hours after O, and 10 to 12 hours after IM administration. If serum is not obtained at these times after administration, they will not reflect myocardial levels and will not be meaningful.

Special problems occur with hyper- and hypothyroidism, renal disease, dialysis, and the laboratory performing the analysis. Patients with hyperthyroidism are apt to be unusually resistant to therapy and the reason appears to be lower serum levels from a comparable dose of digoxin. These patients often have atrial fibrillation also, and serum levels required to block the AV junction are usually higher than those necessary for an optimal inotropic effect. Therefore, doses larger than usual are frequently required in thyrotoxicosis should the physician elect to attempt control with digitalis glycosides in these patients. Patients with myxedema (hypothyroidism), on the other hand, are easily intoxicated with digitalis and the "usual" doses frequently result in higher serum levels. Therefore caution is advised in the use of digitalis in thyroid disease. Serum levels of the glycoside are very useful in monitoring treatment in these individuals (18).

Renal insufficiency, long known to prolong the $T\frac{1}{2}$ of digoxin, because of reduced excretion (9), may easily lead to digoxin intoxication. Serum levels are quite helpful in determining the appropriate dose of the glycoside in patients in whom excretion is compromised. One should be aware, however, that, serum level obtained by radioimmunoassay may be lower than expected because the sample chemoluminesces in the scintillation detector.

Renal failure also causes changes in the metabolism of digitoxin—more is converted to digoxin (21). Since the $T\frac{1}{2}$ of digoxin in the anephric subject and digitoxin in

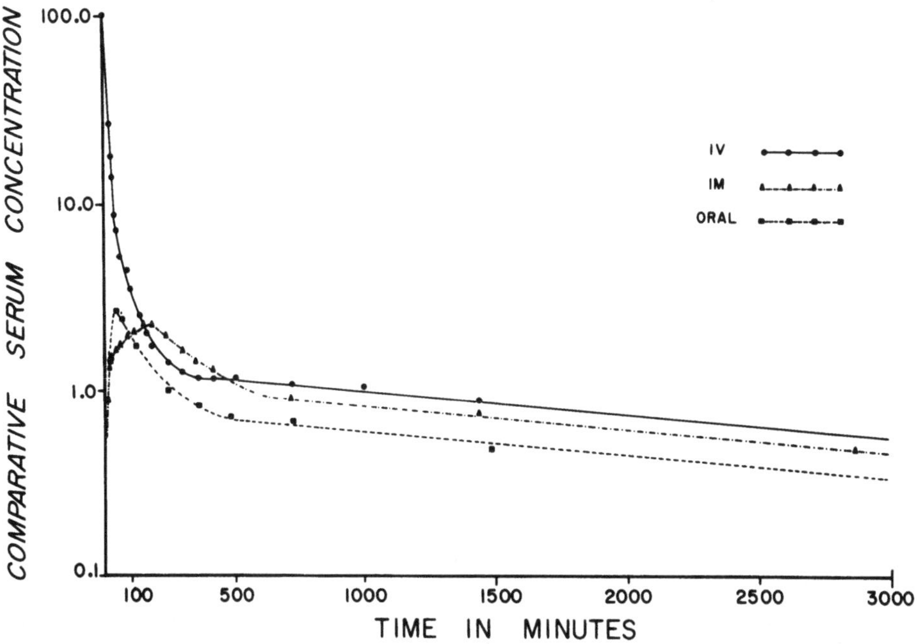

Fig. 6-3. Serum digoxin turnover. Comparative serum digoxin concentration is plotted on the vertical axis, time in minutes on the horizontal. The important feature here is recognition that plateau serum level (straight line function) is not attained after intravenous administration until 120 minutes, oral 300 minutes, and intramuscular 720 minutes. Serum levels should be obtained *after* these times by the appropriate route of administration for a meaningful serum level which approaches equilibration with myocardial level of the drug. Reproduced with permission from Doherty, J. E. and Perkins, W. H. Am. J. Cardiol. 15:170, 1965.

the patient with "normal" renal function are similar, often no change in dosage is necessary when using digitoxin in patients with renal insufficiency.

The increasing use of peritoneal and hemodialysis in renal failure increases the usefulness of serum levels in these patients who may require digitalis. Peritoneal or hemodialysis will not remove excessive amounts of digitalis from the body (1, 21). Digitoxin is not readily dialyzable because it is protein bound (13) and digoxin, although not highly protein bound, is dialyzable, but serum concentrations of digoxin are so low that little is available for dialysis. For these reasons, dialysis is not recommended for digitalis intoxication. The dangers of removing potassium with dialysis may actually precipitate digitalis toxicity.

Increasing use of powerful diuretic agents, such as furosemide and ethacrinic acid, often result in hypokalemia and digitalis toxicity. This is a problem area because normal levels of serum digoxin may be associated with digitalis intoxication in the presence of low serum levels of potassium. Hypomagnesemia produces similar findings.

Table 6-1 outlines problem areas relating to the use of serum glycoside levels in the clinical management of patients. If one is to use serum levels to increase his knowledge of the patient's status, these factors should be borne in mind.

Finally, does the serum level of digitalis glycoside need to be available immediately (4 to 6 hours) for best use? Yes, this is desirable; however, it is not absolutely

Table 6-1. Pitfalls in Interpretation of Digoxin Serum Levels

A. Normal or low serum levels of digoxin *with* toxicity are often seen with:
   1. Hypokalemia
   2. Hypomagnesemia
   3. Lung scans or radioisotopes "on board"
   4. Myocardial infarction
   5. Hypoxia
   6. Myxedema

B. High serum levels of digoxin are sometimes seen *without* toxicity in:
   1. Infants and children
   2. Renal failure (with high serum potassium, uremia, or both)
   3. Antituberculous therapy
   4. Atrial arrhythmia

C. Low serum levels of digoxin with large oral doses may occur with:
   1. Hyperthyroidism
   2. Intestinal malabsorption (sprue) and rapid transit syndromes
   3. Abnormal metabolism

necessary. If toxicity to digitalis is clinically suspect, it would be unwise to be unduly influenced by a low serum level. The serum digoxin level should not carry any more weight than any other laboratory examination. One is measuring nanograms (billionths of a gram), and errors may occur in the laboratory. We have found that serum levels of digoxin useful in patient management (16) even when reports are received several days later. It measures the state of digitalization *at that time* and provides an objective guide to future management.

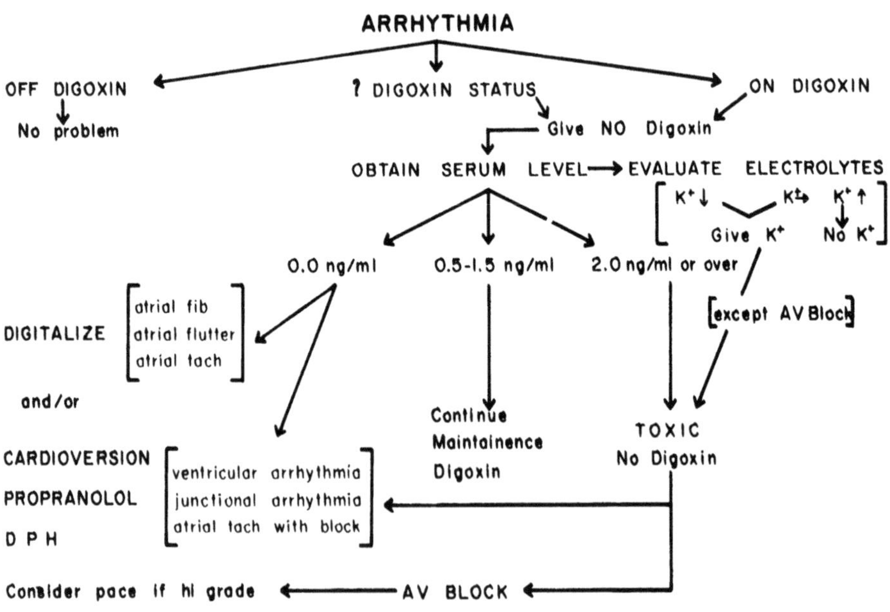

Fig. 6-4. An algorithm which has proved useful in patients with arrhythmia and suspected toxicity to digitalis.

Serum levels of digitalis have been criticized because of the "overlap" of normal, underdigitalized, and toxic patients (Figure 6-2). This is somewhat of a handicap, but if the physician uses the serum level with wisdom and knowledge of the pitfalls associated with the assay, meaningful analysis may be accomplished and will result in improved patient care.

Figure 6-4 is an algorithm that can be used to assist in the evaluation of arrhythmia, which may be associated with digitalis excess. This diagram shows how a rule of procedure may be used when one employs serum levels of digoxin in clinical practice. Naturally, all of the pitfalls of interpretation should be appreciated when one uses this chart.

Finally, we do not recommend a serum level on every patient that is digitalized!

Acknowledgment

Supported in part by United States Public Health Grant 5R01 HL 06642-11 and Veterans Administration Medical Information Systems, grant 1887-01

References

1. Ackerman, G. L., Doherty, J. E., and Flanigan, W. J. Peritoneal dialysis and hemodialysis of tritiated digoxin. Ann. Intern. Med., 67:718–723, 1967.
2. Butler, V. P., Jr. and Chen, J. P. Digoxin-specific antibodies. Proc. Natl. Acad. Sci., 57:71, 1967.
3. Coltart, J., Howard, M., and Chamberlain, D. Myocardial and skeletal muscle concentrations of digoxin in patients on long term therapy. Br. Med. J., 2:318, 1972.
4. Doherty, J. E., Perkins, W. H., and Mitchell, G. K. Serum half-life of tritiated digoxin in congestive heart failure. Clin. Res. 8:43, 1960.
5. Doherty, J. E., Perkins, W. H., and Flanigan, W. J. The distribution and concentration of tritiated digoxin in human tissues. Ann. Intern. Med., 66:116, 1967.
6. Doherty, J. E., Perkins, W. H., Gammill, J., Sherwood, J., and Dodd, C. Tissue concentration and turnover of tritiated digoxin in dogs. Am. J. Cardiol., 17:47, 1966.
7. Doherty, J. E. Digitalis Serum Levels: Clinical Use. Ann. Intern. Med., 74:787, 1971.
8. Doherty, J. E. and Perkins, W. H. Digoxin metabolism in hypo- and hyperthyroidism. Studies with tritiated digoxin in thyroid disease. Ann. Intern. Med., 64:489, 1966.
9. Doherty, J. E., Perkins, W. H., and Wilson, M. C.: Studies with tritiated digoxin in renal failure. Am. J. Med., 37:536, 1964.
10. Duhma, D. W., Greenblatt, D. J., and Koch-Weser, J. Reduction in digoxin toxicity associated with measurement of serum levels. Ann. Intern. Med., 80:516, 1974.
11. Fogelman, A. M., LaMont, J. T., Finkelstein, S., Rado, E., and Pearce, M. L. Fallibility of plasma-digoxin in differentiating toxic from non-toxic patients. Lancet, 2:727, 1971.
12. Lowenstein, J. M. A method for measuring plasma levels of digitalis glycosides. Circulation, 31:228, 1965.
13. Lukas, D. S. Some aspects of the distribution and disposition of digitoxin in man. Ann. NY Acad. Sci., 179:338, 1971.
14. Murphy, M. L. and Doherty, J. E. Comparison of heart size and serum concentration as determinants of digoxin tissue concentration in the normal and hypertrophied rabbit heart. Am. J. Cardiol., 31:47, 1973.
15. Okita, G. T., Talso, P. J., Curry, J. H., Smith, F. D., Jr., and Geiling, E. M. K. Blood level studies of ^{14}C-digitoxin in human subjects with cardiac failure. J. Pharmacol. Exp. Thera., 113:376, 1955.
16. Oliver, G. C., Jr., Parker, B. M., and Brasfield, D. L., *et al.* The measurement of digitoxin in human serum by radioimmunoassay. J. Clin. Invest. 47:1035, 1968.

17. Shapira, W., Narahara, K., Taubert, K. Relationship of plasma digitoxin and digoxin to cardiac response following intravenous digitalization in man. Circulation, 42:1065, 1970.
18. Smith, T. W., Butler, V. P., Jr., and Haber, E. Determination of therapeutic and toxic serum digoxin concentrations by radioimmunoassay. N. Engl. J. Med. 281:1212, 1969.
19. —— Haber, E. Clinical value of the radioimmunoassay of the digitalis glycosides. Pharmacol. Rev., 25:219, 1973.
20. —— —— Digitalis—Medical Progress. N. Engl. J. Med. 289:945, 1010, 1063, 1125, 1973.
21. Sorstein, L. The influence of renal function on the pharmacokinetics of digitoxin, 1973. Oslo, Gyldendal Forlag, O. Sorstein, 1973, p. 1958.
22. Wotman, S., Bigger, J. T., Jr., Mandel, I. D. *et al.* Salivary electrolytes in the detection of digitalis toxicity. N. Engl. J. Med. 285:871, 1971.

Chapter 7 Factors Modifying the Efficacy of Digitalis

EDWARD K. CHUNG, M.D. and LISA S. CHUNG, M.D.

General Considerations

Digitalis is one of the oldest and one of the most commonly used drugs in our practice. Yet, it is not always possible to determine whether digitalis is definitely indicated or not. Needless to say, two major indications for digitalization include (a) the management of congestive heart failure and (b) most supraventricular tachyarrhythmias, particularly atrial fibrillation with rapid ventricular response, provided that the above-mentioned are not digitalis-induced (11). On the other hand, a true contraindication to digitalis is digitalis intoxication (11).

In many clinical situations, the efficacy of digitalis is not satisfactory and consequently, the incidence of digitalis toxicity becomes high. Various factors including electrolyte imbalance, thyroid function, renal function, and so forth, significantly influence the therapeutic result of digitalis (7, 11, 14, 23, 27, 30). In addition, in certain clinical entities, such as idiopathic subaortic stenosis (see Chapter 14), digitalis is not only ineffective but it is also often harmful (11).

The danger of applying a D.C. cardioverter or carotid sinus stimulation to patients with digitalis intoxication has been stressed by many investigators.

Various Clinical Settings

In many clinical situations, the efficacy of digitalis is not fully evident and its dose has to be altered significantly for the best therapeutic outcome (7, 11, 14, 23, 27, 30). In addition, in certain situations, such as in acute myocardial infarction, some physicians consider digitalis contraindicated, whereas others use this glycoside without much hesitation (7, 11, 14, 23, 27, 30).

Such various clinical settings will be discussed in this chapter because significant controversies exist among physicians.

Age

The incidence of digitalis intoxication increases with age in the adult population out of proportion to the increasing incidence of heart disease (13, 18, 19). The reasons for this are considered to be small body size and decreased renal function (18, 19). Therefore it is recommended that the dose of digitalis be reduced according to body weight and degree of renal impairment. Approximately a 50-percent reduction in the dose of digitalis is suggested in elderly patients who weigh less than 100 pounds or have an elevated blood urea nitrogen or serum creatinine level (18, 19).

The danger of digitalis intoxication in the premature, the newborn, and the infant, is greater than that in older children, and digitalis requirements in these groups are much less (29, 33, 34). However, it has been shown that younger children require higher doses of digitalis per unit weight than do adults (33). The factors contributing to the higher dose requirement of digitalis in infants include poorer absorption, more rapid excretion, and greater end-organ resistance (33). Because various factors change rapidly in younger children, such as fluid and electrolyte imbalance, underlying heart disease, degree of absorption and excretion of digitalis, and so forth, a daily requirement of digitalis should be determined carefully. The usual dose of digitalis in different age groups, in children, is described in detail elsewhere by this author (11).

Electrolyte Imbalance

It is well documented that digitalis intoxication is frequently encountered in hypokalemia (11) (Figure 7-1). Hypokalemia alone can cause cardiac arrhythmias as well as predispose to digitalis toxicity (11, 20, 39). The serum potassium level is often normal or near normal in patients with advanced congestive heart failure during digitalization, even when there is marked depletion of potassium in the myocardium and in the total body potassium store (26). The potassium concentration within the myocardial cell is most likely the basic factor in the relationship between hypokalemia and digitalis toxicity. Therefore, electrocardiographic findings (prominent U waves, peaking P waves, or both) should be used in diagnosing intracardiac hypokalemia rather than serum potassium level alone (Figure 7-2).

Potassium is considered the agent of choice in the treatment of various digitalis-induced tachyarrhythmias (11). This is particularly true when there is significant

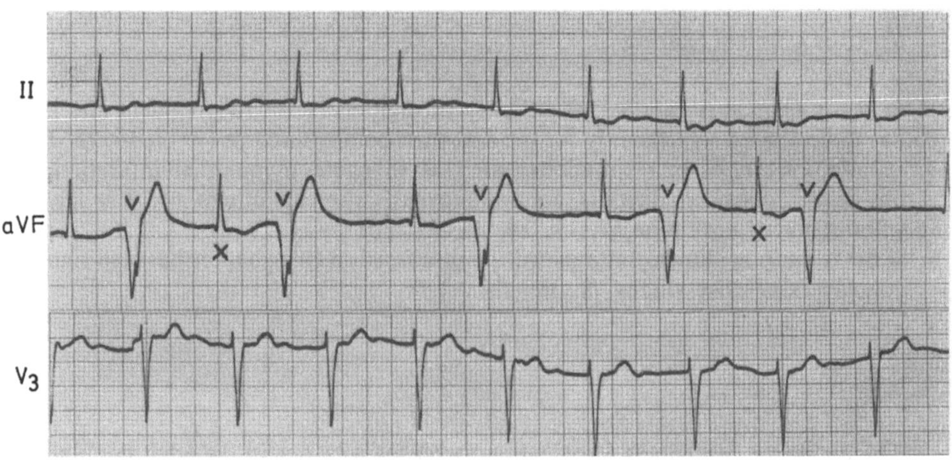

Fig. 7-1. Atrial fibrillation with nonparoxysmal AV junctional tachycardia (rate: 78 beats per minute) producing incomplete AV dissociation and frequent ventricular premature contractions (marked V). The QRS complexes indicated by X are ventricular captured beats. Note prominent U waves suggestive of hypokalemia. Rhythm disturbances in this tracing are induced by digitalis.

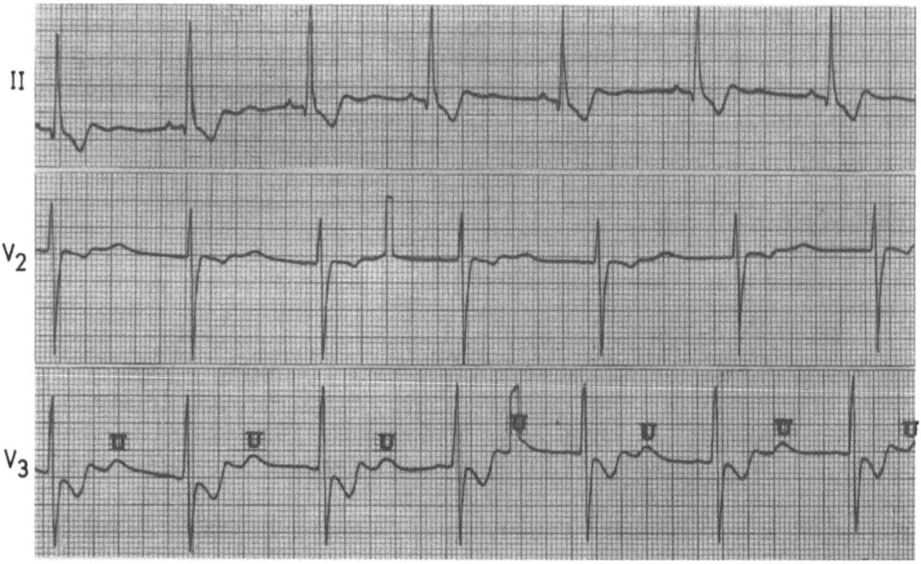

Fig. 7-2. Sinus bradycardia (rate: 57 beats per minute) is the basic rhythm. Marked hypokalemia is manifested by prominent U waves (marked U).

hypokalemia. Potassium may also be effective in terminating digitalis-induced tachyarrhythmias even if the serum potassium level is normal. It should be noted that potassium is capable of producing a prolongation of the refractory period in the AV junction. Thus, potassium administration may increase AV conduction disturbances and is contraindicated in the treatment of digitalis-induced AV block, although there is evidence that it may abolish digitalis-induced AV block associated with marked hypokalemia (11, 26). Hyperkalemia is considered to provide relative protection against digitalis-induced arrhythmias.

Somylo (38) pointed out that magnesium ions have an antiarrhythmic action and are capable of abolishing arrhythmias induced by digitalis. At present, it is evident that hypomagnesemia frequently predisposes to digitalis intoxication (28, 35, 36). The antiarrhythmic action of magnesium is rapid and of short duration. Hypokalemia and hypomagnesemia often coexist, and the latter leads to a decrease in intracellular potassium (36). This combined electrolyte imbalance further predisposes to digitalis toxicity. Hypomagnesemia should be looked for carefully in digitalis intoxication, particularly when in those various clinical situations commonly associated with magnesium deficiency. Such clinical conditions include alcoholic cardiomyopathy, excessive vomiting or diarrhea, diuretic therapy, prolonged magnesium-free intravenous fluid administration, cardiopulmonary bypass, prolonged gastrointestinal drainage and malabsorption.

A synergistic action between digitalis and calcium is well documented (11, 26). Digitalis intoxication may be accelerated by the rapid intravenous infusion of calcium during digitalis therapy, or digitalis toxicity may be induced by a relatively small dose of digitalis if the patient has preexisting hypercalcemia. This synergistic action between digitalis and calcium may even induce sudden death (11).

When hypokalemia, hypomagnesemia, and/or hypercalcemia are present during digitalization, the dose of glycoside should be reduced by one-third to one-half the usual recommended does (11). It is essential to correct electrolyte imbalance as soon as it is detected.

Various Heart Diseases

Any advanced heart disease, regardless of the underlying process, narrows the ratio between therapeutic and toxic doses and increases the incidence of digitalis intoxication (11). If the heart involvement is secondary to, or part of, a systemic or generalized disease, the incidence of digitalis toxicity increases markedly and the efficacy of digitalis is often not satisfactory. Such diseases are acute rheumatic fever, bacterial endocarditis, systemic lupus erythematosus, amyloidosis, beri-beri heart disease, and so forth. Various cardiomyopathies (Chap. 13) are also associated with a high incidence of digitalis toxicity, and the digitalis is often not as effective. This is particularly true in idiopathic cardiomyopathy because the exact etiologic factor is not yet known.

Idiopathic Hypertrophic Subaortic Stenosis

Idiopathic hypertrophic subaortic stenosis (Chap. 14) deserves special comment because there are many controversies among physicians regarding the use of digitalis in this entity. Digitalis is generally considered to be contraindicated in patients with idiopathic hypertrophic subaortic stenosis because the drug improves the contractile state of the left ventricular outflow tract, leading to increased obstruction to left ventircular outflow, left ventricular systolic pressure, left ventricular-aortic pressure gradient, and a diminution of the effective orifice size of left ventricular outflow tract (6). Deterioration in the clinical status by digitalization of this entity was improved when digitalis was discontinued (6). Nevertheless, digitalis may be given with extreme caution to patients with this entity when there is persisting atrial tachyarrhythmias, particularly atrial fibrillation with a very rapid ventricular response (11).

Congenital and Valvular Heart Disease and Mechanical Obstruction

If there is a mechanical obstruction, such as constrictive pericarditis, valvulopathies, subendocardial thickening, and so on, digitalis is not as effective and an increased incidence of digitalis toxicity is expected. Similarly, the efficacy of digitalis is not fully expected when there are significant congenital cardiac or valvular lesions, unless the cardiac lesions are repaired surgically. In many patients with congenital or valvular lesions, digitalis may no longer be necessary after surgical correction.

Prophylactic digitalization even during surgery is probably not indicated in patients with patent ductus arteriosus or coarctation of the aorta without significant cardiomegaly (5). Cardiomegaly itself does not justify digitalization.

Mitral Stenosis

The use of digitalis in patients with mitral stenosis also requires a special discussion because of the significant controversy among physicians. It is generally agreed that digitalis is indicated in all patients with pure mitral stenosis associated with atrial tachyarrhythmias, especially atrial fibrillation, regardless of the presence or absence of congestive heart failure, in order to prevent circulatory embarrassment (2, 40). Digitalis probably has a beneficial value for the patient with mitral stenosis and sinus rhythm, without evidence of congestive heart failure, during pregnancy, infections, or similar conditions, when close daily medical observation is not available (2, 40). On the other hand, digitalis may not be indicated when close medical observation is available, such as in surgical intervention or during delivery, as long as the patient is in sinus rhythm and does not have evidence of heart failure (2, 40). Under this circumstance, digitalis may be given immediately when the need arises.

Acute Myocardial Infarction

The use of digitalis in patients with acute myocardial infarction received much attention because of the significant controversy among many physicians in the past decade. Digitalis is often not used at all or used reluctantly in patients with acute myocardial infarction, which is frequently associated with various cardiac arrhythmias, especially ventricular tachyarrhythmias and various bradyarrhythmias, because it may accelerate or initiate the arrhythmias. In addition, digitalization may possibly worsen the hemodynamic status of patients wih acute myocardial infarction. Nevertheless in the following situations, digitalis is considered definitely beneficial in acute myocardial infarction (12, 32, 37).

1. Atrial fibrillation with rapid ventricular response.
2. Acute congestive heart failure as a result of acute myocardial infarction or as its complication.

On the other hand, the routine use of digitalis in patients with acute myocardial infarction complicated by cardiogenic shock is not justified (Chap. 5). Similarly, prophylactic use of digitalis in asymptomatic patients with myocardial infarction, with or without cardiomegaly, is also not justified. The glycoside may be used in the treatment of atrial flutter or other supraventricular tachyarrhythmias. Under these circumstances, excluding atrial fibrillation, other therapeutic measures, such as D.C. shock, are advised first because often an extremely large amount of digitalis is required, particularly to terminate atrial flutter associated with acute myocardial infarction. A rapid acting digitalis preparation, with a smaller than usual dose by intravenous injection, is advisable in patients with acute myocardial infarction. Rapid intravenous administration of large doses of digitalis may produce pulmonary edema or life-threatening ventricular arrhythmias (12, 24, 37). It has been suggested that the digitalizing dose be reduced to one-third to one-half during the acute phase of myocardial infarction (32).

Cardiac Arrhythmias

When cardiac arrhythmias are present in any form before digitalization, digitalis may accelerate or worsen the preexisting abnormality. This may occur without signs of digitalis intoxication. If new arrhythmias develop after digitalization in patients with preexisting arrhythmias, the total clinical picture may become extremely complicated.

Ventricular Tachyarrhythmias

The use of digitalis in the presence of ventricular tachycardia is also controversial. If it is certain the ventricular tachycardia is a result of congestive heart failure or vice versa, digitalis is indicated and usually is effective (3, 9, 11). Digitalis occasionally terminates ventricular tachycardia even if there is no associated heart failure, although the primary drug of choice in this case is intravenous administration of lidocaine (Xylocaine) or procainaminde (Pronestyl) (see Chap. 2).

AV Block

Although digitalis has been said to be contraindicated in the presence of a partial AV block, which may become complete as a result of digitalis, the drug is not contraindicated if there is evidence of congestive heart failure not due to digitalis (11). Although the treatment of choice for complete AV block is usually the use of artificial pacemaker (Chap. 4), digitalis is not contraindicated in the presence of complete AV block if congestive heart failure is present. Digitalis may not be needed following artificial pacemaker implantation, but the drug should be continued if congestive heart failure persists thereafter. In emergency situations, such as acute pulmonary edema in patients with complete AV block, a clinical trial of rapid intravenous digitalization is justified.

Sick Sinus Syndrome

Digitalis is not contraindicated in the presence of sick sinus syndrome. In fact, when clincially indicated, digitalis may be used successfully for congestive heart failure or supraventricular tachyarrhythmias in sick sinus syndrome, providing that no significant AV conduction defect is present (17). Digitalis produces an increase in automaticity in sick sinus syndrome as evidenced by a shortened sinoatrial recovery time (17).

Wolff-Parkinson-White Syndrome

The use of digitalis in the treatment of various tachyarrhythmias associated with Wolff-Parkinson-White (W-P-W) syndrome deserves special comment because of significant controversies among physicians. It is generally agreed that digitalis is

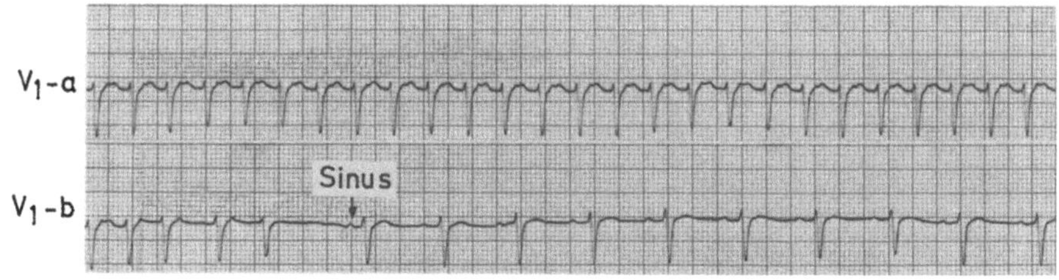

Figure 7-3. Leads V_1-a and b are continuous. Atrial tachycardia (rate: 214 beats per minute) is converted to sinus rhythm (indicated by arrow).

often the drug of choice in the treatment of a regular supraventricular tachycardia in W-P-W syndrome, especially when the QRS complex is normal (9) (Figure 7-3). In this case, propanolol (Inderal) is also equally effective (9). The major difficulty is in the treatment of atrial fibrillation or flutter with anomalous AV conduction in W-P-W syndrome (Figure 7-4). Although digitalis is said to be contraindicated by some physicians in this case, the drug can be given successfully in conjunction with simultaneous administration of other antiarrhythmic agents, such as quinidine or Pronestyl (9). Digitalis alone may terminate atrial fibrillation or flutter in W-P-W syndrome (Figure 7-5), but often a large dose of the drug is required which may lead to digitalis toxicity. Therefore, in this instance combined therapy with digitalis and quinidine (or Pronestyl) is recommended in most cases. In an urgent situation, direct

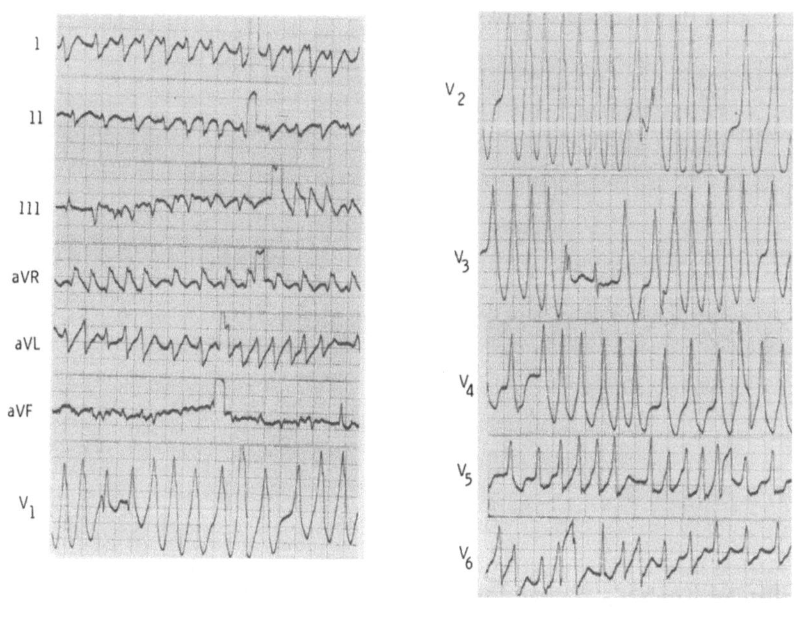

Fig. 7-4. Atrial fibrillation with anomalous AV conduction in Wolff-Parkinson-White syndrome, type A.

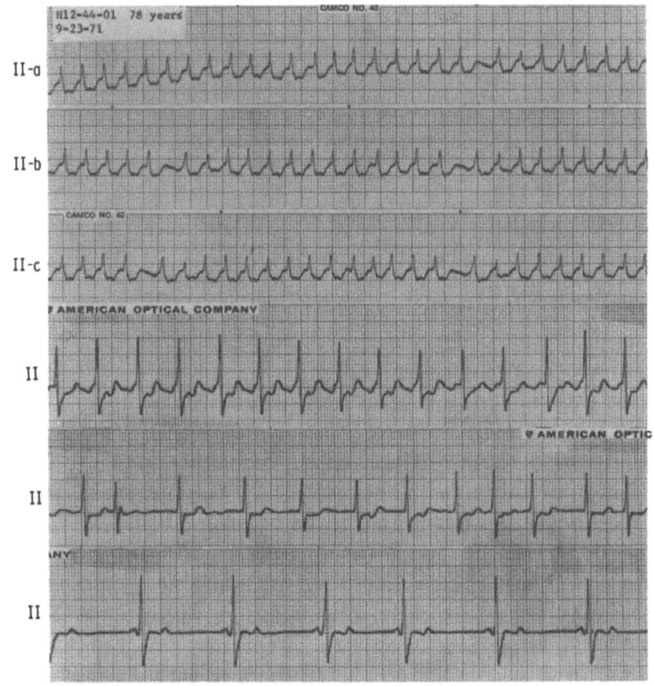

Fig. 7-5. These six rhythm strips were obtained from a 78-year-old male with Wolff-Parkinson-White syndrome. Leads II-a, b, and c are continuous and show atrial flutter, with varying degree and slow progressing Wenckebach AV conduction. The three bottom strips were taken following digitalization. Atrial flutter with 2:1 AV response (fourth strip) is converted to atrial fibrillation (fifth strip) followed by sinus rhythm (bottom strip).

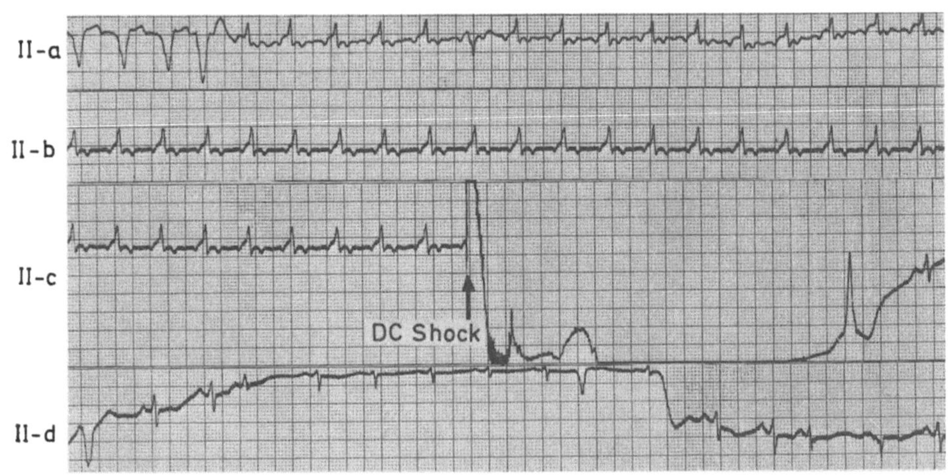

Fig. 7-6. Leads II-a, b, c and d are continuous. Atrial flutter with 2:1 AV response in Wolff-Parkinson-White syndrome is terminated by D.C. shock (indicated by arrow). Note occasional ventricular and atrial premature beats. Two different QRS configurations in lead II-a indicate a dual anomalous AV conduction.

current shock is applied immediately for tachyarrhythmias of any type, particularly atrial fibrillation or flutter with anomalous AV conduction in W-P-W syndrome (Figure 7-6). It is important to remember that many patients with W-P-W syndrome require one or more drugs to prevent tachyarrhythmias following a termination.

Sinus Tachycardia

Sinus tachycardia itself does not require digitalis or any antiarrhythmic agent, but persisting sinus tachycardia deserves full investigation as to the underlying etiologies, including high output states (anemia, beri-beri, AV fistula, hyperthyroidism), infectious processes, myocardial infarction, and pulmonary embolism.

Multifocal Atrial Tachycardia

One of the most malignant and refractory arrhythmias is multifocal atrial tachycardia (10) (Figure 7-7). Since most patients with multifocal atrial tachycardia suffer from chronic cor pulmonale, treatment of the underlying pulmonary disease is much more important than any antiarrhythmic agent (10). For the same reason, digitalis is often ineffective in the treatment of multifocal atrial tachycardia. When digitalis is pushed in this case, a varying degree of AV block is often produced in the presence of multifocal atrial tachycardia (Figure 7-8). Therefore, digitalis should be administered, if clinically indicated, with particular caution. Otherwise, digitalis toxicity may be unavoidable and the clinical picture may deteriorate.

Bundle Branch Block

Digitalis is not contraindicated in the presence of either left or right bundle branch block and hemiblocks (either anterior or posterior, see Chap. 15).

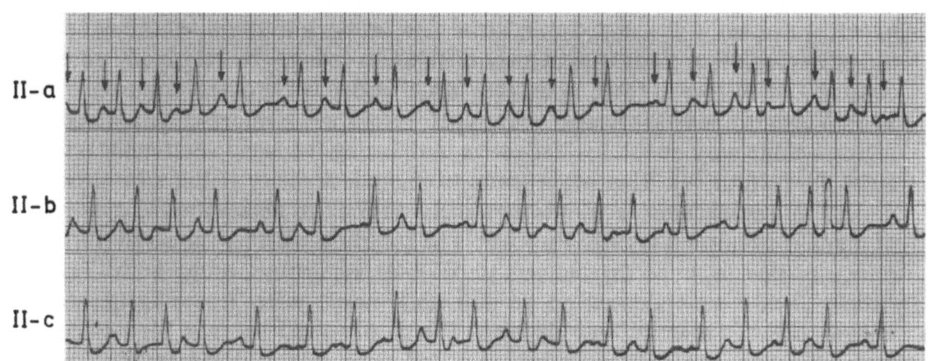

Fig. 7-7. Leads II-a, b, and c are not continuous. Arrows indicate P waves. The rhythm is multifocal atrial tachycardia. Note varying configuration of P waves with varying P-R intervals and P-P cycles. The peaked P waves indicate P-pulmonale.

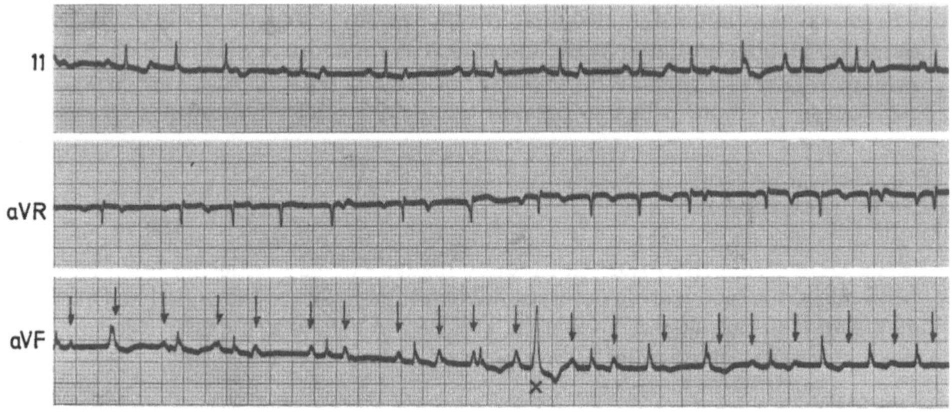

Fig. 7-8. Arrows indicate P waves. The rhythm is multifocal atrial tachycardia with varying degree AV block as a result of digitalis toxicity. Note a ventricular premature contraction (marked V). The evidence of P-pulmonale is also present.

Noncardiac Disorders

There are two major noncardiac disorders that significantly influence the efficacy of digitalis and the incidence of digitalis toxicity: (a) thyroid disease (either hyperthyroidism or hypothyroidism) and (b) renal dysfunction. In addition, various pulmonary diseases (either acute or chronic), various high output states, liver diseases, nutritional disturbances, endocrine disorders, and psychoneurotic disorders also may influence the therapeutic result of digitalis.

Diseases of Thyroid

Hyperthyroid patients often require greater amounts, whereas myxedematous patients usually require much less than the usual digitalizing dose (11, 38). When hyperthyroidism is associated with atrial fibrillation with rapid ventricular response, the physician often finds it extremely difficult to reduce the ventricular rate. This is observed when two to three times the "usual" doses of digitalis are used. When the W-P-W syndrome is associated with hyperthyroidism, a rather common occurrence, digitalis alone may be totally ineffective in reducing the rapid ventricular response in atrial fibrillation (9). This often leads to digitalis toxicity if the treatment is continued. In this circumstance, it is extremely difficult to determine the optimum dose of digitalis because it is often impossible to ascertain whether the atrial fibrillation is primarily due to hyperthyroidism, to W-P-W syndrome, or to both. Thus, each patient should be evaluated on an individual basis. After hyperthyroidism is well treated, digitalis toxicity may develop. This is observed becasue the treated patient requires much less digitalis when rendered euthyroid. By the same token, myxedematous individuals require more digitalis after they are returned to the euthyroid state. In addition, the presence of a pericardial effusion, a frequent complication of myxedema, is another factor that interferes with the efficacy of digitalis and may lead to digitalis toxicity. When there is significant hypothyroidism, the dose of digitalis should be reduced markedly (usually one-third to one-half the usual dose), depending upon the severity of disease (11).

Renal Diseases

It is well documented that digitalis intoxication is frequently observed in patients with renal failure (11). This is due to various factors, including a slowing of digitalis excretion by the kidneys, electrolyte imbalances, anemia, severe hypertension, cardiac tamponade complicating uremic pericarditis and/or myocarditis (16, 39). Doherty *et al.* (16) reported that patients with renal failure, manifested by an elevation of blood urea nitrogen (BUN), and congestive heart failure showed a marked reduction of renal excretion, prolonged digoxin half-life in serum, and higher serum levels of digoxin. They found a reasonably accurate correlation between the excretion of digoxin and the level of BUN (16). The same investigators showed similar results with patients after bilateral nephrectomy prior to renal transplantation (15). We can conclude from clinical and experimental studies that the dose for digitalization should be reduced one-third to two-thirds in patients with significant renal failure (BUN 50 mg/100 ml or more).

Digitalis intoxication is common after peritoneal dialysis or hemodialysis (16). The reason for this is that only very small amounts of digitalis are removed by the procedure compared with large amounts of potassium (16). Therefore, the dose of digitalis should be adjusted after peritoneal dialysis or hemodialysis.

Pulmonary Diseases

The incidence of digitalis toxicity is high in patients with various pulmonary diseases, including pulmonary embolism, chronic lung disease with or without cor pulmonale, bronchitis, and pneumonia (11, 38). In addition to a probable unusual sensitivity to digitalis in patients with lung disease, there are various other reasons for this high incidence of digitalis toxicity. Among the various factors, the most important contributing factor for the high incidence of digitalis toxicity in patients with lung disease is considered to be hypoxia (11, 38). In addition, aggressive attempts to slow persisting sinus tachycardia, which is compensatory for the hypoxia in pulmonary disease, may lead to digitalis toxicity. A high incidence of digitalis toxicity in patients with multifocal atrial tachycardia, which is common in pulmonary diseases, has been stressed in this Chapter. Furthermore, unnecessary digitalization for the treatment of dyspnea caused by the lung disease per se may result in digitalis intoxication. Digitalis has been shown to be of no effect in the treatment of respiratory distress syndrome (4). Congestive heart failure associated with or due to lung disease definitely requires digitalization, but symptomatology should be carefully evaluated and various contributing factors, particularly hypoxia, should be considered in selecting the optimum dose of digitalis. Needless to say, the treatment of underlying lung disease is manditory under these circumstances.

High Output States

Unless the underlying process responsible for the high output heart failure is corrected, the efficacy of digitalis is extremely unsatisfactory. In addition, digitalis may no longer be necessary when the high output states (anemia, AV fistula, beri-beri, and so forth) are corrected in many patients. Therefore, the underlying process should be treated simultaneously, with digitalization for all high output failure. The dose of digitalis should be adjusted frequently, according to the severity of the high output failure, and the true necessity of digitalization should always be evaluated during active treatment of the underlying process.

Diseases of the Liver

It has been frequently stated over the years that there is a high incidence of digitalis toxicity in patients with liver disease. This was attributed to the fact that the metabolic breakdown of digitalis occurred in the liver (41). However, the probable cause for the increasing incidence of digitalis toxicity in these patients is hypokalemia, which often occurs in these patients particularly during diuretic therapy (11, 27).

Cardioversion

Recent studies by different investigators have shown that direct current shock is not only ineffective in abolishing digitalis-induced tachyarrhythmias but may worsen the preexisting arrhythmias or may produce more serious new arrhythmias, such as ventricular fibrillation (11, 25). It is also known that cardioversion may unmask concealed digitalis-induced arrhythmias, even when the electrocardiogram prior to the use of electrical discharge fails to show evidence of digitalis toxicity (11, 8). The reason for this is probably that the threshold of excitability is lowered by electrical stimulation during digitalis therapy, leading to digitalis toxicity (8). Lown *et al.* (25) suggested that loss of intracellular potassium from the myocardium following electrical discharge predisposes to digitalis toxicity.

From the above observations, cardioversion should be applied with great caution during digitalis therapy. Hypokalemia and hypoxia should be aggressively corrected before the procedure. It is preferable to discontinue digoxin for 24 to 48 hours before cardioversion. When cardioversion is urgently needed during digitalis therapy, prophylactic intravenous administration of diphenylhydantoin (Dilantin) 100 to 250 mg, 5 to 10 minutes before the procedure is of great value in preventing postcardioversion arrhythmias. Cardioversion should be used only as the last resort when any tachyarrhythmia is considered to be digitalis-induced (11).

Carotid Sinus Stimulation

Recently, various clinical studies confirmed the danger of provoking serious cardiac arrhythmias and even death by carotid sinus stimulation in patients with suspected digitalis intoxication (1, 21, 22, 31). Therefore, carotid sinus stimulation should be avoided during digitalis therapy, even if the diagnosis of digitalis toxicity is not certain.

Summary

The dose of digitalis varies markedly between individuals, and it also varies significantly even in the same individual depending upon the presence or absence and the severity of various modifying factors. Various factors that modify the efficacy of digitalis and the incidence of digitalis toxicity have been described in detail. When the efficacy of digitalis becomes equivocal and not fully satisfactory in certain clinical situations, needless to say, significant controversial opinions are provoked among many physicians as to indications, nonindications, or contraindications for digitalization. Various controversial opinions have been discussed in different clinical settings and current concepts of digitalization in the presence of various modifying factors have been expressed.

References

1. Alexander, S. and Ping, W. C. Fatal ventricular fibrillation during carotid stimulation. Am. J. Cardiol., 18:289, 1966.
2. Beiser, G. D., Epstein, S. E., Stampfer, M., *et al.* Studies on digitalis. XVII. Effects of ouabain on the hemodynamic response to exercise in patients with mitral stenosis in normal sinus rhythm. N. Engl. J. Med., 278:131, 1968.
3. Bilson, J. S. and Schemm, F. R. Digitalis and ventricular tachycardia. Circulation, 2:278, 1950.
4. Braudo, M. and Keith, J. D. The value of digitalis in the respiratory distress syndrome: A controlled study. J. Pediatr., 74:310, 1969.
5. Braunwald, E., Bloodwell, R. D., Goldber, L. I., *et al.* Studies on digitalis. IV. Observations in man on the effect of digitalis preparations on the contractility of the nonfailing heart and on total vascular resistance. J. Clin. Invest., 40:52, 1961.
6. Braunwald, E., Brockenbrough, E. C., and Frye, R. L. Studies on digitalis. V. Comparison of the effects of ouabain on left ventricular dynamics in valvular aortic stenosis and hypertrophic subaortic stenosis. Circulation, 26:166, 1962.
7. Braunwald, E. and Klocke, F. J. Digitalis. Ann. Rev. Med., 16:371, 1965.
8. Castellanos, A. Jr., Lemberg, L., Cenurion, M. J., and Berkovits, B. V. Concealed digitalis-induced arrhythmias unmasked by electrical stimulation of the heart. Am. Heart J., 73:484, 1967.
9. Chung, E. K. Electrocardiography: Practical Applications with Vectorial Principles. Hagerstown, Harper and Row, 1974.
10. —— Appraisal of multifocal atrial tachycardia. Br. Heart J., 33:500, 1971.
11. —— Digitalis Intoxication. Amsterdam, Excerpta Medica, 1969.
12. Constant, J. Digitalis in myocardial infarction, New York State J. Med., 70:650, 1970.
13. Dall, J. L. C. Digitalis intoxication in elderly patients. Lancet, 2:194, 1965.
14. Doherty, J. E. Digitalis in congestive heart failure. Mod. Treat., 2:278, 1965.
15. —— Flanigan, W. J., Perkins, W. H., *et al.* Studies with tritiated digoxin in anephric human subjects. Circulation, 35:298, 1967.
16. —— Perkins, W. H., and Wilson, M. C. Studies with tritiated digoxin in renal failure. Am. J. Med., 37:536, 1964.
17. Engel, T. R. and Schaal, S. F. Digitalis in the sick sinus syndrome. The effects of digitalis on sinoatrial automaticity and atrioventricular conduction. Circulation, 48:1201, 1973.
18. Ewy, G. A., Kapadia, G. G., Yao, L., Lullin, M., and Marcus, F. I. Digoxin metabolism in the elderly. Circulation, 39:449, 1969.

19. —— Marcus, F. I. Digitalis therapy in the aged. Family Physician, 1:81, 1970.
20. Greenspan, K. and Steinmetz, E. Digitalis and Potassium: pharmacodynamic relationship. In Dreifus, L. S. and Likoff, W. eds. Mechanisms and Therapy of Cardiac Arrhythmias. New York, Grune and Stratton, 1968.
21. Greenwood, R. J. and Dupler, D. A. Death following carotid sinus pressure. J.A.M.A., 181:605, 1962.
22. Hilal, and Massumi, R. Fatal ventricular fibrillation after carotid sinus stimulation. N. Engl. J. Med., 275:157, 1966.
23. Jelliffe, R. W. Factors to consider in planning digoxin therapy. J. Chron. Dis., 24:407, 1971.
24. Karliner, J. S. and Braunwald, E. Present status of digitalis treatment of acute myocardial infarction. Circulation, 46:891, 1972.
25. Kleiger, R. and Lown, B. Cardioversion and digitalis. II. Clinical studies. Circulation, 33:878, 1966.
26. Lown, B., Black, H., and Moore, F. D. Digitalis, electrolytes, and surgical patient. Am. J. Cardiol., 6:309, 1960.
27. McIntosh, H. D. and Morris, J. J., Jr. Problems in the use of digitalis in the management of congestive heart failure. Prog. Cardiovasc. Dis., 7:360, 1965.
28. Neff, M. S., Mendelssohn, S., Kim, K. E., *et al.* Magnesium sulfate in digitalis toxicity. Am. J. Cardiol., 29:377, 1972.
29. Neil, C. A. The use of digitalis in infants and children. Prog. Cardiovasc. Dis., 7:399, 1965.
30. Ogilvie, R. I. and Ruedy, J. An educational program in digitalis therapy. J.A.M.A., 222:50, 1972.
31. Porus, R. L. and Marcus, F. I. Ventricular fibrillation during carotid-sinus stimulation. N. Engl. J. Med., 268:1338, 1963.
32. Rahimtoola, S. H. and Gunnar, R. M. Digitalis in acute myocardial infarction: help or hazard? Ann. Intern. Med., 82:234, 1975.
33. Rutkowski, M. M., Coken, S. N., and Doyle, E. F. Drug therapy of heart disease in pediatric patients. II. The treatment of congestive heart failure in infants and children with digitalis preparations. Am. Heart J., 86:270, 1973.
34. Sedeman, W. A. Current concept—diagnosis and treatment of digitalis toxicity. N. Engl. J. Med., 273:35, 1965.
35. Seller, R. H. The role of magnesium in digitalis toxicity. Am. Heart J., 82:551, 1971.
36. —— Cangiano, J., Kim, K. E., *et al.* Digitalis toxicity and hypomagnesemia. Am. Heart J., 79:57, 1970.
37. Selzer, A. The use of digitalis in acute myocardial infarction. Prog. Cardiovasc. Dis., 10:518, 1968.
38. Somylo, A. P. The toxicology of digitalis. Am. J. Cardiol., 5:523, 1960.
39. Surawicz, B. and Lepeschkin, E. The electrocardiographic pattern of hypopotassemia with and without hypocalcemia. Circulation, 8:801, 1953.
40. Werkö, L. The use of digitalis in mitral stenosis without right heart failure. Prog. Cardiovasc. Dis., 7:284, 1964.
41. Wright, S. E. The Metabolism of Cardiac Glycosides. Springfield, Ill., Charles C. Thomas, 1960.

Chapter 8 Hyperlipidemia and Vascular Disease

Basil M. Rifkind, M.D. and Robert I. Levy, M.D.

General Considerations

There is no doubt that hypercholesterolemia is associated with an increased risk of coronary heart disease. Evidence for this in man has been derived from various sources. Clinicians have long recognized that certain forms of hypercholesterolemia are familial and are often associated with premature vascular disease. In numerous retrospective studies higher lipid levels were observed in subjects with a history of myocardial infarction when compared with control subjects, especially in the younger age groups. The most impressive evidence, however, is derived from the results of prospective population studies (1). Of these the Framingham study is probably the best known. In this study, it was found for example, that in males 34 to 44 years of age, a cholesterol level over 265 mg/100 ml is associated with a five times greater risk that coronary heart disease will develop than levels below 220 mg/100 ml.

An association between triglyceride levels and coronary heart disease is less securely documented but seems to be emerging. Such studies were delayed until a relatively simple method, applicable on a large scale, was developed for the direct determination of triglyceride. Fortunately, suitable automated methods for the determination of plasma triglyceride are now available. However, studies are still hampered by the need for a fasting blood specimen to eliminate the confounding influence of diet-derived chylomicron triglyceride.

Many studies have been reported showing higher triglyceride levels in subjects with myocardial infarction than in age-matched controls, sometimes more so than cholesterol. Prospective data, unfortunately, is quite scanty. Sf 20–400 lipoproteins, but not triglycerides per se, were determined in nonfasting subjects in the Framingham Study and were found to be an independent risk factor in females over 50 years of age, but not in those under 50 years, or in males, irrespective of age. Recently Carlson and Böttiger (2) observed a significant relationship, in their Stockholm prospective study, between triglyceride levels and the risk of coronary heart disease for male subjects under 60 years but not for older subjects. They interpreted triglyceride levels as possibly more closely associated with coronary heart disease than cholesterol and concluded that cholesterol and triglycerides were each independent predictors of coronary heart disease.

Lipids, such as cholesterol or triglyceride, are not in free solution in plasma but circulate, bound to specific proteins, as lipoproteins. Four families of lipoproteins are generally recognized (Table 8-1); *chylomicrons*, almost exclusively composed (Table 8-2) of triglycerides of dietary (exogenous) origin; *VLDL*, rich in endogenously derived triglyceride, cholesterol-rich LDL, and HDL. A fifth lipoprotein, an intermediate density lipoprotein (ILDL) appears to be formed transiently during the conversion of VLDL to LDL (12).

Table 8-1. Operational Classifications of Plasma Lipoproteins

Electrophoretic mobility (paper or agarose gel)	Density class (preparative ultracentrifuge)	Flotation class S_f* (analytical ultracentrifuge)
Chylomicrons (remain at origin)	Chylomicrons <0.95	>400
Pre-beta (α_2)	Very low density liproprotein (VLDL) 0.95–1.006	20–400
Beta	Low density liproprotein (LDL) 1.006–1.063	0–20
Alpha (α_1)	High density liproprotein (HDL) 1.063–1.21	—

*An S_f unit = 10^{-13} cm/sec per dyne per gram in a sodium chloride solution of density 1.063 g/ml (26°C).

Table 8-2. Typical Lipid and Protein Composition of Plasma Lipoproteins

	Chylomicrons	VLDL	LDL	HDL
Cholesterol	5	13	43	18
Triglyceride	90	65	10	2
Phospholipid	4	12	22	30
Protein	1	10	25	50

Results expressed as percentage of total lipid and protein content of each lipoprotein family.

The need to translate hyperlipidemia (Table 8-3) into hyperlipoproteinemia has been emphasized previously. Not all forms of hypercholesterolemia and hypertriglyceridemia are equally associated with an increased risk of coronary heart disease. Risk appears to depend on which lipoprotein is responsible for the hyperlipidemia. Hyperlipoproteinemia is said to be present when abnormal concentrations of one or more of the lipoproteins occur under standardized sampling

Table 8-3. Suggested Normal Limits[a] of Plasma Lipid Concentrations (mg/100 ml) in Subjects 0 to 59 Years of Age

Age (yr)	Total Cholesterol	Triglyceride
0–19	120–230	10–140
20–29	120–240	10–140
30–39	140–270	10–150
40–49	150–310	10–170
50–59	150–310	10–190

[a]Figures are based on 90 percent fiducial limits calculated for small samples. All values are rounded to the nearest 5 mg, and for practical purposes, sex differences have been ignored except for HDL concentrations. The population sampled was from the Washington, D. C. metropolitan area. Limits may differ elsewhere.

Table 8-4. Sampling Conditions for Screening for Hyperlipidemia and for Establishing a Lipoprotein Type

1. Conventional Western diet
2. Steady weight
3. No acute illness
   Defer sampling after myocardial infarction for at least 6 weeks
4. No lipid-lowering drugs
   No lipid-influencing drugs
5. 12 to 16-hour fast prior to sampling

Table 8-5. Types of Hyperlipoproteinemia

I. Fasting chylomicronemia	III. Presence of intermediate lipoprotein form ("floating" beta lipoprotein; $d < 1.006$)
II. Increased LDL concentration when VLDL normal—IIa when VLDL increased—IIb	IV. Increased VLDL only V. Fasting chylomicronemia with VLDL increase

conditions (Table 8-4). The most common classification in use recognized five basic patterns (Table 8-5) of hyperlipoproteinemia occurring either secondary to other disease states or as primary disorders, often displaying characteristic genetic and clinical features and distinct therapeutic requirements. An increased risk of coronary heart disease does not appear to occur in types I and V, but undoubtedly features in the common type II and uncommon type III forms. While type IV seems to occur frequently in subjects with coronary heart disease, which is unusually prevalent in certain kindreds with familial type IV, more reliable evidence of a general association between an increase in VLDL and coronary heart disease is needed.

The Primary Hyperlipoproteinemias

Type I

The lipoprotein abnormality in type I hyperlipoproteinemia consists of chylomicronemia, often severe, in fasting plasma. The plasma is milky and storage overnight at 4°C results in the formation of a creamy layer of chylomicron over an otherwise clear infranate. Marked hypertriglyceridemia with slight-to-moderate hypercholesterolemia results, the plasma triglyceride:cholesterol ratio characteristically being 10 to 20:1. The disorder usually presents in infancy with the development of recurrent attacks of acute abdominal pain with or without potentially fatal pancreatitis. Eruptive xanthomas, lipemia retinalis, and hepatosplenomegaly occur, but accelerated atherosclerotic disease does not.

The disorder may be genetically determined and inherited as a recessive trait. A deficiency of one of the enzymes, collectively known as lipoprotein lipase results in the inability to clear exogenous triglyceride, transported as chylomicrons, from plasma.

Type II

An increased LDL concentration is the hallmark of the type II pattern. When this is the sole abnormality, it is called type IIa; when triglycerides (and VLDL) are coincidentally increased, it is called type IIb. The LDL increase almost always results in hypercholesterolemia; hypertriglyceridemia is also present in the type IIb variety.

Clinical consequences of type II stem from lipid deposition at various sites. Many subjects exhibit tendon xanthomas, characteristically at the elbows, dorsum of the hands and feet, the tibial tuberosities, and in the tendon achilles. Xanthelasma and premature corneal arcus are frequent. These features are mainly of cosmetic significance. Arterial lipid deposition results in coronary heart and, less commonly, peripheral vascular disease.

Primary type II is often familial in occurrence, exhibiting a pattern of autosomal dominant inheritance. So-called sporadic forms also occur. The relative frequency of the familial and sporadic forms remains to be determined. Type II homozygotes are occasionally encountered. These children are severely hypercholesterolemic, exhibit xanthomas at birth or in infancy, develop coronary heart disease, and invariably die during the first or second decades. Recent tissue culture studies using fibroblasts (2) point to an inability to bind LDL to the cell surface as the underlying abnormality leading to failure to normally catabolize LDL.

Type III

Although type III shares several features with type II, and has been confused with it in the past, it appears to be a distinct disorder. It is characterized by the presence of an abnormal lipoprotein, so-called *"floating" beta lipoprotein* (intermediate density lipoprotein), which is identified by the abnormal presence of beta-migrating lipoprotein in the d <1.006 (VLDL) fraction. Current evidence points to plasma LDL as being totally or largely derived from the catabolism of VLDL through the formation of a transient intermediate lipoprotein form not normally detectable in plasma. An abnormality in the catabolism of VLDL, possibly brought on by excess VLDL production, appears to underlie the type III abnormality.

The clinical features of type III include the xanthomas described for type II. In addition, planar (palmar crease) and tuboeruptive xanthomas are often present.

As in type II, coronary heart disease often occurs; peripheral vascular disease is also unusually prevalent. Impaired glucose tolerance, with or without frank diabetes, obesity, and hyperuricemia may coexist.

Primary type III undoubtedly occurs as a familial disorder, but its mode of inheritance is yet to be defined. It is rare to observe it in childhood. A type IV pattern is unusually frequent in first-degree relatives.

Type IV

In type IV the only lipoprotein abnormality consists of an increased concentration of VLDL; hypertriglyceridemia is always present. In only about 20 percent of subjects is the increase in VLDL sufficient to also produce hypercholesterolemia.

Subjects with type IV are often obese, may show abnormal glucose tolerance and hyperuricemia, and occasionally develop eruptive xanthomas. It is not clear whether coronary heart disease is unusually frequent in type IV, although there is considerable evidence in favour of this.

Type IV may be familial and show a dominant mode of inheritance in affected kindreds. It is uncommon in childhood. Defective removal of VLDL from the plasma, by mechanisms yet poorly understood, appears to underlie the disorder.

Type V

Both chylomicronemia and an increased VLDL concentration occur in type V. The chylomicronemia results in features described for type I. Type V differs from type I subjects, however, in their older age at presentation, frequent obesity, normal lipoprotein lipase activity, and frequent coexistence of abnormal carbohydrate tolerance and hyperuricemia. No special tendency to coronary heart disease has been documented. Type V is often clearly familial and shows an autosomal dominant mode of transmission. The basic defect has yet to be described.

Available Therapy for Hyperlipoproteinemia

Diet

It is possible to substantially or totally correct hyperlipidemia in almost all hyperlipoproteinemic subjects by appropriate diet therapy alone or in combination with selected drugs. The first step in the treatment of primary hyperlipoproteinemia is to prescribe a suitable diet, and this is often sufficient. Specific diets are prescribed for different types of primary hyperlipoproteinemia (Table 8-6). A low fat diet diminishes chylomicron formation and hence the chylomicronemia of type I. A low-cholesterol, high-polyunsaturated:saturated (P:S) diet decreases the elevated LDL of type II subjects, although not always into the normal range, apparently by accelerating the removal of LDL. Reduction to and maintaining ideal body weight by a regimen that emphasizes carbohydrate restriction decreases VLDL formation and plasma concentration in type IV. A weight reduction and maintenance program coupled with a low-cholesterol diet is highly effective in correcting the hyperlipoproteinemia of type III. Reduction of both chylomicrons and VLDL is the goal in treating type V and involves both a low fat diet and reduction to and maintenance of ideal weight.

Drug Therapy

Several effective drugs are now available to reduce elevated plasma lipid levels. As was the case for diet, drug therapy is tailored to the patterns of hyperlipoproteinemia being treated.

Drugs reduce lipoprotein levels by decreasing its production or increasing its removal (Table 8-7). Nicotinic acid decreases VLDL and hence the production of LDL and is often useful in types III, IV, V, and IIa and IIb. Troublesome, though usually transient, side effects, such as pruritus and flushing, gastrointestinal symptoms, and abnormal liver function tests, inhibit its use. The primary mode of action of clofibrate, leading to lipid lowering, is unclear but both diminished synthesis of VLDL and increased catabolism may be involved. Levels of VLDL and ILDL usually fall during clofibrate therapy but levels of LDL may rise or fall. The drug is mainly indicated when levels of VLDL or ILDL are high as in types IIb, III, and IV hyperlipoproteinemia. Although occasionally subjects with type IIa show an impressive response, more often its effect is disappointing. Significant side effects, such as acute myositis, are fortunately infrequent. Cholestyramine consistently diminishes levels of LDL in type II and in normal subjects. This exchange resin binds intestinal bile acids, leading to their increased fecal loss. A compensatory conversion of cholesterol to bile acid as well as increased cholesterogenesis occur. By mechanisms still unclear, the catabolism or clearance of LDL is enhanced.

Table 8-6. Dietary Treatment of Hyperlipoproteinemia. From Levy *et al.* Ann. Intern. Med. 77:267, 1972.

Factor	Type I	Type II	Type III[a]	Type IV[a]	Type V
Dietary prescription	Low fat, 25 to 35 g	Low-cholesterol, polyunsaturated fat increased	Low cholesterol approximately: 20% cal. protein 40% cal. fat 40% cal. CHO	Controlled CHO (approximately 40 to 45% calories); moderately restricted cholesterol	Restricted fat (30% calories), controlled CHO (50% calories), moderately restricted cholesterol
Calories	Not restricted	Not restricted, except in type IIb where weight reduction is often indicated	Achieve and maintain "ideal" weight—reduction diet if necessary	Achieve and maintain "ideal" weight—reduction diet if necessary	Achieve and maintain "ideal" weight—reduction diet if necessary
Protein	Total protein intake not limited	Total protein intake not limited	High protein	Not limited other than control of patient's weight	High protein
Fat	Restricted to 25 to 35 g in adults and 10–15 g in children; kind of fat not important	Saturated fat intake limited; polyunsaturated intake increased	Controlled to 40% to 45% calories (polyunsaturated fats recommended in preference to saturated fats)	Not limited other than control of patient's weight (polyunsaturated fats recommended in preference to saturated fats)	Restricted to 30% calories (polyunsaturated fats recommended in preference to saturated fats)
Cholesterol	Not restricted	Less than 300 mg or as low as possible; only source of cholesterol is meat	Less than 300 mg, only source of cholesterol is meat	Moderately restricted to 300 to 500 mg	Moderately restricted to 300 to 500 mg
Carbohydrates	Not restricted	Not restricted (may be controlled in type IIb)	Controlled; most concentrated sweets eliminated	Controlled; most concentrated sweets eliminated	Controlled; most concentrated sweets eliminated
Alcohol	Not recommended	May be used with discretion	Limited to 2 servings (substituted for carbohydrate)	Limited to 2 servings (substituted for carbohydrate)	Not recommended

[a]Cal = calories; CHO = carbohydrate.

Table 8-7. Drug Treatment of Hyperlipoproteinemia in Adults. From Levy *et al.* Ann. Intern. Med. 77:267, 1972.

	Nicotinic Acid	Cholestyramine	D-Thyroxine	Clofibrate
Effect on plasma lipoproteins	↓VLDL, ↓LDL, ↓LDL synthesis	↓LDL, may ↑VLDL, ↑LDL catabolism	↓LDL, little effect on VLDL (?), ↑LDL catabolism	↓VLDL, effect on LDL variable
Initial dose	100 mg orally, three times daily	4 g orally, four times daily	1 mg orally, daily	0.5–1.0 g twice daily
Maintenance dose	1–2 g orally, three times daily with meals	4–8 g orally, four times daily	4–8 mg orally, daily	1 g orally, twice daily
Adverse effects	Flushing, pruritis, hyperuricemia, ↓ glucose tolerance, hepatotoxicity	Constipation, bloating, nausea, malabsorption of fat at doses > 24 to 32 g/day	Signs of hypermetabolism in some patients may ↑ angina	Nausea, weight gain, myositis, alopecia, agranulocytosis. Abnormal liver function
Caution	Peptic ulcer patients. Safe use in pregnancy not established	Drug binds warfarin, digitalis, thyroxin. Safe use in pregnancy not established	Warfarin dose may need ↓ . Avoid in patients with multiple ectopic premature beats. Extreme caution in patients with CAD. Safe use in pregnancy not established	Potential effects of warfarin. Safe use in pregnancy not established
Use	Types III, IV, V, IIb, II	Type IIa, ?IIb	Types II, III	Types III, IV, ?IIb

VLDL = very low density lipoproteins; LDL = low-density lipoproteins.

Triglyceride and VLDL levels show little change and may actually rise. The addition of an adequate dose of cholestyramine to a low-cholesterol diet in subjects with type II consistently produces a total reduction in the plasma cholesterol of 25 to 35 percent. It is not indicated for any other type of hyperlipoproteinemia. A new preparation (Questran[R]) has largely eliminated previous problems of taste and odor but its drawback is it retains bulk. Other bile acid sequestrants, such as colestipol, appear to be effective but have not yet been approved for general use by the Food and Drug Administration. Other lipid-lowering drugs include beta-sitosterol, neomycin, PAS, d-thyroxine and norethisterone acetate. Their use is limited by insufficient evaluation, significant toxicity, or limited efficacy.

Objectives of Lipid Lowering

Lipid lowering is not an end in itself. It is first directed to the elimination of certain established signs and symptoms and second, but most important, to the prevention of premature vascular disease in these types of hyperlipoproteinemia in which it occurs frequently. The first goal can often be achieved; adequate correction of hyperlipidemia leads to (a) the disappearance of superficial xanthomas (eruptive, tuberous, tuboeruptive, planar) variously found in each of the primary hyperlipoproteinemias, which benefit is mainly cosmetic and psychologic, and (b) resolution and subsequent prevention of the attacks of recurrent abdominal pain with or without sometimes fatal pancreatitis observed in the hyperlipoproteinemias characterized by massive chylomicronemia—types I and V.

The second goal, the prevention of premature atherosclerotic disease, cannot yet be said to have been attained. Yes, it is, by far, the main clinical reason we concern ourselves with hyperlipidemia. Four million Americans have symptomatic coronary artery disease. Six hundred thousand deaths attributed to coronary heart disease occur annually, many suddenly and without warning.

Hyperlipoproteinemia is implicated in a considerable fraction of these subjects, assuming much greater proportion when coronary heart disease occurs prematurely. In a recent study (13) the overall frequency of hyperlipidemia in 500 survivors of myocardial infarction was 31 percent. This figure rose to 60 percent in male survivors under age 40 and in females under age 50. The prevalence of hyperlipoproteinemia was similar in subjects with coronary heart disease, having been found to occur in 45 to 65 percent of all subjects who survived myocardial infarction, in 75 percent of those with myocardial infarction or angina, 22 percent of male and 33 percent of female postmyocardial infarction subjects, 54 percent of those who angiographically demonstrated coronary artery disease, and 74 percent of a group with positive coronary arteriograms.

The epidemic scale of morbidity and mortality in coronary heart disease, the high prevalence of hyperlipidemia and hyperlipoproteinemia in victims of coronary heart disease, and the previously cited prospective data relating hypercholesterolemia (and probably hypertriglyceridemia) to coronary heart disease have acted as powerful incentives to the use of lipid-lowering therapy either to prevent further coronary heart disease in subjects who already show manifestations (secondary prevention) or to prevent the development of new disease (primary prevention), especially in those known to be at high risk. To consider lipid lowering a means of preventing coronary heart disease is not, however, confined to subjects with hyperlipidemia. Such subjects merely represent the top end of a continuous distribution of plasma lipids and lipoproteins. Levels exceeding the 95th percentile are usually used to arbitrarily define hyperlipoproteinemia. Subjects whose levels fall below this percentile are by no means free of a risk of coronary heart disease, reflecting a direct relationship between cholesterol levels and risk of coronary heart disease. Such a relationship suggests that potential benefits of lipid-lowering need not be confined to subjects with hyperlipidemia and that a general reduction of plasma cholesterol might have a powerful impact on the incidence of coronary heart disease.

Designing the Clinical Trial

This growing enthusiasm for lipid-lowering has been accompanied by considerable advances in understanding the pathogenesis of hyperlipidemia and hyperlipoproteinemia and by the increasing availability of improved diet and drug regimens. Drug therapy is increasingly and extensively used by clinicians responsible for treating individual patients and has been paralleled by a growing awareness on the part of the general public of the need to lower cholesterol and the demand for low cholesterol products on supermarket shelves.

It is clearly necessary that such therapy be put to the acid test; namely, does a reduction in plasma cholesterol decrease the risk of coronary heart disease? Although many attempts have been made to answer this question, and some have been rewarded with encouraging results, no study has yet provided unequivocal evidence of benefit.

Why, given the abundant circumstantial evidence in favor of lipid-lowering, have such studies left us still in doubt as to whether it is really effective? Several reasons account for this, especially the difficulty in developing a satisfactory study design and the size of the population needed to yield definite conclusions.

The information available to permit design of a study to evaluate the efficacy of lipid-lowering is inadequate in many important respects. Factors taken into account include the:

1. Coronary Heart Disease Event Rate. Considerable information is available from prospective studies to predict the rate at which new coronary heart disease events (fatal or nonfatal coronary infarction) are likely to occur in untreated subjects relative to their cholesterol levels. As mentioned earlier, corresponding data for triglyceride levels is scanty. Although inferences can be drawn regarding the risk associated with levels of certain lipoproteins from knowledge of plasma lipid levels, there is little direct data, a considerable disadvantage when certain high risk groups, such as those with type II, are considered for intervention. In the general population, new coronary heart disease occurs in about 1 of 100 middle aged men each year. The use of high-risk groups reduces the sample size but not to a level free of recruitment and logistic problems.

2. Time to Maximum Therapeutic Benefit. This is based on the predicted degree of lipid-lowering and assumes that a reduction in cholesterol levels reduces the risk of coronary heart disease corresponding to untreated levels to that associated with the new lower levels. There are no data in humans and only scanty data in primates on this, so that it is not known whether it takes weeks or months to achieve a reduction in risk.

3. Drop-Out Rate. Allowances are made for possible study drop-outs (subjects who fail to adhere to treatment) on the basis of such factors as prior experience in clinical trials of the therapy being tested and the nature of the population participating in the study. At best, it can be an approximate estimate.

4. Duration of Trial. The relatively low coronary heart disease rate in high-risk groups, also necessitates lengthy periods of observation measured in years, making it especially troublesome to adhere to prescribed regimens.

The implication of such considerations are well-illustrated by the report of the NHLI Task Force on Arteriosclerosis (19), which on the basis of the Diet Heart Feasibility Study and others concluded that it was not feasible to perform a major national dietary prevention study in a free-living population. Major considerations leading to this decision were the prohibitive size of the study population (24,000 to 115,000), associated managerial and logistic problems, and huge projected expenditures (0.5 to 1.0 billion dollars). The report was also pessimistic as to whether the required degree of lipid-lowering could be achieved in such a free-living population and, most important, was apprehensive that concomitant modification of other major risk factors (smoking, blood pressure, obesity) would be liable to occur and to confound the study. Problems of sample size, duration of observation, and so forth, in such studies are compounded by other considerations, such as the need for a strict double-blind design after subjects were randomized (with or without stratification) into treatment and placebo groups.

In an attempt to bring sample sizes down to manageable proportions, some studies focused on certain high-risk groups. For example, the NHLI-sponsored Lipid Research Clinic Type II Coronary Primary Prevention Trial selected males with type II hyperlipoproteinemia and free of coronary heart disease for their trial; although the risk of coronary heart disease in such a group undoubtedly is high, about 3,600 men are still required, posing major recruitment problems.

A paradox underlying sample-size determinations is the infrequent occurrence of end points used to measure the primary goals of the study, in contrast to the extremely high frequency and often severe nature of the underlying atherosclerotic disease. Undoubtedly, considerable reductions in sample size could be achieved if safe, noninvasive, readily applicable, sensitive, and specific methods were available to evaluate atherosclerotic disease per se. While the development of new techniques offer promise, no satisfactory method is yet available for application in large-scale clinical trials.

Such considerations indicate why an unequivocal answer is still not available to the question as to whether lipid-lowering reduces the risk of coronary heart disease.

Clinical Trials to Date

In 1969 Cornfield and Mitchell (4) reviewed 19 major primary or secondary completed or ongoing prevention studies. They noted disagreement; some reported positive results, of varying magnitude, others did not. The positive results were sometimes achieved with no effects on cholesterol. They attributed much of this inconclusiveness to faults in study design or analysis, such as inadequate numbers, randomization and follow-up, failure to double-blind with possible effects on other risk factors and the exercise of unconscious bias, as well as the use of soft end points, such as angina. They concluded that there was no "clear-cut, generally accepted answer to the question of whether cholesterol-lowering can effectively prevent coronary disease." Further, they cautioned that the statistical treatment employed meant that "no results of intervention studies to date are as statistically significant as the *P* value calculation indicates."

Five years and several clinical trials later, this position is essentially unchanged. A 12-year study of dietary intervention (primary and secondary) was recently reported by Miettinen (18). Performed in two Finnish mental hospitals, the study employed a crossover design and mortality from coronary heart disease was found to be considerably reduced in men who received a cholesterol lowering diet. Cornfield and his colleagues (5) made some important criticisms of the study to the extent that they doubted whether it established that lipid-lowering reduces the risk of coronary heart disease. They drew attention to inadequacies in the crossover design, such as its nonrandom nature and indications that the populations studied during the two observation periods at each hospital were not fully comparable.

Several trials of clofibrate have also been reported recently; two secondary prevention studies were performed in the United Kingdom (1, 20) and both described beneficial effects from the active drug in subjects with angina, with or without myocardial infarction at entry. Both studies randomized subjects and used a double-blind design. However, both contained several important design defects, leading to doubts as to their conclusions. Feinstein (9) and others, in reviewing these trials, drew attention, for example, to the lack of standard entry and end point criteria in one of them and criticized the main method of statistical analysis; alternative results were obtained using other statistical approaches. In a primary prevention trial of clofibrate in the United States (15), benefit was also reported but this study too failed to employ a double-blind design; other major defects severely limit its interpretation. These inconclusive findings pertaining to clofibrate are, in effect, endorsed by distributors of the drug in the United States, who advertise that its effects on mortality from coronary heart disease have not been established.

The National Heart and Lung Institute-sponsored Coronary Drug Project is a secondary prevention trial of several lipid-lowering drugs. Its final results are yet to be published, but interim results describe serious toxicity from two of the drugs. In this study, males with a previous history of myocardial infarction were enrolled and randomized into one of six medication schedules. Certain categories of subjects receiving dextrothyroxine showed an increased mortality from coronary and cardiovascular disease and a high rate of myocardial infarction (7). Subjects on a high dose of estrogens developed an excess number of events of nonfatal coronary infarction, pulmonary embolism, and thromboembolism (9). A low-dose estrogen group was also subsequently withdrawn, partly on the grounds of toxicity, including a suggestive increase in mortality from cancer (6). These Coronary Drug Project observations strongly reinforce the view that widespread use of hypolipidemic drugs to prevent coronary heart disease should be deferred until distinct benefit is demonstrated and significant toxicity ruled out from any given regimen.

Ongoing Studies

Several well-developed clinical trials are now in progress in an attempt to provide some conclusive answers as to the benefits of lipid-lowering. One approach has been to select a relatively homogeneous, high-risk group and powerful lipid-lowering therapy to reduce sample size. Thus, as already mentioned, the National Heart and Lung Institute's Lipid Research Clinics Program initiated a primary prevention study in 3,600 type II males, age 35 to 59, and free of coronary heart disease in which combined diet and cholestyramine is the therapeutic modality. Another study at the Clinical Center of the National Institutes of Health involves 250 type II males with coronary heart disease and uses coronary angiography as its major end point. A less specific, but nonetheless important, approach is to evaluate the simultaneous correction of multiple coronary heart disease risk factors (cholesterol, hypertension, cigarette smoking). Two such major studies, the National Heart and Lung Institute sponsored Multirisk Factor Intervention Trial and a similar European study, are underway.

Recommended Therapy for Primary Hyperlipoproteinemias

With these considerations in mind, we are in a position to describe our personal recommendations.

1. Type I: All are agreed that subjects with type I should be treated to prevent the oft-severe and potentially fatal abdominal attacks, which are a feature of this disorder. The massive chylomicronemia that characterizes type I is readily controlled by rigidly restricting dietary fat. A low fat diet (25 to 35 g per day for an adult; 10 to 15 g per day for a child) is employed. Medium chain triglycerides, a fat, the mechanism of absorption, of which does not involve the formation of chylomicrons, may be used as a supplement to render the diet palatable. This diet results in a substantial reduction in chylomicronemia within several days, and prompt resolution of abdominal pain, eruptive xanthomas, hepatosplenomegaly, and lipemia retinalis. Triglyceride levels are usually lowered to between 500 and 800 mg/100 ml, a level not usually associated with the reappearance of these features. Oral intake is suspended and parenteral fluids administered during acute attacks of abdominal pain, whether or not associated with pancreatitis. No drugs are presently known to be effective in the treatment of type I.

2. Type IIa: A low-cholesterol ($<$ 300 mg per day in adults; $<$150 mg per day in children), high P/S diet should be the initial treatment in all subjects with Type IIa hyperlipoproteinemia. Calorie restriction is not a component of this diet, which typically reduces the total plasma and LDL cholesterol by 10 to 15 percent. In some subjects, normal lipid levels are restored; in most however, additional therapy must be prescribed to achieve this goal. Satisfactory results may be achieved by supplementing the diet with cholestyramine resin. In adult heterozygotes, a dose of 16 to 24 g per day will usually produce an additional drop of 20 to 25 percent in total plasma cholesterol through its effect on LDL cholesterol. Higher doses (up to 36 g per day) may be required in severe type II heterozygotes and homozygotes. A dose of 0.5 to 1.5 g/kg per day is used in homozygous children. The drug is administered in the form of a powder and must always be taken suspended in water or another liquid, or as a puree with a high fluid content. It is usually taken in divided doses four times a day, although twice-a-day regimen recently has been shown to be equally efficacious. Constipation is the leading side effect of cholestyramine and can usually be managed by administering stool softeners. It is generally free from significant and serious toxicity.

Whether or not to administer drugs that, by the nature of the type II disorder, will have to be given on an indefinite basis, is a controversial question in the absence of categoric information regarding the effectiveness of therapy in the prevention or treatment of vascular disease. We take into account factors such as the patient's age, the degree of severity of the cholesterol increase, the presence or absence of coronary heart disease in the patient, and whether there is a history of premature vascular disease (coronary heart disease, peripheral vascular disease, cerebral vascular disease) in near relatives. In heterozygous children with mild to moderate hyperlipoproteinemia, especially if the family history is not adverse, only diet is prescribed, for it is in children especially that the potential consequences of long-term treatment must be especially guarded against. In children with a more severe degree of hyperlipoproteinemia, especially in the presence of an adverse family history and in whom diet has not corrected the hyperlipidemia sufficiently, cholestyramine is added to the regimen. We tend to employ combined diet and cholestyramine therapy in most adult heterozygotes in whom diet alone has proved insufficient. Aggressive therapy is justified in severe heterozygotes and in type II homozygotes in view of the adverse prognosis. In such subjects, combined nicotinic acid and cholestyramine treatment is employed in addition to the low-cholesterol, high P/S diet. Most severe heterozygotes show a considerable response to this regimen, but some homozygotes do not; a satisfactory hypolipidemic regimen is still to be developed to treat the latter. It is much too early to assess the role of portacaval shunting for the treatment of type II homozygotes, since this procedure has only been reported to date in one case and much more information is required on its mechanism of action, long-term consequences, and efficacy.

We also do not employ the ileal bypass procedure for the treatment of type II since most of our subjects are successfully managed by combined diet and drug regimens, and the means by which cholestyramine reduces cholesterol levels is not dissimilar to that of the surgical procedure.

3. Type IIb: Indications for the treatment of type IIb are similar to those for type IIa. Cholestyramine is often unsuitable for the treatment of type IIb since it does not correct the hypertriglyceridemia and may indeed aggravate it. The same regimen described for the correction of type III abnormality is customarily used.

4. Type III: We are motivated to treat type III hyperlipoproteinemia because of its frequent association with peripheral and coronary vascular disease, the consistent and uniform reductions in plasma lipids that can be achieved by a combined diet and drug regimen, the resolution of superficial xanthomas, which accompanies such treatment, and the suggestive evidence that peripheral blood flow improves as a result.

The diet for type III consists of a reduction to, and maintenance of, ideal weight and restricting cholesterol to less than 300 mg per day. The drug of choice is clofibrate (Atromid-S) 1.0 mg twice daily. This drug has few side or toxic effects. Nicotinic acid is also effective but more prone than clofibrate to produce troublesome side effects. The lipid-lowering effects of these drugs are additive to the effect of the diet.

5. *Type IV*: Since an association between triglyceride (and VLDL) levels and coronary heart disease is less securely established, it is less easy to indicate when therapy is justified. We advocate reduction to and maintenance of ideal weight.

In those subjects in whom triglyceride levels are not reduced below 300 mg/100 ml by such a diet, clofibrate can be considered. Although we personally have not been impressed with this drug for the correction of type IV, many competent investigators advocate its use. Nicotinic acid can also be effective. The use of alcohol should be curtailed because it contributes excess calories.

6. *Type V*: Few would disagree that it is necessary to treat type V hyperlipoproteinemia as in type I, to prevent the adverse consequences of severe chylomicronemia. The diet consists of fat restriction to deal with this element, as well as carbohydrate restriction to reduce the levels of VLDL. The resulting high protein diet is somewhat expensive. Fortunately, prior reduction to ideal weight and its maintenance is often sufficient to reduce lipid levels and to clear the chylomicronemia of such subjects to the extent that recurrent abdominal pain is not a threat. Alcohol is absolutely forbidden because it has the ability to precipitate abdominal emergencies. Treatment of the acute emergency is similar to that for type I, i.e., restriction of oral intake and the administration of parenteral fluids.

When diet alone does not correct the hyperlipidemia of type V sufficiently, drugs are necessary. Nicotinic acid is often the most effective agent in a dose of 3 to 6 g per day. The risk of aggravating coexisting hyperglycemia or hyperuricemia, however, may preclude its use. Clofibrate is sometimes of benefit but can lead to a troublesome rebound of hyperlipidemia after it is discontinued. Norethisterone acetate is an investigational drug sometimes effective in female patients but less so in males at a daily dose of 2.5 to 5.0 mg.

Summary

An association between hypercholesterolemia and an increased risk of coronary heart disease risk has been established securely, based principally on findings of prospective epidemiologic studies. Hypertriglyceridemia may also carry an increased risk, but this association needs confirmation. From the pathophysiologic standpoint, hyperlipidemia is best translated into hyperlipoproteinemia. The risk of coronary heart disease appears to depend on which lipoprotein family is responsible for hyperlipidemia. Five types of hyperlipoproteinemia are conventionally recognized. Each type may be secondary to another disease state or primary. The primary hyperlipoproteinemias are often familial and display characteristic genetic, biochemical, pathologic and clinical features, and distinct therapeutic responsiveness. It is possible to substantially or totally correct most hyperlipoproteinemias by appropriate therapy. Diet is the cornerstone of therapy and must be tailored to the type of hyperlipoproteinemia. Four basic diets—low-fat, low-cholesterol high P:S, reduction diet, and a balanced maintenance regimen, alone or in combination are employed. Drug therapy is used as a supplement to, and not as a substitute for, diet. It is similarly tailored to the pattern of hyperlipoproteinemia. Several effective drugs are now available to correct hyperlipidemia. Nicotinic acid, clofibrate, and cholestyramine are the most useful. Appropriate hyperlipidemic therapy can lead to resolution of some of the xanthomas and attacks of abdominal pain, with or without pancreatitis, characterizing certain of the hyperlipoproteinemias. The most important objective of therapy, prevention of coronary heart disease, has not yet been verified. Many difficulties stand in the way of designing an adequate clinical trial of primary or secondary coronary heart disease prevention. Information bearing on sample-size requirements is inadequate. Clinical trials to date in man have not yet provided a definitive answer as to whether lipid-lowering is beneficial in the prevention of coronary heart disease. Some of this inclusiveness derives from faulty study design. Recent trials have provided encouraging results. Several studies are presently designed to provide a conclusive answer within a reasonable period of time. Meanwhile, hyperlipidemic therapy directed to the prevention of coronary heart disease should probably be confined to the use of diet, except in certain high-risk subjects, such as type II homozygotes and severe heterozygotes, in whom more aggressive measures may be justified.

References

1. Arthur, J. B., *et al.* Trial of clofibrate in the treatment of ischemic heart disease. Br. Med. Jr., 2:767, 1971.
2. Brown, M. S. and Goldstein, J. L. Expression of the familial hypercholesterolemia gene in heterozygotes: Mechanism for a dominant disorder in man. Science, 85:61, 1974.
3. Carlson, L. A. and Böttiger, L. E. Ischaemic heart disease in relation to fasting values of plasma triglycerides and cholesterol. Lancet, 1:865, 1972.
4. Cornfield, J. and Mitchell, S. Selected risk factors in coronary disease. Possible intervention effects. Arch. Environ. Health, 19:382, 1969.
5. Cornfield, J. Halperin, M., and Mitchell, S. Effect of diet on coronary heart disease mortality. Lancet, 2:438, 1973.
6. The Coronary Drug Project. Findings leading to discontinuation of the 2.5 mg/day estrogen group. J.A.M.A., 226:654, 1973.
7. The Coronary Drug Project. Findings leading to further modifications of its protocol with respect to dextrothyroxine. J.A.M.A., 220:996, 1972.
8. The Coronary Drug Project. Initial findings leading to modifications of its research protocol. J.A.M.A., 214:1303, 1970.
9. Feinstein, A. R. The clofibrate trials: Another dispute about contratrophic therapy. Clin. Pharmacol. Ther., 13:953, 1972.
10. Fredrickson, D. S. and Levy, R. I. Familial hyperlipoproteinemia. *In* Stanbury, J. B., Wyngaarden, J. B., and Fredrickson, D. S. eds. Metabolic Basis of Inherited Disease, 3rd Ed. New York, 1972, pp. 545–614.
11. Fredrickson, D. S., Levy, R. I., Jones, E., Bonnell, M., and Ernst, N. The Dietary Management of Hyperlipoproteinemia: A Handbook for Physicians. Washington, D.C., U.S. Dept. of Health, Education and Welfare, Public Health Service, U.S. Government Printing Office, 1970.
12. Fredrickson, D. S., Levy, R. I., and Lees, R. S. Fat transport in lipoproteins—an integrated approach to mechanisms and disorders. N. Engl. J. Med., 276:32, 94, 148, 215, 273, 1967.
13. Goldstein, J. L., Hazzard, W. R., Schrott, H. G., Bierman, E. L., and Motulsky, A. G. Hyperlipidemia in coronary heart disease. I. Lipid levels in 500 survivors of myocardial infarction. J. Clin. Invest., 52:1533, 1973.
14. Kannell, W. B., Castelli, W. P., Gordon, T., and McNamara, P. M. Serum cholesterol, lipoproteins and the risk of coronary heart disease. Ann. Intern. Med., 74:1, 1971.
15. Krasno, L. R. and Kidera, G. J. Clofibrate in coronary heart disease. Effects on morbidity and mortality. J.A.M.A., 219:845, 1972.
16. Levy, R. I., Bonnell, M., and Ernst, N. D. Dietary management of hyperlipoproteinemia. J. Am. Dietetic Assoc., 58:406, 1971.

17. Levy, R. I. and Rifkind, B. M. Lipid lowering drugs and hyperlipidemia. Drugs, 6:12, 1973.
18. Miettinen, M., Turpeinen, O., Karvonen, M. J., Elosuo, R., and Paavlainen, E. Effect of cholesterol-lowering diet on mortality from coronary heart disease and other causes. A twelve-year clinical trial in men and women. Lancet, 1:835, 1972.
19. National Heart and Lung Institute Task Force on Arteriosclerosis. Washington, D.C., U.S. Dept. of Health, Education and Welfare, Public Health Service, U.S. Government Printing Office, 1971.
20. Oliver, M. F., *et al.* Ischemic heart disease: A secondary prevention trial using clofibrate. Br. Med. J., 2:775, 1971.

Chapter 9 Antianginal Agents for Coronary Heart Disease

MATTHEW T. MONROE, M.D. and EWARD K. CHUNG, M.D.

General Considerations

Drug therapy is an acceptable mode of management in angina pectoris, with three therapeutic objectives of clinical importance (8, 9, 27). Historically, the first purpose of antianginal drug therapy, which is still justified, is relief of chest pain during an acute attack of angina pectoris. The second is to prevent recurrent anginal attacks. To achieve this goal, a drug is needed that will reduce the frequency of spontaneously occurring anginal attacks. The third therapeutic goal is to prevent myocardial infarction and its complications.

It is extremely difficult to evaluate antianginal drug therapy because anginal pain is a subjective complaint and the response to treatment requires an even more subjective evaluation.

At present, there are two major opposing views with respect to the nature and natural history of angina pectoris (27). One is that angina pectoris is a highly lethal disorder with a high mortality rate that requires vigorous and immediate treatment. This treatment includes both antianginal drug therapy and, at times, surgery (27). An opposing view is that angina pectoris is a benign disorder compatible with long survival in most cases. This long survival was observed in patients whose angina was treated. Furthermore, it was proposed that, at times, angina pectoris may be aggravated by treatment (27).

The ultimate goal in treatment must be its favorable effect upon the mortality of the disease, although symptomatic relief of angina pain can be considered a sufficient therapeutic result. Therefore, the natural history of angina pectoris will be discussed briefly, emphasizing annual mortality. Some authors have reported that the annual mortality from angina pectoris in a large series of untreated patients from clinical presentation was 3 to 6 percent (3, 16, 23, 32). The validity of these clinical investigations may be challenged because the diagnosis was based on clinical symptoms alone, without objective supportive evidence from coronary arteriography. Kannel *et al.* (16) reported in the Framingham study that the annual mortality rate from angina pectoris was 4 percent. This figure is similar to that reported by Parker (23), by Block (3), and by Zuckel (32).

Recently, the natural history of angina pectoris has been studied by coronary arteriography and clinical data (5, 15, 20). Thus, the investigative results are more reliable in terms of diagnostic accuracy relative to the mortality rate in angina pectoris.

As shown in Table 9-1, obstructive coronary lesions documented by coronary angiography are usually a reliable index in predicting death among patients with angina pectoris (5, 14, 15, 20). In a recent study (5) of 590 cases of coronary artery disease during a 5- to 9-year follow-up period, annual mortality among patients with one-vessel disease was 2.9 percent; with two-vessel disease, 7.5 percent; and with three-vessel disease, 10.7 percent, respectively. Mobert *et al.* (20) also presented data supporting these findings. They studied the natural history of severe proximal coronary artery disease, as defined by angiography, in 200 patients followed for 7 years. They found that single-vessel anterior descending disease has a 4-percent annual mortality rate and a 30.5-percent 7-year mortality, whereas a single circumflex or right coronary lesion has a 1.8-percent yearly death rate and a 12.5-percent 7-year mortality. In two-vessel disease the annual mortality was 6.7 percent, while in three-vessel disease it was 10.5 percent during 7 years of observation.

Table 9-1. Annual Mortality in Angina Pectoris

Number of patients	Year of study	Authors	Annual mortality (%)
3,440	1946	Parker *et al.* (23)	6
6,682	1952	Block *et al.* (3)	6
2,234	1969	Zukel *et al.* (32)	3
303	1972	Kannel *et al.* (16)	4
200	1972	Moberg *et al.* (20)	6.4
			3.3 (1-vessel disease)
			6.7 (2-vessel disease)
			10.5 (3-vessel disease)
133	1974	Russek (27)	4.0
			1.2 (102 patients with good ventricular function)
			25.0 (31 patients with poor ventricular function)
140	1973	Gazes (14)	18.0 (preinfarction angina)
590	1973	Bruschke *et al.* (5)	6.9
			2.9 (1-vessel disease)
			7.5 (2-vessel disease)
			10.7 (3-vessel disease)
224	1974	Humphries *et al.* (15)	2.5 (mild disease)
			9.4 (severe disease)
Annual mortality in the United States (24) (56 years old)			1.24

A sudden increase in the frequency of angina pain or prolonged and more severe cardiac pain is termed *preinfarction* or *unstable angina* (12, 14, 15). Annual mortality among patients with unstable angina is much higher and approached 18 percent in a study by Gazes *et al* (14). Among patients with preinfarction angina, Fulton *et al.* (12) reported an annual mortality rate of 11 percent. The lower mortality in this group was thought to be due to the different patient population compared with that of other studies. Using their own scoring technique to assess the degree of arteriographic abnormality, Humphries and his co-workers (15) reported that the annual mortality among patients with mild coronary disease was 2 percent and among those with severe obstructive disease 9.4 percent.

Various factors influence prognosis in patients with angina pectoris. Valvular heart disease, hypertension, atrial fibrillation, diabetes mellitus, cardiac enlargement, and congestive heart failure are major factors that contribute to risk in angina pectoris. Annual mortality among high-risk patients has been shown to approach 25 percent (27). On the other hand, mortality among patients with angina, who do not have these risk factors, is no greater than that among the control population (24, 27).

That acute myocardial infarction is often preceded by angina pectoris of varying duration is well known (14, 15, 27). During an 8-month period of observation, 21 percent of patients with angina pectoris developed myocardial infarction, whereas 35 percent of the high-risk group sustained myocardial infarction within 3 months following the onset of preinfarction angina (14).

Various Antianginal Agents and Their Efficacy

Since its introduction by Murrell (21), nitroglycerin has been the drug of choice in the treatment of acute attacks of angina pectoris for almost a century. The rationale for the use of longer-acting nitrate compounds was considered to be their prophylactic value, and as a consequence large numbers of organic nitrates have been synthesized and tested as antianginal agents (1). Despite extensive clinical and pharmacologic evaluation, the value of these agents has still remained controversial and various opinions concerning the efficacy of long-acting nitrates as prophylactic antianginal agents have ranged from negative to enthusiastic.

Representative clinical trials of drugs commonly employed in the treatment of angina pectoris will be summarized briefly. Group 1 presents clinical observations in which authors found nitrates and other drugs effective in the treatment of angina, whereas in Group II, studies are cited in which authors found various drugs ineffective.

Group I: Clinical Trials of Drugs Found Effective

Isosorbide Dinitrate, Pentaerythritol Trinitrate, Erythrityl Tetranitrate

In a study of 10 hospitalized patients with angina pectoris, the efficacy of isosorbide dinitrate, pentaerythritol trinitrate, and erythrityl tetranitrate were evaluated using multiple exercise tests (17). The patients were exercised to the point of myocardial ischemia manifested by typical angina pain and/or a 1.0-mm or more S-T segment depression. Placebo did not influence the duration of exercise needed to induce ischemia. However, mean durations of exercise, 45 minutes after erythrityl tetranitrate, isosorbide dinitrate, and pentaerythritol trinitrate, were much longer and all were different from that after a placebo. The study indicated that each long-acting nitrate is effective for at least 45 minutes and that these drugs should not be given on a fixed dose schedule but taken prophylactically whenever an angina-provoking situation is anticipated.

The influence of nitroglycerin on myocardial metabolism and hemodynamics during angina induced by atrial pacing was studied in 15 patients before and after the administration of 0.5 mg of chewable nitroglycerin (6). This preparation effectively abolished chest pain in 8 patients and, at the same time, 5 had less pain during pacing. Mean lactate production, an indicator of anaerobic cardiac metabolism, was abolished; S-T segment became less depressed; and mean left ventricular end-diastolic pressure was reduced during pacing in patients treated with nitroglycerin.

Results of this study indicate that nitroglycerin may prevent or reduce pacing-induced angina; improve the exercise electrocardiogram and hemodynamics; and, in some patients, decrease myocardial ischemia.

Propanolol and Isosorbide Dinitrate

Medical treatment of angina pectoris with propanolol and isosorbide dinitrate was evaluated in 133 patients with severe angina pectoris (27). In each case, slight-to-moderate physical or emotional stress regularly evoked classic episodes of angina pectoris which, until the time of study, could not be prevented despite the use of nitroglycerin, long-acting nitrates, sedatives, and other measures. Medical treatment consisted of the combined administration of propanolol and isosorbide dinitrate. The daily dose of propanolol varied from 10 mg twice daily to 160 mg four times daily, and the dose was sufficient to reduce resting heart rate to 55 or 60 beats per minute. Isosorbide dinitrate was administered sublingually in a dose varying between 2.5 and 10 mg, according to individual tolerance and response. In 90 percent of the patients, angina was improved and exercise tolerance increased; the frequency of anginal episodes was reduced 50 percent or more. Favourable clinical responses correlated closely with improved ischemic ECG changes induced by the standard exercise ECG test. The average annual mortality among *good-risk* patients was 1.2 percent, which is not different from that of the general population in the same age groups. A *good-risk* patient was defined as one in whom left ventricular function was normal at the time he entered the study. In sharp contrast, the anticipated annual mortality among *poor-risk* patients was approximately 25 percent. A *poor-risk* patient was defined as one who had signs of left ventricular dysfunction, such as congestive heart failure, cardiomegaly, gallop rhythm, hypertension, or other complicating factors, including diabetes mellitus, atrial fibrillation, previous myocardial infarction, stroke, or cerebrovascular insufficiency. The prospects for 5-year survival were found to be excellent in patients with good left ventricular function. The results suggested that severe angina pectoris responds well to an intensive program of optimal medical care.

Propanolol and Nitroglycerin

Studies of the rationale for beta-blocking agents in antianginal therapy included measurements of arterial and left ventricular pressure, indocyanine green cardiac output, and arterial and coronary sinus oxygen content in patients treated with propanolol and nitroglycerin (31). Hemodynamic measurements were recorded for a total of 27 subjects. At rest, the average heart rate dropped, left ventricular end-diastolic pressure was lowered, cardiac index decreased, and brachial artery pressure fell. During exercise with a bicycle ergometer, mean heart rate, left ventricular external work, and cardiac index in the 6 patients studied fell to lower levels during exercise performed after propanolol was administered. The average myocardial oxygen consumption fell after propanolol, as did coronary flow. When nitroglycerin was given sublingually after propanolol, left ventricular end-diastolic pressure fell even further, cardiac index declined, and myocardial oxygen consumption decreased. Systemic pressure was reduced by nitroglycerin, but the reflex tachycardia usually associated with this drug was abolished by propanolol. These results supported the clinical impression that the effects of propanolol and nitroglycerin in relieving anginal symptoms are additive.

Another aspect of this study was the 3-year clinical trial of propanolol in patients with angina pectoris documented by coronary angiography. Of 104 patients treated with this drug, 90 improved significantly. While control of anginal symptoms alone is a sufficient goal for therapy, the ultimate end point for treatment must be its impact on mortality. Results of the study suggest that survival in patients treated with propanolol and observed for a 24-month period was better than that of a control group that had not been treated with this drug.

Propanolol

Warren *et al.* (29) studied 63 patients with severe angina pectoris treated with propanolol and followed for 6 to 8 years to assess the incidence of complications and the long-term effectiveness of this drug after an initial control period. Each patient had a dose threshold (between 160 to 480 mg) at which maximum benefit was obtained. Average yearly mortality in this group was 3.8 percent. There was no evidence of tachyphylaxis. Congestive heart failure developed in 25 percent and acute myocardial infarction in 15 percent of the patients. All, except 1 patient who died after sustaining a myocardial infarction, suffered from cardiogenic shock. Propanolol was judged to be effective in the treatment of angina pectoris, although it could increase the risk of cardiogenic shock in acute myocardial infarction. More than a 50-percent reduction in anginal pain by propanolol therapy predicted a low mortality group.

Isosorbide Dinitrate and Placebo

The hemodynamic response to sublingual isosorbide dinitrate in unstable angina pectoris was compared to that of a sublingual placebo in 15 patients (30). The reduction in systolic arterial pressure and pulmonary end-diastolic pressure was six times

Table 9-2. Clinical Trials on Antianginal Agents Found to be Effective

No. of patients	Year	Author	Drug	Effectiveness
10	1973	Klaus *et al.* (17)	Isosorbide dinitrate,	(+)
			pentaerythritol .tetranitrate	(+)
			Erythrityl tetranitrate	(+)
15	1972	Chiong *et al.* (6)	Nitroglycerin	(+)
133	1974	Russek (27)	Isosorbide dinitrate	(+)
			Propranolol	(+)
27	1970	Wolfson *et al.* (31)	Propranolol	(+)
			Nitroglycerin	(+)
63	1974	Warren *et al.* (29)	Propranolol	(+)
15	1974	Willis *et al.* (30)	Isosorbide dinitrate	(+)
			Placebo	(−)

longer in patients treated with isosorbide dinitrate than in those who received sublingual nitroglycerin. Sublingual isosorbide dinitrate caused a prolonged decrease both in left ventricular preload and afterload in patients with unstable angina.

The results of studies supporting the efficacy of antianginal drugs are summarized in Table 9-2.

Group II: Clinical Trials in Which Drugs Were Found To Be Ineffective

Nitroglycerin

Ganz and Marcus (13) studied the efficacy of intracoronary nitroglycerin on angina pectoris induced by pacing. In 25 patients, 0.075 mg of nitroglycerin in 1 ml of 5 percent dextrose was injected into the left coronary artery through an angiographic catheter during angina induced by pacing. In 20 patients this procedure was repeated, injecting the same amount of nitroglycerin into the right coronary artery. No relief of pain was observed during a 1-minute observation period whether the drug was injected into the artery supplying collaterals to the obstructed artery or into the obstructed artery itself. The injection was ineffective despite a significant increase in coronary sinus blood flow. Results could suggest that the increase in blood flow did not occur in the ischemic area, but an increase did take place where arterioles were normal. The study seems to indicate that the action of nitroglycerin on coronary blood flow does not play a significant role in its antianginal effect.

Isosorbide Dinitrate, Nitroglycerin, and Placebo

In a double-blind crossover study designed to investigate the possibility that isosorbide dinitrate may interfere with the effectiveness of sublingual nitroglycerin on exercise-induced angina, 17 male patients with angina pectoris were treated (2). The results failed to show a significant difference in the duration of angina following nitroglycerin whether or not the patients were given a sublingual placebo, sublingual isosorbide dinitrate, or no medication. The data indicated that long-acting nitrates do not influence the effectiveness of nitroglycerin administered sublingually to relieve anginal pain.

Nitroglycerin, Isosorbide Dinitrate, and Mannitol Hexanitrate

Studies of the biotransformation of orally administered organic nitrates, nitroglycerin, isosorbide dinitrate, and mannitol hexanitrate (22) revealed that organic nitrates were degraded rapidly in the liver, so that little or no compound was available to relax vascular smooth muscle. Human liver contains the enzyme, glutathione-organic nitrate reductase, which promptly and efficiently degrades organic nitrates, so that their pharmacologic activity disappears almost completely. These results have led authors to conclude that there is no rational basis for the use of long-acting nitrates in the prophylactic therapy of angina pectoris, since the drugs studied were completely degraded in the liver within a short period of time.

Nitroglycerin, Peritrate, Isosorbide Dinitrate, Nilatil, and Placebo

In one study, nitroglycerin was not superior to a placebo in either shortening the duration of angina or in improving preanginal work output (11). Nine patients were subjected to multiple quantitative standard bicycle tests performed to the point of inducing angina. By double-blind random assignment, nitroglycerin or a placebo was administered sublingually at the onset of exercise-provoked angina; the duration of chest pain was timed with a stop watch. Ten minutes after treatment, the patients underwent a similar second test to assess the prophylactic value of nitroglycerin on angina, as determined by changes in work capacity. Statistically, nitroglycerin was not superior to the placebo. The same group of authors reported that pentaerythritol tetranitrate, isosorbide dinitrate, and itramine tosylate (Nilatil) were not superior to a placebo, administered by blind procedures in standard as well as maximally tolerated doses, in reducing the frequency of anginal attacks.

From a study by Lange *et al.* (19), it may be concluded that chronic administration of long-acting nitrates should be avoided, and treatment with nitrates should not be stopped abruptly after they had been used frequently and regularly because an ischemic event may develop when the chronic use of nitroglycerin is discontinued. Recently, Aronow (1) summarized the results of studies in which long-acting nitrates were found to be ineffective in the treatment of angina and concluded that their efficacy as anti-anginal agents has not been adequately established.

Group III: Miscellaneous Drugs Used to Treat Angina Pectoris

Although nitrates alone or combined with beta-blocking agents are commonly used to treat angina and are the focus of existing controversy, other drugs used in the treatment of angina will be discussed briefly (1). *Digitalis* and *diuretics* have been used routinely by many physicians for nocturnal angina accompanying radiographic evidence of left ventricular enlargement. Numerous *coronary vasodilators* have been advocated, and although some of them, such as Dipyridamole, are powerful *coronary vasodilators*, there is almost universal agreement that they are not effective in the treatment of angina (1).

Hypotensive drugs can reduce the frequency of angina by reducing cardiac work and, hence, myocardial oxygen consumption. *Antithyroid drugs and radioiodine*, by

Table 9-3. Clinical Trials of Antianginal Agents Found to be Ineffective

No. of patients	Year	Author	Drug	Effectiveness
25	1972	Ganz and Marcus (13)	Nitroglycerin	(–)
17	1970	Aronow *et al.* (2)	Isosorbide dinitrate	(–)
			Placebo	(–)
			Nitroglycerin	(+)
—	1972	Needleman *et al.* (22)	Isosorbide dinitrate	(–)
			Mannitol hexanitrate	(–)
9	1963	Fisch and DeGraff (11)	Nitroglycerin	(–)
			Placebo	(–)
24	1957	Cole *et al.* (7)	Peritrate	(–)

reducing metabolism, diminish the work of the heart and may prevent transient myocardial ischemia. Prevention and treatment of obesity and hyperlipidemias are usually considered an important aspect of the management of angina. *Alcohol* has been completely discredited as a coronary vasodilator, but it provides a sedative effect for many patients so that alcohol may reduce tensions that precipitate anginal attacks. Other *sedatives* and *MAO inhibitors* can contribute to the management of anginal episodes, and their action will be discussed later.

Discussion

Since angina pectoris is a subjective complaint recognized by the patient's history and its response to treatment is also subjective, antianginal therapy is extremely difficult to evaluate. The accurate assessment of drugs for the treatment of angina pectoris is further complicated by many factors that not only influence their efficacy but the disease itself (26). Angina pectoris may be aggravated by exposure to a cold, humid atmosphere. Therefore, seasonal factors should be considered in planning a drug evaluation study. In some patients the frequency and severity of angina pectoris fluctuates spontaneously; symptoms may be constant for weeks or months then change suddenly without apparent cause. The placebo effect should also be considered carefully, because symptoms of angina may improve significantly with a placebo alone in 50 percent or more of the patients (18, 26).

Some of the practical problems that occur even in a well-designed therapeutic trial have been described by Cole and his associates (7). Only about one-fourth of the patients referred for angina were acceptable for the trial. Some of those rejected had chest pain from other causes or had conditions, in addition to angina pectoris, that made it impossible to analyze the results. Others were suffering primarily from anxiety and were unable to differentiate minor chest discomfort from true anginal attacks. Still others were unwilling or unable to keep records of the daily incidence of angina attacks or the number of nitroglycerin tablets used. Some patients had angina attacks too infrequently to permit a valid comparison of antianginal drug and placebo. A surprising, but not unexpected, feature of this study was that half of the placebo-treated patients reported a decrease in the frequency of attacks over the first 2 to 4 months of treatment. This illustrates the potent effect of the patient–doctor relationship and of the placebo on manifestation of an illness such as angina pectoris. It should be noted that none of the long-acting preparations evaluated in this study were more effective than a placebo. This point was stressed by the Panel of the National Academy of Sciences (Division of Medical Sciences, National Research Council) in their formal report entitled *Drug Efficacy Studies*, which has been sent to the Commissioner of Food and Drug Administration (26). It soon became apparent to the nearly 200 panel members and consultants after the pertinent literature was reviewed that many claims of therapeutic effectiveness for antianginal drugs were based on rather doubtful evidence (8). In the opinion of the panel, well-controlled and well-designed clinical studies were nonexistent for several categories of drugs; supporting clinical evidence consisted, at times, of nothing more than a few testimonials in which little or no attempt had been made to control observer bias or to evaluate the placebo effect. These deficiencies were quite striking, according to the panel, in the case of drugs promoted for the treatment of disease in which the principal measure of effectiveness was relief of a symptom, such as anginal pain. In the conclusion of the report it was suggested that a prerandomization trial period of several months' duration would be sufficient to establish a reasonably stable baseline for the frequency of anginal attacks. This time interval would serve to eliminate additional unreliable, uncooperative, or unsuitable patients. During this period, the patient would continue to take nitroglycerin and a placebo.

The postrandomization period could be interspersed with additional control periods as check points on the long-term fluctuations in the severity and frequency of anginal attacks. However, it has been pointed out elsewhere that the report of the panel may not have been carefully edited and proofread (9). Unfortunately, the opinions of the panel were not identified as to authorship, but it was evident that many of the authorities apparently had not been directly involved with the care of patients. This was reflected by their ignorance of prescribing practices and evidence of drug effectiveness used on an everyday basis. It has been suggested that some of the panelists could have been helped in their task by an experienced pharmacist from a large university hospital who was familiar with prescribing practices. It should be recognized that even complex research employing double-blind conditions affords no guarantee of infallible conclusions.

Some evaluations have frequently used an experimental design in which the test drug was administered without regard for its known pharmacologic action. The timing of drug administration was established arbitrarily without considering pain experience, and the choice of patients was seriously limited by the opportunity for identifying prophylactic response. It could be argued that the drug was ineffective. On the other hand, one may conclude that because the study was improperly designed, the drug was ineffective.

Many patients who experience angina only in the morning, on arising, and in the evening when they return from work may obtain no relief from a potent drug administered three times a day after meals. These patients are unprotected during their most vulnerable periods. Similar negative responses could be expected when patients with postprandial angina receive a long-acting preparation. Another poor therapeutic response could be expected in the case of nocturnal angina treated with a routine, four times a day, therapeutic regimen. These individual variations of the disease in the evaluation of antianginal drugs have not been considered in many studies.

The importance of emotional factors that influence the frequency and intensity of anginal pain has been stressed (18). The patient's mood and mental state are known to alter his perception of and ability to tolerate pain. In angina pectoris the frequency and intensity of pain may be affected by many factors, including anger, fear, anxiety, guilt, sexual feelings, body image, and dependency motivations. In this context one can understand why angina can be favorably influenced by placebo, whiskey, sedatives, tranquilizers, suggestion, hypnosis, monoamine oxidase (MAO) inhibitors, and some surgical procedures. It has been suggested that surgery has a powerful placebo effect in patients with angina pectoris that makes it very difficult to evaluate symptomatic improvement following revascularization procedures.

Recently, two methods for reevaluating the effects of short-term antianginal drug therapy were proposed: (a) the electrocardiographic response to treadmill exercise and (b) the response to atrial pacing (28). There is no evidence that repeated testing results in improved exercise tolerance attributable to conditioning. Blomquist (4) reported, in a review of exercise testing, results in patients with arteriosclerotic heart disease, that can provide information necessary to advise patients about occupational activity. It would appear, from a study by Redwood *et al.* (25), that an acute study, such as an exercise protocol, is more reliable and reproducible than a chronic study in which many other variables are introduced. The result of the investigation in which the order of exercise, with and without placebo, was randomized showed that the placebo did not affect exercise-induced angina pectoris. It was also found that the work load required to precipitate angina is constant, regardless of the amount of preceding exercise performed at submaximal work load. Thus, exercise testing can be employed to evaluate the efficacy of a therapeutic intervention with drugs in the treatment of angina pectoris.

Summary

The complexities of evaluating antianginal agents are well documented, as discussed above, and the efficacy of long-acting nitrates remains to be settled. There is no sound conclusion or agreement regarding their efficacy in the treatment of angina. Furthermore, the subjective nature of anginal pain makes it more difficult to determine the efficacy of antianginal therapy in conjunction with multiple contributing factors and problems.

Much less is known about the effectiveness of drug treatment in preventing anginal attacks and very little is known about the influence of this treatment on the natural history of the disease and its complications. Although there are reports in which the progress of the disease has been said to have been prevented, these reports are controversial.

Despite the controversy surrounding the evaluation and effectiveness of antianginal therapy, the authors have a choice of measures to select from for the management of angina pectoris. Treatment consists of two parts: (a) general measures and (b) specific drug therapy.

In the first part weight reduction and maintenance of ideal weight should be advised. The diet should restrict saturated fats and increase polyunsaturated fats. Patients should be advised to stop smoking. If hypertension is a contributing factor in the patient with angina pectoris, it should be treated and attempts made to maintain blood pressure at normal levels. This will reduce cardiac work and, hence, myocardial oxygen consumption. A sedative can be prescribed for the patient in whom angina attacks are precipitated by uncontrollable emotional tension.

Antianginal drug therapy is the second important measure. A dose of 0.4 to 0.6 mg of nitroglycerin sublingually will reduce the duration and frequency of anginal pain. It is recommended that this drug be taken when any angina-provoking situation is anticipated. Nitroglycerin ointment rubbed into the chest wall before bedtime may be used in the treatment of angina decubitus (10). If physical exertion, such as walking up a hill, a flight of stairs, sexual relations, or walking on the street, consistently produces pain, sublingual nitroglycerin should be used before such activity is undertaken.

None of the long-acting nitrates are as active as nitroglycerin in preventing or terminating acute anginal pain. However, they can be used as sublingual or chewable preparations to prolong the time interval between attacks. A recommended long-acting nitrate is isosorbide dinitrate, 2.5 to 10 mg sublingually two to four times daily. The dose can be adjusted according to the patient's needs and response. If angina occurs in spite of treatment with isosorbide dinitrate, the additional use of sublingual nitroglycerin can be helpful.

Long-acting nitrates can be administered alone but they are preferably used in conjunction with a beta-blocking agent, such as propanolol. In stable angina, propanolol reduces heart rate, myocardial contractility, cardiac output, and myocardial oxygen consumption, thereby reducing the incidence of angina. The recommended initial dose of propanolol is 10 mg two to three times daily, which may be increased gradually, as tolerated, to a maximum of 320 mg per day. Therapy is monitored by heart rate, which should be maintained faster than 55 beats per minute. The patient should be examined for signs of congestive heart failure. Treatment with long-acting nitrates and propranolol in stable angina without heart failure should never be discontinued abrubtly because the oxygen demand of the myocardium may increase suddenly, leading to myocardial oxygen deficit and resulting in acute myocardial infarction. Since propranolol decreases myocardial contractility, it can precipitate congestive heart failure. If a patient treated with propranolol develops myocardial infarction and congestive heart failure, mortality may reach to 100 percent in severe cases. Because of this, propranolol in doses that reduce myocardial contractility to a significant degree is not recommended in patients with preinfarction angina and/or borderline congestive heart failure.

The authors stress the importance of individualizing therapy for the successful treatment of angina pectoris.

References

1. Aronow, W. S. Drug therapy, management of stable angina. N. Engl. J. Med., 289:516, 1973.
2. Aronow, W. S. and Chesluk, H. M. Evaluation of nitroglycerin in angina in patients on isosorbide dinitrate. Circulation, 42:61, 1970.
3. Block, W. J., Crumpacker, E. L., Dry, T. J., *et al.* Prognosis in angina pectoris. Observations in 6,682 cases. J.A.M.A. 150:259, 1952.
4. Blomquist, C. G. Use of exercise testing for diagnostic and functional circulation of patients with arteriosclerotic heart disease. Circulation, 54:1120, 1971.
5. Bruschke, A. V. G., Proudfit, W. L., and Sones, F. M. Progress study of 590 consecutive non-surgical cases of coronary disease followed 5–9 years. Circulation, 47:1154, 1973.
6. Chiong, M. A., Roxroy, O. W., and Parker, J. O. Influence of nitroglycerin on myocardial metabolism and hemodynamics during angina induced by atrial pacing. Circulation, 45:1044, 1972.
7. Cole, S. L., Kaye, H., and Griffith, G. C. Assay of antianginal agents: Q curve analysis with multiple control periods. Circulation, 15:405, 1957.
8. Editorial. Cardiovascular drugs: experience of the drug efficacy study. (DES) Circulation, 41:3, 1970.
9. Editorial. Comment on drug efficacy study. Circulation, 41:9, 1970.
10. Epstein, S. E., Kent, K. M., Goldstein, R. E., *et al.* Reduction of ischemic injury by nitroglycerin during acute myocardial infarction. N. Engl. J. Med., 292:29, 1975.
11. Fisch, S. and DeGraff, A. C. Coronary vasodilators. Dis. Chest. 44:533, 1963.
12. Fulton, M., Lutz, W., Donald, K. W., *et al.* Natural history of unstable angina. Lancet, 1:860, 1972.
13. Ganz, W. and Marcus, H. S. Failure of intracoronary nitroglycerin to alleviate pacing induced angina. Circulation, 46:880, 1972.
14. Gazes, P. C., Mobley, E. M., Faris, H. M., *et al.* Preinfarction (unstable) angina—a projective study—ten year follow-up. Circulation, 48:331, 1973.
15. Humphries, T. O., Kuller, L., Ross, R. S., *et al.* Natural history of ischemic heart disease in relation to arteriographic findings. A twelve year study of 224 patients. Circulation, 49:489, 1974.

16. Kannel, W. B. and Feinlieb, M. Natural history of angina pectoris in the Framingham study. Am. J. Cardiol. 29:154, 1972.
17. Klaus, A. P., Zaret, B. L., Pitt, B. L., *et al.* Comparative evaluation of sublingual long-acting nitrates. Circulation, 48:519, 1973.
18. Lane, F. M. Mental mechanisms and the pain of angina pectoris. Am. Heart J., 85:563, 1973.
19. Lange, R. L., Reid, M. S., Trescu, D. D., *et al.* Nonatheromatous ischemic heart disease following withdrawal from chronic industrial nitroglycerin exposure. Circulation, 46:666, 1972.
20. Moberg, C. H., Webster, J. S., and Sones, F. M. Natural history of severe proximal coronary disease as defined by cineangiography (200 patients, seven-year follow-up). Am. J. Cardiol., 29:282, 1972.
21. Murrel, W. Nitroglycerin as a remedy for angina pectoris. Lancet, 1:80, 113, 151, 224, 1879.
22. Needleman, P., Lang, S., and Johnson, E. M. Organic nitrates: Relationship between biotransformation and rational angina pectoris therapy. J. Pharmacol. Exp. Ther., 181:489, 1972.
23. Parker, R. L., Dry, T. J., Willius, F. A., *et al.* Life expectancy in angina pectoris. J.A.M.A., 131:95, 1946.
24. Public Health Service Life Table in Vital Statistics of the U.S. Dept. of H.E.W., Vol. II, Sec. 5, 1969.
25. Redwood, D. R., Rosing, D. R., Goldstein, R. E., *et al.* Importance of the design of an exercise protocol in the evaluation of patients with angina pectoris. Circulation, 43:618, 1971.
26. Report of the Panels on Cardiovascular Drugs from the Drug Efficacy Study. Circulation, 41:149, 1970.
27. Russek, H. J. The "Natural" history of severe angina pectoris with intensive medical therapy alone. A five-year prospective study of 133 patients. Chest, 65:46, 1974.
28. Sowton, E. E., Balcon, R., Cross, D., *et al.* Measurement of the anginal threshold using atrial pacing. New technique for the study of angina pectoris. Prog. Cardiovasc. Dis., 1:306, 1967.
29. Warren, G., Brewer, D. L., and Orgain, E. S. Propranolol in the long-term treatment of angina pectoris. Am. J. Cardiol., 33:176, 1974.
30. Willis, W. H., Russel, R. O. Jr., Mantle, J. A., *et al.* The hemodynamic response to sublingual isosorbide dinitrate in unstable angina pectoris. Am. J. Cardiol., 33:179, 1974.
31. Wolfson, S., Amseterdam, E., and Gorlin, R. Rationale for the use of beta-blockage as therapy for angina pectoris. In Russek, H. I. and Zohmaid, B. L., eds. Coronary Heart Disease. Philadelphia, J. B. Lippincott, 1970.
32. Zukel, W. J., Cohen, B. M., Mattingly, T. W., *et al.* Survival following first diagnosis of coronary heart disease. Am. Heart J., 78:159, 1969.

Chapter 10 Anticoagulation Therapy for Coronary Heart Disease

LOUIS A. PAPA, D.O. and EDWARD K. CHUNG, M.D.

General Considerations

Although the best approach to atherosclerosis is prevention, all modalities for management must be examined by the physician confronted with the problem of coronary artery disease. Much of the controversy concerning anticoagulation and coronary artery disease results from the poor methodology used in the design of many of the early investigative efforts. Even with better design after 1961 all the questions have not been answered. The fact that we are treating arterial occlusive disease, which has a poorly understood etiology, by using drugs which do not have their main usefulness on the arterial side, has also perpetuated the confusion. Our objective in this brief review is to present a theory as to the etiology of occlusive arterial disease, and just touch on the problem of thrombosis and what occurs in myocardial infarction. Finally, we take the emperic approach and examine the investigative trials to determine the efficacy, if any, of anticoagulation in coronary artery disease.

Physiologic Considerations

The theory that atheroma may be derived from plasma constituents (mainly fibrin) was first formulated by Rokitansky (36), but the work of Duguid (7–9) further delineated the process. Duguid postulated that arterial thrombosis progressed to atheroma formation in an orderly fashion. After a thrombus is formed, it initially retracts and recanalizes so that circulation is restored. Organization of this mass occurs and the canal becomes lined with endothelium. Hence the mass becomes incorporated into the arterial wall. Fatty changes first make their appearance as lipid droplets within the thrombotic elements and eventually become a prominent feature of it. This process has been confirmed experimentally in the pulmonary artery (16). Washed fragmented clots were injected intravenously into rabbits, and pulmonary emboli were produced. Some animals died and others were examined at intervals to observe the progression of the pulmonary artery lesions. It was shown that the lesions went through stages of organization similar to that described by Duguid.

Hence, although not all atherosclerosis is thrombotic in origin, the characteristic features can be products of mural thrombi. The process was recently discussed again by Roberts and Buja (35).

In general, venous thrombi (so-called red thrombi) have a large coagulation component (fibrin), are related to retarded blood flow, and therefore would be more susceptible to the action of anticoagulant drugs. Thrombi on the arterial side (white thrombi) have less fibrin composition and therefore, in theory, are less susceptible to anticoagulants (30) and more related to platelet action.

In arteries, thrombi develop in relation to exposed collagen or collagen-like material (42). Also, rupture of an atherosclerotic plaque may cause platelets to aggregate (5, 42).

The mechanism of platelet aggregation can be devided into three parts:

1. Release of platelet factors
2. Adherence of platelets to each other induced by adenine diphosphate (ADP)
3. The influence of blood coagulation on platelet aggregates and the stabilization of these aggregates by fibrin (30, 31, 42).

Because platelet adhesiveness is so important in the early stages of thrombosis, the effects of anticoagulant drugs on platelet action should be examined. It was shown, in a well controlled in vitro study (22) that ADP-induced platelet aggregation was actually prolonged in the majority of well-anticoagulated patients (Coumadin). On the other hand, using a high-flow pulsatile chamber (28), thrombosis formation was not completely suppressed by Dicumarol (even in high doses). It was also pointed out that when prothrombin time was only slightly prolonged, there was an increase in artificial thrombus formation. Another important finding was that the fibrin component of thrombi could be reduced by therapy. It was concluded that Dicumerol seemed to block the later stages of thrombus formation but had a lesser effect on platelet clumping.

In rats large doses of warfarin sodium, which reduced prothrombin levels considered unsafe for man, did reduce ADP-induced platelet aggregation (32).

Microscopic examination of wounds made during bleeding-time tests were performed on 2 patients who were treated with heparin (21). These exminations demonstrated small, friable platelet aggregates and showed the need for intact coagulation and thrombin in the genesis of thrombi.

The initiation of the arterial thrombus has been discussed for about 100 years and several studies have delineated the process somewhat (19, 20). A good model was demonstrated by Jorgensen *et al.* (19) to study the arterial thrombotic process: they produced mural thrombi in the carotid arteries of swine by placing a silk suture or a collagen fiber intraarterially. The arteries were studied at intervals of 1 hour to 4 months.

At 1 hour the thrombi were composed of dense aggregates of platelets with some fibrin at the periphery of this mass. At 2 to 3 hours the platelets were not as tightly packed and by 7 to 24 hours there was more fibrin present. Later, endothelium started to grow on the luminal surfaces. Smooth muscle cells later appeared in the thrombus. They concluded that what appears to be a fibrin thrombus in an artery could have started as a platelet thrombus. This shows the importance of platelets in initiating the arterial thrombus, and the role fibrin plays in arterial thrombosis.

The next problem to be considered is what happens with acute myocardial infarction. It has been stated by Harland (14) that "It seems remarkable that there is still uncertainty about the sequence of events that lead to infarction." Much of the controversy concerns the role of the acute lesion in myocardial infarction. It should be mentioned that although many studies show moderate to severe coronary athersclerosis in most coronary deaths (11, 18, 35, 41) the precipitating event is still in question. In a study by Mitchell (27), he lists various reports that show the incidence of thrombosis in myocardial infarction varies between 0 and 96 percent. Certainly this wide variability may reflect the technical difficulty encountered. Harland and Holburn (15) report coronary thrombosis in 90 percent of recent myocardial infarctions, with multiple thrombi being seen in 28 percent of the cases. Their conclusion was that "thrombosis was the decisive event in the natural history of coronary atheroma" and that myocardial infarction, in many cases, is caused by coronary thrombosis. In a study by Roberts and Buja (35) thrombi were found in 54 percent of the patients with transmural infarctions. It was interesting that there were no thrombi in 9 patients with subendocardial infarctions. Jorgenson *et al.* (18) found acute lesions in 79 percent of patients who died from presumed coronary causes within 48 hours after the clinical onset and it was possible to study the acute lesions in a treated (anticoagulated) versus an untreated group. The major acute lesions found were:

1. Ruptured necrotic plaques in which the intima of the plaque was interrupted (with or without hemorrhage or thrombosis)
2. Thrombosis of nonruptured plaques
3. Hemorrhage into a fibrous (nonnecrotic) plaque.

Ruptured plaques (necrotic) were not usually associated with thrombosis if the patient died within 15 minutes after the onset of clinical symptoms, but the longer the survival the greater the probability of thrombosis. This showed that rupture itself could be enough to cause cardiac death (without thrombosis). Hemorrhage into ruptured plaques was more frequent in treated patients, but the frequency with which enlargement as the result of the hemorrhage was not different in the treated as compared with the untreated group. Thrombosis of nonruptured plaques was not related to the length of survival, but the incidence of this type of acute lesion was found with less frequency in patients treated with anticoagulants; however the difference was only significant at the 10 percent level. Hemorrhage into a fibrous (nonnecrotic) plaque, the least common lesion, usually was not associated with thrombosis, but the hemorrhage was large enough to cause the lumen to narrow. The incidence of hemorrhage into a fibrous plaque was not increased by anticoagulation.

In treated patients ruptured plaques predominated, whereas in untreated patients there was an equal frequency of ruptured plaques and thrombosis of nonruptured plaques. Hence anticoagulants appeared to reduce the incidence of thrombosis of nonruptured plaques (significantly only at $P = 0.10$ level).

Another view to be examined is that of Spain and Bradess (41). They stated that the frequency of coronary thrombi was related to the length of time between the onset of symptoms and death. There was only a 16-percent frequency of thrombi in cases surviving less than 1 hour, but the frequency rose to 37 percent if the patient survived for up to 24 hours; the percentage rose to 54 when the patient survived longer. They concluded that thrombi were purely a secondary event. This was reconfirmed by this same group in 1970 (40). They also considered the question of postmorten lysis of thrombi and concluded, like Jorgensen *et al.* (18), that it probably did not occur.

Friedman *et al.* (11) divided cardiac deaths into instantaneous (in which cardiac arrest appeared to occur within 30 seconds of any symptoms) and sudden-death groups (in which death occurred from minutes to 24 hours). They found that with instantaneous death no acute lesion was usually found, although extensive atherosclerosis was usually present. They postulated that instantaneous death was most likely caused by an electrical phenomena in a diseased heart and not to an acute lesion. Conversely, in the sudden-death group 28 of 37 specimens contained probable recent thrombi, but only 7 of the patients exhibited an acute infarction.

Walston *et al.* (44) studied patients who had myocardial infarctions associated with "power failure" (inability of the myocardium to maintain the cardiac output necessary for visceral perfusion). At autopsy they found a high percentage (88) of recent acute lesions.

Some mention of the action of commonly used anticoagulants will be discussed briefly. Heparin affects almost all stages of the clotting sequence but, more specifically, it inhibits the action of thrombin, inhibits thromboplastin generation, and interferes with the prothrombin to thrombin mechanism (1). Coumarins act by decreasing the synthesis of factors II, VII, IX, and X (1).

Although the initiating factor in arterial thrombosis is generally related to the action of platelets, it is obvious that the use of anticoagulants in coronary artery disease is not totally unphysiologic.

Clinical Investigations

The question as to the value of anticoagulants must only be answered after pertinent clinical trials are examined. Most of the early (1948 to 1966) studies on the benefit of anticoagulation and acute myocardial infarction were examined in depth by Gifford and Feinstein (12). They scrutinized 32 reports, most of which compared anticoagulated patients with a control group. Eight methodologic standards were set up to evaluate each study. The first standard examined was whether the study included a statement of criteria used to diagnose myocardial infarction. Only 25 percent of the studies gave precise criteria.

The next factor examined was whether the study was a survey of medical records as opposed to a new clinical trial. Only 41 percent of the 32 reports were performed as an experimental investigation.

An attempt was made to discover whether the control groups were formed during approximately the same time period as the treated groups. Only 72 percent of the studies stated that they used concurrent controls. The authors felt that if the study used patients from different hospitals, some attempt should have been made to coordinate ancillary treatment received by the different groups. Of eight studies performed in more than one hospital, only two reported inter-hospital coordination. Random allocation of treatment is necessary to avoid bias on the part of the investigator. Only four of 32 reports used a random method to assign treatment. Other categories included "stratified prognostic correlation" and "diagnostic criteria for thromboembolism" in which many of the studies did not come up to the authors' standards.

Two studies (3, 45) that met most of the above criteria should be examined in more detail. Carleton *et al.* (3) compared a heparin-treated and a control group in the acute phase of myocardial infarction. There was no significant difference in survival between the two groups. Thromboembolic manifestations (mural thrombi, arterial emboli, lower extremity thrombophlebitis, pulmonary emboli, and recurrent infarctions) occurred with similar frequency in the two groups. They concluded that heparin was of no value in the early postinfarction period.

A study by Wasserman *et al.* (45) compared a control group with a warfarin-treated group with respect to acute myocardial infarction. The groups were comparable in many parameters except for an increased incidence of previous heart failure in the untreated group. The results showed no significant decrease in mortality with treatment. Hence, during the immediate post-infarction period there does not appear to be any benefit with anticoagulation.

Long-term Anticoagulation Trial

Manchester (24) reported a study of 204 patients on oral anticoagulants and 200 control patients. The results showed that the incidence of subsequent infarction in the anticoagulant group was 29 (14.2 percent), with a 20.6 percent mortality. In the control group infarcts occurred in 68 (34 percent), of whom 36 (54 percent) died. The incidence of bleeding was 2.9 percent, with no mortality.

About this time a study by Bjerkelund (2) showed that in anticoagulated patients under 60 years of age, mortality was significantly ($P = 0.05$ level) lower as compared to a control group treated by long-term anticoagulation following myocardial infarction. The treated patients were on Dicumerol. The results were only significant for up to 1 year of treatment. The reinfarction rate was significantly lower ($P = 0.05$ level) in the treated group over this same period of time.

The report of the *Working Party on Anticoagulant Therapy* (46) showed that in males under the age of 55 years, who were treated with phenindione in doses large enough to double the one-stage prothrombin time, there was a statistically significant decrease in the reinfarction rate as compared to controls receiving long-term anticoagulation. The difference in mortality was not significant.

In the second report of the Working Party (39) more patients were added to the above study and the original sample was followed further. Again the difference in mortality was not significant, however, the difference was significant in patients under or over 55 years with respect to reinfarction. Studies in females showed no benefit with anticoagulation, although the numbers were small.

One of the first studies to show that long-term anticoagulant therapy was of no benefit was done by Harvald *et al.* (17). These investigators found no significant differences with respect to reinfarction or mortality in patients on oral anticoagulants. Another of the principal studies to show no value in long-term anticoagulation was done by Seaman *et al.* (37). During this 7-year double-blind controlled study it was demonstrated that there were no differences in mortality between controls and in patients receiving phenindione.

The Veterans Administration Cooperative study (43) compared patients (males only) anticoagulated with bishydroxycoumarin. Some hospitals used sodium warfarin. The therapeutic range for prothrombin time was 2 to $2\frac{1}{2}$ times the normal value. The difference in survival between controls and treated patients was significant at the $P = 0.05$ level. The difference occurred most often during the first 2 years of therapy. Mortality in patients over 55 years of age did not appear to be reduced significantly with treatment. Control patients had a significantly higher rate of reinfarction.

In a double-blind study by Loeliger *et al.* (23) differences in the rate of cardiovascular deaths between the treated group (phenprocoumon) and the placebo group were not significant. The results were significant with respect to reinfarction rate and favorable results were maintained for the duration of the follow-up period

($16\frac{1}{2}$ months). The authors thought that the results may have been due to the intense anticoagulation achieved. In patients who were only moderately anticoagulated the results were not nearly as favorable.

In the papers reviewed from 1969 to the present, the report of the Working Party on Anticoagulant Therapy (34) deserves special attention. Although the results showed no significant reduction in survival in the treated group with acute myocardial infarction, there seems to have been a valid criticism of the study. In the report phenindione was used to maintain the thrombotest between 10 and 20 percent, but using this as an adequate level has been questioned by Wright (48). He maintained that a therapeutic level should be in the 5 to 10 percent range. This casts some doubt on the interpretation of these results.

In the final report of the Veterans Administration Cooperative Study (10) in 1969 (original report in 1965) long-term oral anticoagulation was found to have reduced the death rate ($P<0.01$) during the first 3 years after a myocardial infarction. However, by 5 years there was no significant difference between the treated (bishydroxycoumarin mainly) and untreated groups. Anticoagulation seemed to have a more beneficial effect on patients who had previous infarctions before they were admitted into the study. The difference between the groups reached the $P=0.05$ level with regards to reinfarction. It was demonstrated, in this study, that by 5 years the death rate between the two groups was similar; however, treatment appeared to favor survival for the first 3 years after infarction. Methodology in this study appeared to be acceptable.

Meuwissen *et al.* (26) demonstrated benefit from long-term anticoagulation with respect to survival; however, the sample size and follow-up period were considerably less than in the Veterans Administration study.

The final report by Seaman *et al.* (38) agreed with their earlier investigation (37), that no benefit could be accrued by long-term anticoagulation. The study used a double-blind technique; however, the sample size was relatively small.

In the most recent study reviewed here (6) the effect of anticoagulants in acute myocardial infarction on a large group of females and of males was assessed in detail. Also an attempt was made to divide the groups with respect to the severity of infarction. Criteria for the diagnosis of infarction were used as follows:

- Group I Showed classic Q-wave evolution on the electrocardiogram
- Group II Showed only ST-T wave evolution
- Group III The diagnosis was made by history and laboratory changes only.

The results showed that mortality was significantly higher for the female control group as compared to the treated females ($P<0.01$). Overall mortality in treated men was not significantly changed by treatment. Our objection to the study was that the Group I patients were the only patients who undoubtedly had an infarction by strict ECG standards. Although many patients in Groups II and III (criteria for infarction) may have actually sustained an infarct, this could have had an unknown effect on overall mortality data. Thus when only Group I patients are studied mortality among females must be questioned because there were not enough in this group for adequate statistical analysis. In Group I mortality was not significantly reduced between treated and untreated men, but when men over 75 years of age were excluded, those with moderate infarction (presence of one or two of the following:

recurrent chest pain, congestive heart failure, or hypotension without shock) showed a significant decrease in mortality with treatment. This confirmed earlier studies which demonstrated significant benefits in younger males.

Comments and Conclusions

1. The majority of trials generally have failed to show significant benefit with anticoagulation in the acute infarction period. However, we feel heparinization is indicated in the hospital during the first 72 hours, since recent reports (13, 25, 29, 33, 47) show a high incidence of deep vein thrombosis (using [^{125}I] labeled fibrinogen) in patients with acute myocardial infarction, and its beneficial treatment with heparin (13, 33, 47).

2. Long-term anticoagulation appears to be of value in myocardial infarction in male patients under age 55 years for a period of approximately 2 years. Although there was no universal agreement, an international review group (4), which analyzed nine major trials, generally favored long-term anticoagulation.

3. If anticoagulation is to be used, a vigorous approach to hypocoagulation should be followed. For example, prothrombin time should be 2 to 2.5 times the control value.

4. Since thrombi are more likely to occur during cardiogenic shock and these patients are immobilized for greater periods, we feel that anticoagulation should be used.

5. The value of anticoagulants in women has not been evaluated fully and their use remains equivocal.

6. We agree with the contraindictions as set forth by Drapkin and Mersky (6): the presence or history of gastrointestinal hemorrhage; a known hemorrhagic diathesis; acute alcoholism; significant hepatic disease, significant azotemia, or uremia; malignant or accelerated hypertension; a recent cerebrovascular accident. We might add that the patient should be able to follow instructions with regard to follow-up and laboratory control.

In conclusion, our main concern should be in prolonging survival, and whether anticoagulation works by reducing thromboembolic phenomena, coronary thrombi, or an unknown mechanism is only of secondary importance.

References

1. Anticoagulant drugs. Br. Med. J., I: 365–367, 1969.
2. Bjerkelund, C. J. The effect of long-term treatment with dicourmoral in myocardial infarction. Acta Med. Scand. Suppl., 330:1–212, 1957.
3. Carleton, R. A., Sanders, C. A., and Burack, W. R. Heparin administration after acute myocardial infarction. N. Engl. J. Med., 263:1002, 1960.
4. Collaborative analysis of long-term anticoagulant administration after acute myocardial infarction. An International Anticoagulant Review Group. Lancet, 1:203, 1970.
5. Constaninides, P. Plaque fissures in human thrombosis. J. Atherosclerosis Res., 6:1, 1966.
6. Drapkin, A. and Merskey, C. Anticoagulant therapy after acute myocardial infarction. J.A.M.A., 222:541, 1972.

7. Duguid, J. B. Mural thrombosis in arteries. Br. Med. Bull., 2:36, 1955.
8. Duguid, J. B. The arterial lining. Lancet, 2:207, 1952.
9. Duguid, J. B. Pathogenesis of atherosclerosis. Lancet, 2:925, 1949.
10. Ebert, R. V., Borden, C. W. and Hypp, M. R. Long-term anticoagulant therapy after myocardial infarction. Final report of the Veterans Administration Cooperative Study, J.A.M.A., 207:2263, 1969.
11. Friedman, M., Manwaring, J. H., Rosenman, R. H., Donlon, G., Ortega, P., and Grube, S. M. Instantaneous and sudden deaths: Clinical and pathological differentiation in coronary artery disease. J.A.M.A., 225:1319, 1973.
12. Gifford, R. H. and Feinstein, A. R. A critique of methodology in studies of anticoagulant therapy for acute myocardial infarction. N. Engl. J. Med., 280:351, 1969.
13. Handley, A. J., Emerson, P. A., and Fleming, P. R. Heparin in the prevention of deep vein thrombosis after myocardial infarction. Br. Med. J., 2:435, 1972.
14. Harland, W. A. Pathogenesis of myocardial infarction and coronary thrombosis. In Sherry, S., Brinkhouse, K. M., Genton, E., and Stengle, J. M. eds., Thrombosis. Washington, D.C., National Academy of Sciences, 1969.
15. —— Holburn, A. M. Coronary thrombosis and myocardial infarction. Lancet, 2:1158, 1966.
16. Harrison, C. V. Experimental pulmonary atherosclerosis. J. Pathol. Bacteriol., 60:289, 1948.
17. Harvald, B., Hilden, T., and Lund, E. Long-term anticoagulant therapy after myocardial infarction. Lancet, 2:626–30, 1962.
18. Jorgensen, L., Chandler, A. B., and Borchgrevink, C. F. Acute lesions of coronary arteries in anticoagulant treated and in untreated patients. Atherosclerosis, 13:21–44, 1971.
19. —— Rowsell, H. C., Hoving, T., and Mustard, J. F. Resolution and organization of platelet-rich mural thrombi in carotid arteries of swine. Am. J. Pathol., 51:681, 1967.
20. —— Experimental platelet and coagulation thrombi: A histological study of arterial and venous thrombi of varying age in untreated and heparinized rabbits. Acta Pathol. Microbiol. Scand., 62:189, 1964.
21. —— Borchgrevink, C. F. The haemostatic mechanism in patients with haemorrhagic diseases. A histological study of wounds made for primary and secondary bleeding time tests. Acta Pathol. Microbiol. Scand., 60:55, 1964.
22. Knieriem, H. J. and Chandler, A. B. The effect of warfarin sodium on the duration of platelet aggregation. Thrombos. Diathes. Haemorrhage, 18:766, 1967.
23. Loeliger, E. A., Hensen, A., Kroes, L. M., Van Diyk, L. M., Fekkes, M., DeJorge, H., and Hemker, H. C. A double-blind trial of long-term anticoagulant treatment after myocardial infarction. Acta Med. Scand., 182:549, 1967.
24. Manchester, B. The value of continuous (1 to 10 years) long-term anticoagulant therapy. Ann. Itern. Med., 47:1202, 1957.
25. Maurer, B. J., Wray, R., and Shillingford, J. P. Frequency of venous thrombosis after myocardial infarction. Lancet, 2:1385, 1971.
26. Meuwissen, O. J. A. T., Vervoorn, A. C., Cohen, O., Jordan, F. L. J., and Nelemans, F. A. Double-blind trial of long-term anticoagulant treatment after myocardial infarction. Acta Med. Scand., 186:361, 1969.
27. Mitchell, J. R. A. The role of thrombosis in myocardial infarction. In Sherry, S., Brinkhouse, K. M., Genton, E., and Stengle, M. J. eds., Thrombosis. Washington, D.C., National Academy of Sciences, 1969.
28. Murphy, E. A., Mustard, J. F., Rowsell, H. C., and Downie, H. G. Quantitative studies on the effect of Dicumarol on experimental thrombosis. J. Lab. Clin. Med., 61:935, 1963.
29. Murray, T. S., Lorimer, A. R., Cox, F. C., and Lawrie, T. D. V. Legvein thrombosis following myocardial infarction. Lancet, 2:792, 1970.
30. Mustard, J. F. and Packham, M. A. Thromboembolism. Circulation, 42:1, 1970.
31. —— Roswell, H. C., Murphy, E. D., Robinson, G. A., and Downie, H. C. The role of platelets in the etiology of myocardial infarction. In Nichol, E. S. ed., Anticoagulant Therapy in Ischemic Heart Disease. New York, Grune and Stratton, 1965.
32. Newland, H. and Nordoy, A. Effect of large doses of warfarin sodium on haemostasis and on ADP-induced platelet aggregation in vivo in the rat. Cardiovasc. Res., 1:362, 1967.
33. Nicolaides, A. N., Kakkar, V. V., Renney, J. T. G., Kidner, P. H., Hutchinson, D. S. C., and Clarke, M. D. Myocardial infarction and deep-vein thrombosis. Br. Med. J., 1:432, 1971.
34. Report of the Working Party on Anticoagulant Therapy in Coronary Thrombosis to the Medical Research Council. Assessment of short-term anticoagulant administration after cardiac infarction. Br. Med. J., 1:335, 1969.

35. Roberts, W. C. and Buja, L. M. The frequency and significance of coronary arterial thrombi and other observations in fatal acute myocardial infarction. Am. J. Med., 52:425, 1972.
36. Rokitansky, C. A Manual of Pathological Anatomy. Translated by George Day. London: Sydenham Society, Vol. 4, 1852, pp. 251, 275.
37. Seaman, A. J., Greswold, H. E., Reaume, R. B., and Ritzman, L. W. Prophylactic anticoagulant therapy for coronary artery disease. J.A.M.A., 189:183, 1964.
38. ———————— Long-term anticoagulant prophylaxis after myocardial infarction. Final Report. N. Engl. J. Med., 281:115, 1969.
39. Second Report of the Working Party on Anticoagulant Therapy. An assessment of long-term anticoagulant administration after cardiac infarction. Br. Med. J., 2:837, 1964.
40. Spain, D. M. and Bradess, V. A. Sudden death from coronary heart disease. Chest, 58:107, 1970.
41. ———— The relationship of coronary thrombosis to coronary athersclerosis. Am. J. Med. Sci. Dec., 1960 pp. 701–710.
42. Thomas, D. P. The role of platelets in arterial and venous thrombosis. In Mannucci, P. M. and Giorini, S. eds., Advances in Experimental Medicine and Biology, New York, Plenum Press, Vol. 34, 1972.
43. Veterans Administration Cooperative Study. Long-term anticoagulant therapy after myocardial infarction. J.A.M.A. 193:157, 1965.
44. Walston, A., Hackel, D. B., and Estes, E. H. Acute coronary occlusion and the "Power failure syndrome". Am. Heart J., 79:613, 1970.
45. Wasserman, A. J., Gutterman, L. A., Yoe, K. B., Kemp, V. E. and Richardson, D. S. Anticoagulants in acute myocardial infarction: The failure of anticoagulants to alter mortality in randomized series. Am. Heart J., 71:43, 1966.
46. Working Party on Anticoagulant Therapy. An assessment of long-term anticoagulant administration after cardiac infarction. Br Med. J., I:803–810, 1959.
47. Wray, R., Mauer, B., and Shellingford, J. P. Prophylactic anticoagulant therapy in the prevention of calf-vein thrombosis after myocardial infarction. N. Engl. J. Med., 288:815, 1973.
48. Wright, I. S. Anticoagulants after myocardial infarction. Br. Med. J., I:188, 1969.

Chapter 11 When to Operate on Congenital Heart Disease

AMNON ROSENTHAL, M.D.

General Considerations

During the past decade, great advances in the surgical therapy of congenital cardiovascular malformations have taken place and techniques continue to change and improve. Mustard (21) described the correction of transposition of the great arteries using an intraatrial baffle, hypothermia was utilized in repair of cardiac malformation in infancy, a prosthetic conduit with interposed valve was used in cases with pulmonary atresia or truncus arteriosus, and Fontan (10) devised an operation for physiologic correction of tricuspid atresia. With each new solution, however, new problems emerged; some were anticipated and others, unforeseen. The cardiologist caring for the child with congenital heart disease must decide in each case what the indications for surgery are and the optimal time for operation. The decision and recommendations for surgery will be dictated by considering the patient's symptoms and the anticipated benefits and risks of operation. The indications will have to be balanced against the long-term results of various operative procedures, operative and postoperative mortality and morbidity, and the uncertain fate of some of the prosthetic devices now in use.

A better understanding of the problems will be gained by an initial discussion of the general considerations in the timing of cardiac surgery, which are applicable to many lesions or procedures. This will be followed by specific controversial decisions and appropriate recommendations. In reviewing the general considerations, it should be remembered that while many of them are important, medical indications for surgery often militate against postponement that may be justified on other grounds.

Various Factors to be Considered

Age

During the neonatal period, only infants in danger of dying should be operated on. Surgery in infancy is reserved for symptomatic patients or those at high risk for the development of pulmonary vascular obstructive disease. Elective surgical procedures are best delayed until after 6 years of age when hospitalization and surgery are psychologically less traumatic (separation anxiety, regressive reactions, negative attitudes). Older children follow instructions better and are more cooperative during the postoperative period. The adolescent is usually a better surgical patient than the young adult because he has greater tolerance and is free from the financial and family responsibilities that all too often dominate the life of the married person. In general, whenever feasible, it is advisable to have all elective cardiac surgery performed before marriage.

Repair of lesions associated with a high risk of complete heart block and, therefore, the possible need for a permanent pacemaker or lesions that may require a prosthetic valve replacement should be postponed as long as possible or until an appropriate age and adequate growth are achieved. Increasing age in childhood is associated with an increase in physical maturation. When inspection of the growth curve indicates a declining or flat weight maturation, it may be pointless to delay surgery in the hope the child will "get bigger".

Surgical Skill

The successful outcome of surgery is directly related to the cardiovascular surgeon's skill and experience. These are, perhaps, the most important factors in determining survival and morbidity. Timing of surgery must consider the surgical experience at any given institution with a particular lesion and at a given age. Many cardiovascular malformations are rare and sufficient experience in their management is limited to few major medical centers with a large volume of patients with congenital heart disease. Some residual or undesirable sequelae are inherent in the procedure, but many complications can be avoided by expert preoperative, operative, and postoperative management.

Cardiovascular Status and Type of Malformation

Appropriate surgical intervention before hemodynamic or anatomic changes have occurred will improve the patient's prognosis. In the presence of severe cardiac compromise, surgery, where feasible, may be urgent and undue delay can cause death. The delicate timing of surgery will depend on (a) the type of cardiovascular malformation present; (b) the patient's symptoms; (c) cardiac status determined by thorough hemodynamic evaluation and the use of ancillary laboratory tests; (d) the natural history of the lesion; and, (e) anticipated dynamic cardiac and extracardiac changes. When symptoms are difficult to evaluate, objective studies, such as standardized exercise tests, peripheral arterial oxygen saturation, vital capacity, and so forth, should be obtained. Cyanotic lesions may remain stable but are usually progressive and do not improve spontaneously. Ventricular septal defects, however, often close or diminish in size spontaneously, particularly during the first year of life. Valvar pulmonary stenosis rarely becomes more severe, whereas valvar aortic stenosis commonly does. Irreversible pulmonary vascular obstructive disease develops during the first 2 years of life in infants with transposition of the great arteries and in the third to fourth decade of life in patients with atrial septal defect. In general, greater emphasis may need to be placed on objective findings and consequences of the lesion (for example, cardiomegaly or ventricular hypertrophy) and less on potential or poorly documented hazards.

Surgical Procedures and Techniques Required

The surgical procedure or technique (hypothermia, cardiopulmonary bypass, inflow occlusion) required or contemplated for the repair of a particular lesion may dictate the timing of surgery. This is particularly true for corrective surgical procedures and to a lesser extent for palliative surgery. A Blalock-Taussig shunt is preferable to a Waterston (36) anastomosis, but the former can usually be successfully carried out only after 3 to 6 months of life. If possible, therefore, palliative therapy in the infant who requires a shunt should be delayed until the Blalock-Taussig anastomosis can be performed. Relief of valvar pulmonary stenosis by inflow occlusion is preferable to cardiopulmonary bypass. Repair of complex intracardiac lesions is greatly facilitated by a bloodless field achieved by deep hypothermia, which in turn is best tolerated in early infancy. If a prosthetic conduit is anticipated, it is best to delay surgery until the child is 6 to 9 years of age. A sufficiently large conduit, that may not need replacement can then be employed. Transatrial closure of a ventricular defect is preferable to a right ventriculotomy because the latter may result in a right bundle branch block electrocardiographic pattern, an ectopic focus, free wall aneurysm, or area of dyskenesis. An incision in the systemic ventricle is potentially more damaging than one in the "pulmonary" ventricle.

Palliative Versus Corrective Surgery

In the treatment of some cardiovascular malformations (ventricular septal defect, transposition of the great arteries or tetralogy of Fallot), the physician may have to decide between two alternatives. Palliative surgery (for example, pulmonary artery banding in an infant with ventricular septal defect) followed at a later date by corrective surgery or early one-stage correction of the malformation. The latter has the advantage of avoiding (a) double jeopardy, (b) the undesirable sequelae of palliative surgery, (c) the psychologic trauma, and (d) the financial burden of a second operation. The disadvantages of early correction are related to (a) the unknown long-term effects of deep hypothermia on the central nervous system. Limited studies have shown that neurologic defects are not uncommon in the immediate postoperative period but persistent significant neurologic damage or measureable change in intelligence quotient are uncommon (4, 30). (b) Limitation imposed by size (margin of safety in the postoperative infant may be smaller than in the child), and (c) the possible increased mortality of the procedure. Whether indeed, the mortality and morbidity of early single corrective operation is lower than the combined risk of palliative and corrective surgery at a later date, remains to be established. Nor does it necessarily follow that a single stage operative correction will be the appropriate option for all patients or lesions. As experience accumulates, indications and contraindications for each option and a variety of lesions will become better defined. The alternatives present in some lesions and appropriate recommendations are discussed under *Specific Controversies.*

Developmental and Psychologic Factors

Delayed height and weight maturation are common in infants with cyanotic congenital heart disease and those with congestive heart failure due to large left to right shunt. Evidence suggests that surgery at an early age may reverse this trend (29). Cyanotic congenital heart disease is often associated with delayed developmental milestones and a lower preceptual and intellectual quotient (28). It is unclear whether these are related to hypoxemia, the physical limitations associated with severe illness or to psychologic factors such as limited educational and social opportunities or parental overprotection. Many of these possible etiologic factors may be remedied by surgery and improvement in performance can be demonstrated following surgery (18). The psychologic and physical benefits to the child who is able to partake in all educational, recreational, and physical activities of his peers are obvious and must be considered in the early school years. A chest scar is of particular concern to girls. It is likely to be less noticeable when surgery is performed at an early age. Hospitalization and surgical procedures are psychologically less traumatic to older than to younger children (1).

Ethics

Ethical questions about the care and therapy of infants with severe and complex congenital heart disease (uncorrectable lesions), those with associated severe extracardiac congenital malformations that offer little or no hope of a functional existance are, in my opinion, best decided by the family and the physician most familiar with the situation. Considerable variation will be present among cases and much latitude in decision-making is to be expected and tolerated (7, 27). Decisions regarding major surgical undertakings (transplants, artificial devices) or innovative procedures (repair of single ventricle, Fontan for pulmonary atresia with intact ventricular septum) should be made after extensive consultation between pediatric cardiologist and surgeon. A full and complete explanation of risk and benefit must be given to the patient, family, or both. The parents should participate in any decision about treatment and must be fully informed of the consequences of consenting and withholding consent. Surgery may need to be delayed pending further experience with other patients in different institutions or in the animal laboratory. After deciding that the operation can be done, one should ask the question: should it be done? The decision should not be predicated on technical considerations alone but must consider the quality of life as a value that must be balanced against a belief in the sanctity of life. All too often, a palliative procedure and extensive cardiac and ventilatory support system result in failure to thrive, severe limitations, an enormous financial burden, and the anticipation of further surgical procedures.

Geographic, Seasonal, and Economic Considerations

It may be desired to postpone elective surgery in school age children until the summer so that school work is not compromised. While this is not a major consideration in most children, those with marginal performance may ill afford a long absence from school, which may result in the loss of an entire semester or academic year. Complex surgical procedures, however, are best not scheduled in July in institutions where a new surgical crew begins its rotation during that part of the year.

Geographic and economic considerations may often dictate the timing of surgery. Financial help from the state may be available in some locations only up to a given age or from an insurance policy while the father is employed. A patient seeking help from a foreign country with inadequate facilities for cardiac care, or from a great distance within the continental United States, particularly if of limited financial resources, may require an adjustment in the timing as well as the type of procedure performed. A porcine xenograft may be the valve of choice if the patient lives in an area where therapy with anticoagulants cannot be monitored. All too often, patients from inaccessible geographic areas have had a palliative operation (for example, Pott's procedure or pulmonary artery banding) and have not returned for further therapy. In many of these cases, an attempt at a one-stage procedure is probably preferable.

Specific Controversies

Should the Infant with a Large Ventricular Septal Defect Have Pulmonary Artery Banding or Primary Closure of the Defect?

The indications for surgery in patients with ventricular septal defect in infancy are: intractable congestive heart failure, persistent pulmonary artery hypertention, or both. The protagonists for primary closure claim all the advantages outlined above for a one-stage procedure. It is also pointed out that pulmonary artery banding, particularly if present for many years, is associated with a variety of complications (Table 11-1) (11, 15, 19). Pulmonary artery band may be placed too tightly, resulting

Table 11-1. Sequelae and Complications Following Pulmonary Artery Banding

1. Hypertrophy of right ventricular infundibulum	8. Inadequate band with persistent hypertension
2. Thickening and deformity of pulmonary valve	9. Migration of distal placement with obstruction or right pulmonary artery
3. Subaortic stenosis	10. Persistent stenosis after band removal or angioplasty
4. Valvar pulmonary regurgitation	11. Suprasystemic right ventricular pressure (with spontaneous closure of ventricular defect)
5. Right to left intracardiac shunting	
6. Pulmonary artery thrombosis	
7. Erosion and/or rupture of pulmonary artery	

in early development of right to left shunting with its various consequences, or too loosely, resulting in an ineffective reduction in pulmonary artery pressure. If the ventricular septal defect closes or decreases in size spontaneously, suprasystemic right ventricular pressure may result. The risk of bacterial endocarditis is probably greater than if the patient had primary repair for ventricular defect.

Advocates of pulmonary artery banding followed later by primary repair, point to the low mortality of pulmonary artery banding in patients with a simple ventricular septal defect (Table 11-2), the advantages of avoiding hyperthermia and the relative ease with which repair is performed under cardiopulmonary bypass when the child is older and not as ill. In many cases presurgical definition of the anatomy by cardiac catheterization may be better in the older, less acutely ill, patient. Should the ventricular septal defect close spontaneously, only relief of the pulmonary artery band may be necessary and an intracardiac procedure avoided. The ligation or division of a coexistent patent ductus arteriosus is technically easier when pulmonary

Table 11-2. Results of Palliative Surgery at the Children's Hospital Medical Center, Boston

	No. of patients	Mortality
Atrial septal defect creation[a] (1966–1973)	35	8 (23)[d]
Ascending aorta to pulmonary artery shunt[b] (Waterson; 1965–1974)	206	49 (24)
Pulmonary artery banding[c] (1958–June 30, 1973)	64	5 (8)

[a] D-transposition of the great arteries and intact ventricular septum with prior balloon septostomy (6).
[b] In 80/206 patients (40 percent) procedure done in newborn period. Includes patients with tetralogy of Fallot (51 percent), pulmonary atresia with intact septum (13 percent), tricuspid atresia (11 percent) and complex cyanotic congenital heart disease (25 percent) (14).
[c] For simple ventricular septal defect.
[d] Figures in parentheses are percentages.

artery banding is performed through a left thorocotomy than via the midline if primary repair is done. Intraoperative electrocardiographic mapping of the conduction system in cases with large defects that may border the conduction system (for example, those in the endocardial cushion position) cannot be performed under hypothermia.

Conclusion

Infants with isolated ventricular septal defect and intractable congestive heart failure, persistent pulmonary artery hypertension, or both should undergo primary transatrial closure of the septal defect provided precise preoperative catheterization and angiography data are obtained and the necessary surgical skill and postoperative care is available. At our institution, the mortality for primary repair (Table 11-3) is similar to the combined mortality of banding and subsequent closure (Tables 11-2

Table 11-3. Deep Hypothermic Circulatory Arrest in Infancy

Cardiac lesion	No. of patients	Age (days)	Weight (kg)	Hospital mortality
Ventricular septal defect	24	20–340	2.0–7.5	3 (12%)
Tetralogy of Fallot	13	12–355	2.2–8.5	0
D-transposition of the great arteries				
Intact ventricular septum	21	60–354	4.0–9.0	1 (6%)
Complex	6	60–320	4.0–8.5	2 (33%)

Children's Hospital Medical Center, Boston, Massachusetts, January 1, 1973 to September 1, 1974.

Table 11-4. Repair of Ventricular Septal Defect and Pulmonary Artery Band

	No. of patients	Mortality
Ventricular septal defect closure and pulmonary angioplasty	29	1
Pulmonary angioplasty only (spontaneous closure of defect)	2	0
Total	31	1 (3.2%)

Children's Hospital Medical Center, Boston, Massachusetts, July 1, 1971 to December 31, 1973.

and 11-4). The criteria for surgical closure are the same as those for pulmonary artery banding. Pulmonary artery banding should be reserved for (a) infants with multiple ventricular septal defects or virtual absence of the interventricular septum, (b) prematures (under 5 pounds) with or without a patent ductus arteriosus, and (c) when significant parenchymal pulmonary disease such as pneumonia or atelectasis are present.

Should Symptomatic Infants with Tetralogy of Fallot Have a Systemic to Pulmonary Artery Anastomosis or Primary Repair?

The indications for surgery in an infant with tetralogy of Fallot are (a) hyperpneic spells and (b) significant or progressive hypoxemia. Palliative surgery in infants under 3 to 6 months is performed by an ascending aorta to right pulmonary artery shunt (Waterston) and after 6 months of age, by subclavian to pulmonary artery anastomosis (Blalock-Taussig shunt). Advocates of palliative surgery during infancy maintain that a systemic to pulmonary anastomosis has a number of advantages. It is an effective and simple operation that relieves symptoms and has a lower morbidity and mortality than repair and none of the disadvantages inherent in early corrective surgery. Adequate repair can then be performed when the child is older. The presence of a Blalock-Taussig shunt does not contribute significantly to the mortality or morbidity of repair (Table 5).

Table 11-5. Repair of Tetralogy of Fallot

	No. of patients	Hospital Mortality
Previous shunt	63	4 (6.3)
Blalock-Taussig	27	1 (3.5)
Waterston	23	2 (8.5)
Potts	13	1 (7.5)
No previous shunt	54	2 (3.7)
Total	117	6 (5.1)

Children's Hospital Medical Center, Boston, Massachusetts, January 1973 to July 1974.

Some of the advantages of primary repair in infancy are listed under *Palliative Versus Corrective Surgery*. It is also pointed out that the low mortality for shunt procedure in infancy is a misconception. The mortality for Waterston shunt at our institution is 24 percent (Table 11-2). Results of Blalock-Taussig shunt, usually done in older infants, are considerably better (4 to 12 percent). Furthermore, complications following a Waterston anastomosis are common and may make repair more difficult (Table 11-6). Tetralogy of Fallot is a progressive lesion (2) and if repair is delayed for years acquired pulmonary atresia may develop and more extensive surgery required. Resection of the outflow tract in infancy is easier and more effective, since the tissue is more pliable and there is less hypertrophy and fibrosis. Technically, repair is easier in the bloodless field achieved by hypothermia and,

Table 11-6. Sequalae and Complications of Ascending Aorta to Right Pulmonary Artery Shunt

1. Congestive heart failure (early and late)	5. Left ventricular dysfunction
2. Unilateral pulmonary edema or hemorrhage	6. Pericardial and thoracic adhesions
3. Pulmonary artery hypertension and pulmonary vascular obstructive disease	7. Progression of infundibular pulmonary stenosis
4. Deformation or obstruction of right pulmonary artery	

therefore, more satisfactory. The physical and psychologic handicaps of chronic hypoxemia may be avoided (18, 28, 29) and many of the complications associated with right to left shunt (8, 9, 23, 26) prevented.

Conclusion

The operation of choice for symptomatic infants with tetralogy of Fallot is primary repair in infancy provided precise preoperative anatomic and physiologic definition by catheterization, skilled surgical staff, and appropriate postoperative care are available. The results of primary repair in infancy at our institution are most gratifying (Table 11-3). Repair is indicated in infants with hyperpneic spells and/or severe hypoxemia (resting systemic oxygen saturation below 75 percent). Palliative surgery is indicated in infants with (a) origin of the anterior descending coronary artery from the right coronary artery, (b) infundibular atresia, (c) atresia of the main pulmonary artery and/or severely hypoplastic main and branch pulmonary arteries (less than 30 percent of the diameter of the ascending aorta), and (d) prematures weighing less than 5 pounds.

Systemic to pulmonary artery anastomosis should not be performed in infants with (a) hyperpneic spells associated with adequate systemic arterial oxygen saturation but due to hyper-reactive infundibulum, (b) suprasystemic right ventricular pressure (tricuspid valve or endocardial tissue adherent to the ventricular septal defect). Surgery in infants with a dominant left to right shunt or mild hypoxemia should be delayed into early childhood.

Treatment of D-Transposition of the Great Arteries: Is Atrial Septectomy Obsolete? When should the Mustard Operation be Performed?

Without medical or surgical intervention, less than 5 percent of neonates with transposition of the great arteries survive to one year of age (13). Creation of an adequate interatrial communication to improve mixing between the systemic and pulmonary circulation is essential to survival. With the introduction of balloon atrial septostomy performed during cardiac catheterization, the need for immediate surgical intervention has lessened. What are the indications for surgical intervention in infants with D-transposition of the great arteries and intact ventricular septum if balloon septostomy is ineffective? What surgical procedures should be performed—atrial septectomy of Mustard procedure? If hypoxemia is severe and is associated with metabolic acidosis, surgical intervention is manditory. Repeat balloon atrial septostomy is often ineffective. A decision must then be made regarding surgical atrial septal defect creation (24) or the Mustard procedure (5).

Surgical septectomy, a palliative procedure followed later by a corrective operation, is felt by many to have the disadvantages inherent in an additional operation. When hypoxemia is severe, complete physiologic correction can be achieved by the Mustard procedure and, therefore, why use a palliative operation associated with a considerable mortality (Table 11-2). Other disadvantages of atrial septectomy are the resultant thoracic and pericardial adhesions which (a) make the definitive operation more difficult, (b) may eliminate use of the pericardium in the construction of the intra-atrial baffle, and (c) obscure the anatomy and distribution pattern of the coronary arteries.

The advantages of atrial septal defect creation, however, are its usefulness in early infancy (under 3 to 6 months of age) when Mustard procedure may be associated with a greater incidence of systemic or pulmonary venous obstruction by the intraatrial baffle (32). To delay the Mustard procedure until approximately 9 to 12 months of age, will also lessen the likelihood the baffle may have to be revised as the patient grows. Systemic arterial oxygen saturation after balloon septostomy is relatively low (approximately 55 to 70 percent) whereas after atrial septectomy it is significantly higher (approximately 65 to 80 percent). Reluctance to perform atrial septectomy and permitting relatively lower oxygen saturation level for months until a Mustard operation is performed, exposes the infant to a considerable risk of cerebrovascular accident (23) and other motor psychologic and developmental hazards.

Conclusion

All infants with transposition of the great arteries should undergo a balloon septostomy. If systemic blood oxygen saturation level is maintained at the high 60s or better, clinical course is satisfactory, and there is no evidence of pulmonary artery hypertension, Mustard procedure should electively be performed at approximately 9 to 12 months of age. Further delay increases the risk of pulmonary vascular obstructive disease (24). In the newborn with persistent hypoxemia, watchful waiting, therapy with oxygen, and maintaining hemoglobin at approximately 16 to 18 g/100 ml, will often result in improvement. Pulmonary vascular resistance falls, pulmonary blood flow increases, and correction of the anemia increases systemic venous oxygen content. If after initial balloon septostomy persistent hypoxemia is associated with bradycardia, lethargy, poor feeding, or metabolic acidosis, surgical septectomy is indicated. Atrial septectomy should probably be performed in infants under 3 to 6 months of age with moderately severe hypoxemia (saturation under 65 percent). The Mustard operation is then performed at about 9 to 12 months of age (Table 11-3).

Is Pulmonary Valvotomy Indicated in Patients with a Resting Right Ventricular Pressure of 50 to 75 mm Hg?

Opinion is almost unanimous that surgery is indicated in patients with valvar pulmonary stenosis and right ventricular pressure at or above systemic level with or without symptoms or right to left shunt. It is in the asymptomatic child with a resting right ventricular peak systolic pressure of 50 to 75 mm Hg and systemic pressure of

100 mm Hg or more that the advisability of surgery is in doubt. The temptation to perform surgery is great because the surgical procedure is relatively simple (can be done under inflow occlusion or cardiopulmonary bypass and does not require a ventriculotomy) and safe (mortality less than 1 percent). Morbidity is low and the operation is usually curative. Available evidence indicates that pulmonary valvar restenosis does not develop and when pulmonary regurgitation occurs, it is mild and not hemodynamically significant. Furthermore, it is pointed out that (a) during exercise (17), work, emotional stress, or pregnancy, the right ventricular pressure is considerably higher than that demonstrated during cardiac catheterization at rest, (b) over decades such pressure may result in myocardial fibrosis and hypertrophy, and (c) recommendations regarding participation in competitive athletics and vocational planning can be given without reservations and with the assurance that no hemodynamically significant abnormality is present.

Persuasive as the arguments for surgery are, no evidence is currently available that significant or irreversible cardiac complications develop in patients with mild to moderate pulmonary stenosis. The lesion does not appear to be progressive. While surgical morbidity and mortality are, indeed, very low, complications can and do occur. These complications are related to the hospitalization, anesthesia, thorocotomy and cardiopulmonary bypass (Table 11-7). Symptoms such as fatigability or

Table 11-7. Some Sequalae and Complications of Thorocotomy and Cardiopulmonary Bypass

1. Air embolism (coronary artery, central nervous system)	8. False aneurysm (aortotomy site, suture line)
2. Serum hepatitis	9. Toxicity or hypersensitivity reaction to medications
3. Infective Endocarditis	10. Phrenic nerve injury
4. Wound infection	11. Hemorrhage
5. Wound dehiscence	12. Tamponade
6. Post perfusion syndrome	13. Chest deformity
7. Post pericardiotomy syndrome	14. Keloid formation
	15. Pneumonia and/or atelectasis

decreased exercise tolerance in many of these patients are often out of proportion to the degree of compromise and may be unrelated to the cardiac lesion. Objective exercise studies may be helpful in selecting those patients with symptoms due to heart disease.

Conclusion

I, for one, do not believe that the evidence indicates that surgery is necessary or advisable for most patients with valvar pulmonary stenosis and right ventricular pressure of 50 to 75 mm Hg. Some of the reasons are outlined above. Valvotomy should be reserved for patients in this category (a) who become symptomatic, substantiated by objective exercise testing, (b) have right ventricular hypertrophy on the electrocardiogram disproportionate to the measured pressure, and (c) have cardiac catheterization evidence of significantly reduced right ventricular compliance. Young children with mild pulmonary stenosis should be recatheterized after the adolescent growth spurt (preferably with an exercise study) and decision regarding surgery be considered at that time.

When should a Child with Valvar Aortic Stenosis be Operated On?

The decision regarding surgery in patients with valvar aortic stenosis, is often the most difficult one of all. No surgical therapy is required in patients with gradients under 50 mm Hg, absence of symptoms, or myocardial ischemic changes on ECG. Surgery, on the other hand, is clearly indicated in patients with peak systolic ejection gradient of 50 mm Hg or more and symptoms (angina, syncope) or the appearance of ischemic electrocardiographic changes. This is true regardless of age or need for prosthetic valve, because the risk of sudden death under these circumstances is very high.

The problem that needs to be faced all too often is: whether surgery should be recommended for the asymptomatic child with a gradient of 50 to 100 mm Hg in the absence of ischemic myocardial changes on the electrocardiogram? Proponents for surgery argue that relief of the stenosis will avoid the development of severe myocardial hypertrophy, infarction of papillary muscles and subendocardial ischemia (20, 35). Ischemic changes are often irreversible and persist depite relief of the obstruction. A more compliant, less fibrotic and better perfused systemic ventricle will increase the patient's longevity. If a tricuspid valve is demonstrated at cardiac catheterization, a more favorable surgical result is likely.

Reluctance to recommend surgery stems from the following considerations: (a) aortic valvotomy is a palliative procedure; a second operation is often required. Restenosis may occur, the annulus become relatively smaller with the patient's growth or calcification may develop in early adulthood; (b) incomplete relief of the stenosis or excessive surgical zeal resulting in significant aortic regurgitation is not uncommon (3); (c) a prosthetic valve may be required. The size of the valve may be limited by the aortic valve annulus. The prospect of anticoagulation therapy and need to replace the valve in the future.

Conclusion

In the absence of clear guidelines, I would recommend relief of aortic stenosis in the asymptomatic older child or adolescent with a gradient of 80 to 100 mm Hg (in the absence of ECG ischemic changes) and would be inclined to procrastinate in the younger child (age 1 to 5 years). In the preschool child, the cardiac catheterization study should be repeated in 3 to 4 years. Systolic resting gradients greater than 100 mm Hg should be relieved regardless of age because of the potential damage to the systemic ventricle. In patients with a resting gradient of 50 to 80 mm Hg, the appearance of ST-segment depression (one millimeter or more) in the left chest or inferior ECG leads on exercise (treadmill or ergometer) may be considered a valid indication for surgery.

Should One Operate on Asymptomatic Patients with an Isolated Small Ventricular Septal Defect or Atrial Septal Defect and Normal Pulmonary Artery Pressure?

To provide an appropriate answer to this common dilemma, one must first define what constitutes a small defect. Since the size of the defect cannot be accurately measured preoperatively, it is usually estimated from the magnitude of the left-to-right shunt, determined at cardiac catheterization. A pulmonary to systemic flow ratio of 1.5:1 is usually considered small, 1.6 to 1.9:1, intermediate and 2:1 greater, a large shunt. These criteria are arbitrary and estimates of the shunt magnitude should consider the accurancy of the methodology employed and the physiologic conditions present at the time the measurements were taken. For example, anxiety or exercise may result in an increased left-to-right shunt, whereas hypoventilation may diminish its magnitude.

Decisions regarding surgical closure of small or intermediate ventricular and atrial septal defects (pulmonary to systemic flow ratio of 1.9:1 or less) should be based not only on thorough evaluation of the catheterization data but on clinical evidence of the hemodynamic significance of the defect, natural history of the lesion, and the numerous factors listed in *Various Factors to be Considered.*

Advocates of surgery contend that closing the defect will eliminate the risk of infective endocarditis, prevent congestive heart failure (particularly during pregnancy) and pulmonary vascular obstructive disease in adulthood, and eliminate the possibility of parodoxic embolism. Surgery for the simple lesion is safe and associated with a very small mortality and morbidity.

Proponents of conservative management contend that surgery is not indicated in patients with small defects because they usually do not have nor are prone to the development of a hemodynamically significant cardiac compromise as a consequence of the shunt. There is no evidence that pulmonary vascular obstructive disease develops in association with small left to right shunt. Congestive heart failure as a consequence of small left-to-right shunts must be exceedingly rare even with the added volume overload that occurs in pregnancy. Patients with an isolated atrial septal defect secundum are not susceptible to endocarditis and the risk in those with small ventricular defects is very small (16). Moreover, the infection is amendable to treatment and no data are available concerning the risk of endocarditis in postoperative patients with ventricular septal defect. While surgical results for closure of small ventricular or atrial defects are indeed excellent and morbidity low, it behooves us to remember that surgery for small defects may not even qualify as prophylactic surgery. Serious consideration should, therefore, be given to the potential sequalae and complications of hospitalization, thorocotomy and cardiopulmonary bypass (Table 11-7). Complete heart block requiring a pacemaker may occur with ventricular septal defect closure and atrial arrhythmias are not uncommon after surgical close of atrial septal defect, particularly of the sinus venosus type. When partial anomalous pulmonary venous connection to the superior vena cava is associated with atrial septal defect, repair may result in infarction of the corresponding lung segment.

Conclusion

The great majority of children with small ventricular septal defects and atrial septal defects do not require surgery. Since spontaneous closure or diminution in size is common, particularly with ventricular septal defect, a decision should be deferred until the child is an adolescent. Surgical closure of small defects is indicated, however, in patients with evidence of hemodynamic compromise or embarrassment of the circulation. Such evidence in asymptomatic patients consists of associated cardiomegaly on chest x-ray, ventricular hypertrophy on the electrocardiogram or clearly demonstrated decreased ventricular compliance on exercise or other stress testing. A greater reluctance to advise surgery should exist in patients with (a) atrial septal defect of the sinus venosus variety, (b) when the atrial defect is associated with partial anomalous pulmonary venous connection to the superior vena cava, (c) if transventricular closure of a ventricular septal defect is contemplated, or (d) if the surgery is likely to be accompanied by major psychologic or socioeconomic trauma. On the other hand, anticipation of possible congestive heart failure during pregnancy and the potential for parodoxic embolism should lower the threshold to surgery in females. The benefits of surgery should be carefully weighted against the risk involved and an appropriate recommendation then made.

When is Surgery Indicated for Patients with Ventricular Septal Defect and Associated Aortic Regurgitation?

Aortic regurgitation in patients with ventricular septal defect may be the result of deficiency of conal musculature (subpulmonary defect) which usually supports the annulus of the aortic valve or from a congenital defect of the lower margin of the sinuses of valsalva or valve commissures associated with an infracristal ventricular septal defect (33). The degree of aortic regurgitation is variable and it may be accompanied by prolapse of the coronary sinus of valsalva into the ventricular septal defect. The left-to-right shunt through the ventricular septal defect is usually small. Hemodynamic changes are nearly always due to significant aortic regurgitation and less often due to the left-to-right via the ventricular septal defect. Treatment is clearly indicated in patients with (a) symptoms (dyspnea, angina and so forth), (b) congestive heart failure, (c) progressive cardiac enlargement or (d) evidence of serious

Table 11-8. Ventricular Septal Defect and Aortic Regurgitation

Number of patients		72
Age at discovery of aortic regurgitation (median) (yr)		8.4
Pulmonary to systemic flow ratio (mean)		1.8:1.0
Location of ventricular septal defect	Subaortic	36
	Subpulmonary	12
	Muscular	2
	Not defined	22
Incidence of infective endocarditis (410 patient-year follow-up)		9/72 patients
Severity of aortic regurgitation at detection	Mild	47%
	Moderate	33%
	Severe	20%
Severity of aortic regurgitation at follow-up (median = 5 yr)	Mild	41%
	Moderate	17%
	Severe	38%
	Dead	4%
Results of surgery in survivors ($n = 27$; median follow-up 8 yr)	"Cured"	26%
	Improved	26%
	Unchanged	41%
	Deteriorated	7%

Children's Hospital Medical Center, Boston, Massachusetts, 1972.

left ventricular dysfunction. Ventricular septal defect closure and valvuloplasty or valve replacement are usually required (12, 31).

Controversy exists concerning the treatment of asymptomatic patients with ventricular septal defect and trivial or mild aortic regurgitation (12, 22, 31, 33, 34). Whether closure of the septal defect with or without plication of the aortic valve abolishes or prevents aortic insufficiency is yet to be established. Long-term results of surgery in these patients are not yet available. Proponents of ventricular septal defect closure point to excellent operative results in patients with ventricular septal defect and mild aortic regurgitation; disappearance or diminution of the aortic insufficiency, prevention of sinus of valsalva prolapse, and avoidence of valve replacement at a later time (31, 33). The volume overload of the left ventricle from both the left to right shunt and valvular insufficiency are eliminated.

It has been our experience, however, that mild aortic regurgitation in association with a ventricular septal defect (regardless of type) is a very slowly progressive lesion and often stable for decades (22) (Table 11-8) and that the left ventricular volume overload is not excessive since both the shunt and the insufficiency are mild. Furthermore, in a number of well studied and followed patients, aortic regurgitation first appeared 1 to 4 years after successful closure of an isolated ventricular septal defect. The patients continue to be susceptible to infective endocarditis after surgery because the aortic valve remains abnormal. Plication of the valve if unsatisfactory may aggravate the aortic regurgitation and require early prosthetic valve insertion. This is of particular concern in the younger child subjected to surgery.

Conclusion

Surgery in patients with ventricular septal defect and aortic regurgitation should be performed for the same indications commonly used in patients with isolated aortic regurgitation. In these cases, treatment will involve closure of the ventricular septal defect and aortic valve replacement or less often plication of the aortic valve. In the asymptomatic child with mild aortic regurgitation, careful medical follow-up and conservative management are preferable. The lesion in most patients remains stable for many years. Closure of the defect with or without plication of the aortic valve is a "palliative" procedure whose long-term effectiveness has not been established. Early closure of the ventricular defect is not likely to eliminate the aortic regurgitation in many patients because of inherent abnormalities in the aortic valve. Considering the operative mortality, morbidity, probable need for further surgery in the future, and a continued susceptibility to infective endocarditis, I do not feel that prophylactic surgery is warranted in these patients.

Summary

The treatment of hemodynamically significant congenital cardiac malformations is, with few exceptions, surgical repair or palliation. The indications for surgery are well established for most cardiovascular malformations. However, in many instances clear guidelines to management are lacking. The rapid advances in surgical techniques during the last decade have altered significantly the pattern of care and quality of life in patients with complex cardiovascular lesions. Information regarding the long term prognosis of operated patients is still limited and one must, therefore, rely primarily on results measured by mortality and short-term gain. Decision or recommendation regarding surgery should be dictated by the anticipated benefits and the risk of operation. The potential benefits must be weighted against mortality, complications, sequalae, and residua of the proposed surgical procedure. In deciding the appropriate timing for an elective operation in any patient, consideration should be given to a variety of factors including: age of the patient, available surgical skill, type of malformation and cardiovascular status, surgical procedure and technique required, developmental and psychologic factors present, ethical and moral issues involved, and occasionally, to geographic, seasonal, and economic circumstances. Some major currently contested surgical therapeutic problems are reviewed and relevant data from our institution provided. To those who would disagree with my conclusions and recommendations for specific controversial subjects, I would like to quote from Maimonides physician's prayer: "If wiser men wish to teach and correct me, may I follow them and be grateful: for the compass of our art is large and wide."

Acknowledgment

I am indebted to Dr. Aldo R. Castaneda for much of the recent surgical data and to Drs. Alexander S. Nadas and Donald C. Fyler for reviewing the manuscript. Supported in part by Program Project Grant HL10436 and Training Grant HL05855 from the National Institute of Health.

References

1. Aisenberg, R. B., Wolff, P. H., Rosenthal, A., and Nadas, A. S. Psychological impact of cardiac catheterization. Pediatrics, 51:1051, 1973.
2. Banchek, I. L., Starr, A., Sunderland, C. V., and Menashe, V. D. Natural history of tetralogy of Fallot in infancy. Circulation, 48:392, 1973.
3. Bernhard, W. F., Keane, J. F., Fellows, K., Litwin, S. B., and Gross, R. E. Progress and problems in the surgical management of aortic stenosis. J. Thorac. Cardiovasc. Surg., 66:404, 1973.
4. Braunberg, J. A., Reilly, E. L., and Doty, D. B. Central nervous system consequences in infants of cardiac surgery using deep hypothermia and circulatory arrest. Circulation, 50: Suppl. 2:60, 1974.
5. Champsaur, G. L., Sokel, D. M., Trusler, G. A., and Mustard, W. T. Repair of transposition of the great arteries in 123 pediatric patients. Circulation, 47:1032, 1973.
6. Dooley, K. J., Freed, M. D., Parisi, L. F., and Nadas, A. S. Review of transposition of the great arteries and intact ventricular septum. Circulation, 49-50: Suppl. 3:169, 1974, (abstr.).
7. Duff, S. R. and Campbell, A. G. M. Moral and ethical dilemmas in the special care nursery. N. Engl. J. Med., 289:890, 1973.
8. Fellows, K. E. Jr. and Rosenthal, A. Extracardiac roentgenographic abnormalities in cyanotic congenital heart disease. Am. J. Roentgenol. Radium. Ther. Nucl. Med., 114:371, 1972.
9. Fischbein, C. A., Rosenthal, A., Fischer, E. G., Nadas, A. S., and Welch, K. Risk factors for brain abscess in patients with congenital heart disease. Am. J. Cardiol., 34:97, 1974.
10. Fontan, F. and Bandet, E. Surgical repair of tricuspid atresia. Thorax, 26:240, 1971.
11. Freed, M. D., Rosenthal, A., Plauth, W. H. Jr., and Nadas, A. S. Development of subaortic stenosis after pulmonary artery banding. Circulation, 48: Suppl. 3:7, 1973.
12. Freed, M. D. and Bernhard, W. F. Prosthetic valve replacement in children. Progr. Cardiovasc. Dis., 17:487, 1975.

13. Fyler, D. C. and Rosenthal, A. Neonatal heart disease. In Avery, G. B. ed. Neonatology. In press, 1975.
14. Greenwood, R. D., Rosenthal, A., Nadas, A. S., Freed, M. D., and Castaneda, A. R. Ascending aorta—Pulmonary artery anastomosis for cyanotic congenital heart disease. Am. J. Cardiol., 35:141, 1975.
15. Griepe, E., French, J. W., Shumway, N. E., and Baum, D. Is pulmonary artery banding obsolete? Circulation, 50: Suppl. 2:14, 1974.
16. Johnson, D. H., Rosenthal, A., and Nadas, A. S. Bacterial endocarditis in infancy and childhood. A forty year review. Circulation, 51:581, 1975.
17. Jonsson, B. and Lee, S. J. K. Haemodynamic effects of exercise in isolated pulmonary stenosis before and after surgery. Br. Heart J., 30:60, 1968.
18. Linde, L. M., Rasof, B., and Dunn, O. J. Longitudinal studies of intellectual and behavioral development in children with congenital heart disease. Acta Paediatr. Scand., 59:169, 1970.
19. Mesko, G. Z., Jones, E. J., and Nadas, A. S. Diminution and closure of large ventricular septal defects after pulmonary artery banding. Circulation, 48:847, 1973.
20. Moller, J. H., Nakib, A., and Edwards, J. E. Infarction of papillary muscles and mitral insufficiency associated with congenital aortic stenosis. Circulation, 34:87, 1966.
21. Mustard, W. T. Successful two-stage correction of transposition of the great arteries. Surgery, 55:469, 1964.
22. Nadas, A. S. and Fyler, D. C. Pediatric Cardiology, 3rd ed. Philadelphia, W. B. Saunders Co., 1972, pp. 379.
23. Phornphutkul, C., Rosenthal, A., Nadas, A. S., and Berenberg, W. Cerebrovascular accidents in infants and children with cyanotic congenital heart disease. Am. J. Cardiol., 32:329, 1973.
24. Plauth, W. H., Nadas, A. S., Bernhard, W. F., and Fyler, D. C. Changing hemodynamics in patients with transposition of the great arteries. Circulation, 42:131, 1970.
25. Rashkind, W. J. and Miller, W. W. Creation of an atrial septal defect without thorocotomy. A palliative approach to complete transposition of the great arteries. J.A.M.A., 196:991, 1966.
26. Rosenthal, A., Button, L. N., Nathan, D. G., Miettinen, O. S., and Nadas, A. S. Blood volume changes in cyanotic congenital heart disease. Am. J. Cardiol., 27:162, 1971.
27. Shaw, A. Dilemmas of "informed consent" in childhood. N. Engl. J. Med., 289:885, 1973.
28. Silbert, S., Wolff, P. H., Mayer, B., Rosenthal, A., and Nadas, A. S. Cyanotic heart disease and psychological development. Pediatrics, 43:192, 1969.
29. Souninen, P. Physical growth of children with congenital heart disease. Acta Paediatr. Scand. Suppl., 225:1-50, 1971.
30. Stevenson, G. J., Stove, E. F., Dillard, D. H., and Morgan, B. Intellectual development of children subjected to prolonged circulatory arrest during hypothermic open heart surgery in infancy. Circulation, 50: Suppl. 2:54, 1974.
31. Spencer, F. C., Doyle, E. F., Danilowicz, D. A., Bahnson, H. T., and Weldon, C. S. Long term evaluation of aortic valvuloplasty for aortic insufficiency and ventricular septal defect. J. Thorc. Cardiovas. Surg., 65:15, 1973.
32. Stark, J., Tynan, M. J., Ashcraft, K. W., Aberdeen, E., and Waterston, D. J. Obstruction of pulmonary veins and superior vena cava after the Mustard operation for transposition of the great arteries. Circulation, 45-56: Suppl. I:1-116, 1972.
33. Tatsuno, K., Kouro, S., Ando, M., and Sakakibara, S. Pathogenetic mechanisms of prolapsing aortic valve and aortic regurgitation associated with ventricular septal defect. Circulation, 48:1028, 1973.
34. Trusler, G. A., Moes, C. A. F., and Kidd, B. S. C. Repair of ventricular septal defect with aortic insufficiency. J. Thorac. Cardiovasc. Surg., 66:394, 1973.
35. Vincent, W. R., Buckberg, G. D., and Hoffman, J. I. E. Left ventricular subendocardiac ischemia in severe valvar and supravalvar aortic stenosis. Circulation, 49:326, 1974.
36. Waterston, D. J. Treatment of Fallot's tetralogy in children under 1 year of age. Rozhl. Chir., 41:181, 1962.

Chapter 12 Indications for Coronary Artery Surgery and Patient Selection

RICHARD T. SHORE, M.D. and W. DUDLEY JOHNSON, M.D.

General Considerations

Coronary bypass surgery is now a common procedure in many hospitals, but indications for coronary surgery vary from one center to another and at any hospital are influenced by such factors as previous experience of the surgical team, operative survival, symptomatic improvement following surgery, and long-term graft patency. The following discussion will, of necessity, be based on the authors' experience.

Without a doubt, the greatest limitation in the selection of patients for surgery has been our lack of knowledge concerning the natural course of coronary disease. The advent of coronary surgery has been a great stimulus in the search to establish the natural history, and the evidence now accumulating on nonsurgical therapy will probably further stimulate surgery (4). From the Framingham and other studies in which large population groups were sampled, it became clear that symptoms do not always correlate with risk. Many persons may have repeated infarcts without pain. At St. Luke's Hospital in Milwaukee severe symptoms are not a prerequisite to angiographic studies. As one cardiologist expressed it, angiography is indicated on the reasonable suspicion of coronary disease. Therefore, regardless of age or sex, patients who can reasonably be assured of at least a moderate period of productive life and present with a reasonable suspicion of coronary disease should be studied.

Not every patient advised to have surgery accepts this recommendation, and groups of these patients have been followed since the early years of bypass surgery. One hundred and twelve such patients advised to have surgery, but never operated upon were reviewed (6). The data available from the time of catheterization correlated poorly with subsequent death or survival in these unoperated patients (61 of 112 were dead in 2 years). Only the symptom complex of crescendo pain related to outcome, and this pattern was associated with higher mortality. Other symptom categories, including no symptoms or number of previous infarcts, showed no correlation with subsequent survival or death. There was a highly significant correlation between the number of arteries involved and risk of subsequent death without surgery. Single-artery disease, particularly nondominant right, was not associated with increased attrition rates; while the yearly risk of death rapidly increased in double- and triple-artery disease. Even more significantly associated with early death was a major impediment to flow in the left main or proximal anterior descending artery. Regardless of the total number of other arteries involved or the degree of ventricular malfunction, the major stenosis of the proximal left coronary was the most significant predictor of early death. Essentially the same conclusions evolved from studies of similar groups of patients at other institutions (3) and provide the basis for the evolution of our philosophy of patient selection for surgery.

While most patients referred for catheterization are symptomatic, symptoms have played less and less of a role in the selection of patients for surgery. The obvious exception is the patient with crescendo anginal pattern in whom surgery may be urgently indicated, as in severe triple or proximal left disease (5). The mortality rate in these patients waiting for surgery is higher than the surgical risk, and the operation should be performed without delay.

Most patients suffering an infarction should subsequently be considered for catheterization. Myocardial infarction is the strongest indicator of coronary artery disease, short of death and autopsy. Many of these patients had no symptoms prior to the infarct and it seems irrational to avoid surgery assuming that the patient would subsequently develop a warning sign and symptoms prior to a second and possibly fatal infarct. In many patients who have had an infarct the stage of coronary artery disease plays a more important role in the decision for surgery than does the degree of symptoms.

Maximal stress testing should be considered part of a periodic checkup in patients falling into higher risk coronary prone groups. When the stress test is positive, cine angiograms should be performed. Occasional patients have been found with severe coronary artery disease and no symptoms. Despite the absence of symptoms, surgery has been performed because of the life-threatening nature of the coronary lesions.

Angina can be controlled or relieved with vigorous medical therapy in many patients but there is no effective medical therapy for coronary insufficiency. Relieving angina does not relieve coronary insufficiency. Nitrates and beta-blocking agents relieve symptoms by depressing the workload on the heart, and this approach to symptom control is very safe and preferred in certain circumstances. For example, a totally occluded artery in the presence of good collateral rarely represents a major threat to the patient. The patient has demonstrated that he can live without the vessel, and the total block can not get worse and further compromise circulation. Significant angina associated with an occluded artery is strong indication for vigorous medical therapy. Such a patient would be considered a candidate for surgery only after prolonged medical therapy fails.

However, when the collateral to an occluded artery is poor or arises from an artery in jeopardy, surgery should be considered. Our studies, plus others, have indicated anatomic situations that are a threat to life. In the authors' opinion, tight stenosis of the proximal left system (left main, proximal anterior descending) or severe three-vessel disease with good myocardial function does not deserve a trial of medical therapy. No known medical therapy affects patency of stenotic arteries and none improves coronary flow. With reasonably good ventricular function, the surgical risk in triple-coronary disease is in the 1 percent range. What can be accomplished surgically for this patient, in terms of vascular patency, preservation, and improved myocardial function, and survival is much better established than what can be accomplished with medical therapy. With our present knowledge, medical therapy for triple artery disease is more experimental than surgical therapy. Symptoms per se are not the only indication for surgery, but must be considered along with the angiographic findings. Likewise the lack of symptoms is not necessarily a contraindication to surgery.

Age

Age is only relative when surgery is considered. The age of patients who have undergone coronary revascularization, in the authors' experience, ranged from 19 to 79. Increasing caution is used with increasing age, and with increasing age, less and less enthusiasm is shown for the patient in the salvage category. Women patients do as well as men. Since angina plays a greater role in the symptoms of women, immediate clinical improvement often exceeds that noted in many men, although postoperative psychologic depression may be more frequent in women.

Obesity

Obesity is a common problem. Some patients are encouraged to lose weight by the time they see the surgeon, but vigorous weight reduction may still be in order. How long surgery can be delayed for weight reduction depends, of course, on the coronary situation.

Smoking

Smoking presents a significant hazard to the patient, not only as a catalyst for progression of coronary disease, but more germanely as the single most critical variant in pulmonary complications in the immediate postoperative period. The amount of time and effort required to care for these patients increases exponentially with the frequency and duration of smoking in the preoperative period. The increased respiratory problems also contribute to more frequent sternal disruptions. On the authors' service elective surgery is not performed on patients who continue to smoke.

Associated Problems

Certain diseases are frequently noted in association with coronary heart disease. With refined techniques of surgery and postoperative care, primary cardiac problems such as rhythm disturbances and pump failure no longer are the major causes of early postoperative mortality. Other associated problems have become the prime factor and critical evaluation of these problems may induce one to consider these as the limiting factor in consideration for surgery. However with severe threatening coronary disease, controlled chronic problems are rarely a contraindication to surgery. Certain diseases are frequently present in coronary patients, such as diabetes mellitus and hypertension. Almost as frequently seen are chronic pulmonary disease and moderate to severe renal disease. Diabetes mellitus (including juvenile type) presents no particular problem either with surgery or with pre- and postoperative management. However, with diffuse disease at times it extends well into secondary and tertiary branches of the coronary artery system, and one must be prepared to deal with quite fine vascular anastomoses. We have been gratified by our efforts in these patients with juvenile diabetes mellitus, but there is no doubt that their care requires extra time and caution. A particularly treacherous combination is juvenile diabetes mellitus and type II hyperlipidemia. While seen rarely, its combination has produced the most diffuse disease. The hyperlipidemias themselves have not presented any particular problems so far as surgery or postoperative care is concerned. For the best long-term effect after surgery, dietary and medical management of the underlying lipidemia is strongly advised.

Severe hypertension increases the risk factor for surgery, but again we have not allowed this to challenge the decision for surgery. These patients require careful management in the pre- and postoperative period. With ventricular hypertrophy we prefer to keep the heart beating as much as possible during surgery. The chance for subendocardial damage appears to be reduced if the heart is kept beating most of the time. With these precautions hypertension rarely contraindicates surgery.

Other conditions have also rarely contraindicated surgery. For example, patients with creatinine clearances as low as 30 ml/min. have undergone revascularization. With the use of pulsatile flow on bypass, further deterioration of renal function usually does not occur.

Associated Surgical Problems

Extracoronary atherosclerotic vascular disease is frequently seen in association with coronary disease. Carotid stenosis demands equal priority to coronary revascularization, while vascular problems in other areas may be taken care of at a later date. When symptoms of cerebral insufficiency are present or if a carotid bruit is present, appropriate angiographic studies are obtained preoperatively. When significant carotid stenosis is demonstrated, it is corrected initially while the chest is being opened. As soon as the artery is repaired, the coronary revascularization proceeds in the usual manner. When severe stenosis involves both carotid vessels, the side most severely involved is done first. This procedure is followed in 1 week by the combined procedure, as outlined above. Facilities for coronary surgery are available at the initial carotid endarterectomy in case acute coronary insufficiency develops. This combined approach has been used since early 1970 and is clearly preferable to staging carotid and coronary surgery (1). Thoracic or abdominal aneurysm resection or peripheral arterial surgery is delayed to a second procedure after the coronary disease is corrected. When severe intra-abdominal problems coexist, such as gall bladder or ulcer disease, simultaneous abdominal and heart surgery are performed. This combined surgery is reserved only for patients with very acute abdominal and coronary problems.

Anatomic Variance—Single-Vessel Disease

A number of studies suggested that mortality associated with single-artery disease is extremely low with medical therapy (left main and proximal anterior descending arteries excluded (2). As a general policy, we do not advise surgery for all patients with stenosis in a single artery. In centers where a 25 or 30 percent graft closure rate has occurred, these patients clearly should not be operated upon. Where patency rates are much higher and the surgical risk is known to be low, many of the patients can benefit from surgery. In our center each patient is evaluated in terms of his age, symptoms, stress-test response, and so on. Some with single-artery disease are operated upon.

Multiple-Vessel Involvement

As the number of vessels involved increases, the yearly attrition rate also increases, and the advisability of surgery becomes more emphatic. Patients with three-vessel disease, significant stenosis of the proximal arteries, and good left ventricular function are never refused surgery. Special circumstances that deserve mention arise in coronary disease. We continue to see patients with patterns of diffuse involvement of the coronary arterial tree who have been declined surgery elsewhere. It has been the policy on this service not to refuse surgery to any patient who has reasonably good ventricular function because no matter how diffuse their disease, one or more good arteries can be found and successfully bypassed. This does not imply that all areas can be bypassed that may be in need, but usually several grafts can be inserted. In our practice patients with the diffuse type of disease prevail and many grafts are routinely performed. During the past 2 years over 50 percent of our patients have received from four to seven bypasses. Arteries used for bypass include the anterior descending, one or two diagonal branches, the interventricular septal artery, one to three marginal branches of the circumflex, the posterior descending, distal branches of the right coronary artery, the main right coronary artery, and, on occasion, a large right marginal branch. Any or all of these arteries may be suitable for grafting when significant disease is present in these secondary branches. With good surgical techniques, patency rates in these secondary branches are nearly equal to patency rates in the large main arteries.

Three factors in our experience are the important determinants of graft patency and hence are important in patient selection for surgery. These determinants include flow rates, the use of mammary arteries for direct anastomoses, and the surgical team. Intraoperative flow measurements are recorded routinely on most bypass grafts. Subsequently, these bypass flows and other information from surgery are matched with postoperative catheterization studies and have been correlated with the patency or closure of the bypass. Intraoperative flows bear a relationship to the patency rate of the bypass graft (Figure 12-1). The relationship of the flow appears to vary depending upon the surgeon involved and flow/graft patency curves seem to follow two patterns. On curve B, the bypass patency is relatively constant down to approximately a flow range of 20 ml/min and below that point the patency rate falls rapidly. On curve B the flow is important, but there is no statistically significant level at which the flow becomes critical in the graft patency. On curve A the patency rates

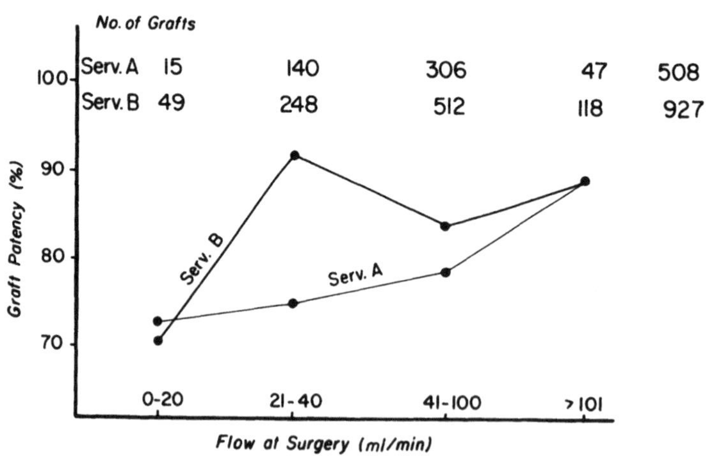

Fig. 12-1. Graft patency by flow and surgical service; 1435 grafts, 1968 to 1973, 0 to 24 months post-surgery.

of bypass grafts is high for the high flow ranges, but the rate steadily falls with declining flows. One must question where surgery should be performed when the patency rate falls much below 80 percent. This type of information, correlating flow with patency, should be obtained routinely; it helps the surgeon to learn his own technical ability and also helps him to select those patients upon whom he can operate with reasonable success.

Overall patency rates, besides being related to flow, are clearly related to the type of bypass used. Mammary artery bypasses continually show a much higher patency rate, and are usually considered preferable when they can be used. Its small size, the time required to mobilize it, or damage to the artery does limit the versatility of mammary bypass. Nevertheless, in at least 90 percent of our patients one or both mammary arteries are used as part of the bypass procedure.

In addition to vein-graft flow and use of the mammary artery as significant determinants of graft patency, the other most significant determinant is the surgical team. These three factors may have little to do with the presenting patient, but all of them are critical and do influence the selection of that patient for an operative procedure. In patients with diffuse disease, the authors' experience with patency rates has been extremely satisfactory, with flows down to 20 ml/min. For this reason patients are continued to be accepted for surgery with multiple obstructions in secondary branches, and mammary bypasses are used where feasible. Only continued experience by a given surgical service, correlated with subsequent catheterization studies, and good clinical follow-up justify this approach.

Surgery for Poor Ventricular Function

Another area of controversy concerns the patient with poor ventricular function, who is perhaps the most difficult to evaluate in terms of suitability for bypass surgery. In reviewing our experience during the past 18 months, it is apparent that a number of factors have clearly influenced our selection of the patient with poor ventricular function for surgery. A high percentage of these patients still have significant angina. It has long been thought that angina is a very favorable sign for surgery in patients with poor ventricular function, based on the premise that angina is due to ischemic, but viable muscle. The patient who has had severe angina, which disappeared after one or more infarcts, is probably not a candidate for surgery. When the angina disappears, it usually implies that the muscle has infarcted. Over 80 percent of our patients with poor ventricular function presented with significant angina during this recent 18-month experience. Only a small percentage had symptoms of frank congestive heart failure.

Evaluation of left ventricular performance is inconsistent, and a grading system may be difficult to define. Hypokinesis is far more favorable for surgery than total akinesis. In general, we define a poor ventricle as a chamber with at least two major areas of gross malfunction on right and left oblique ventriculography. This still leaves considerable variation in the degree of ventricular malfunction within a class.

Some patients with severely hypo- or akinetic areas throughout most of the ventricle have been selected for surgery. The major criteria for these types of patients have been angina and severely stenotic but bypassable coronaries jeopardizing the remaining myocardium. A patient with obviously diffuse disease in all major and many secondary arteries who has poor ventricular function is usually not considered a candidate for surgery. While diffuse disease with good ventricular function has rarely contraindicated surgery, it is clearly a relative contraindication for surgery in patients with a failing myocardium. Once again the experience of a given surgical team must be considered in selecting this type of patient for surgery.

During this 18-month period, the operative mortality was 6 percent in this series of patients with relatively severe ventricular malfunction. Surprisingly only one late death occurred throughout this time period. The fact that surgery was helpful is suggested because 90 percent of the patients were relieved of most or all of their symptomatology. Amongst the patients who had gone 6 months or longer, 75 percent returned to full- or part-time work. This experience has prompted us to perform surgery on many of these less than ideal patients. Marked improvement in ventricular performance should not be anticipated in this group. These patients are not operated on because of their poor ventricle, but because their severe, threatening, coronary disease places the remaining myocardium in great jeopardy. More than half of these patients presented with severe left main or proximal left anterior descending stenosis and 90 percent had severe three-vessel disease, each of which constitutes a high risk in the natural course of the disease.

Rhythm Disturbance

Rhythm disturbances often are encountered preoperatively in coronary revascularization patients. The most common problem is chronic premature ventricular contraction. This condition is rarely corrected by surgery, and patients should be advised of this preoperatively. Premature ventricular contractions are not a contraindication to surgery however. Episodic rhythm problems, including bouts of atrial tachyarrhythmias or, more commonly, runs of ventricular rhythm disturbances usually disappear after full revascularization. Runs of ventricular tachycardia associated with stress is considered a life-threatening situation. This condition subsides after successful bypass and, therefore, we consider this problem among the most urgent requiring surgical intervention. In adult patients with valve disease, coronary cine angiograms are routinely performed. When significant coronary lesions coexist with or without symptoms combined surgery is performed.

Other Complications of Coronary Disease

Ventricular aneurysms of sufficient size to jeopardize cardiac output is a long established indication for surgery. Infrequently, a patient with a ventricular aneurysm has normal coronary vessels in other areas. Less than 5 percent of patients with ventricular aneurysm have an aneurysmectomy alone. One to several bypass grafts are often inserted, along with the aneurysm resection. An aneurysm is a dynamic situation because the area of scar progresses from small to larger areas and as the scar molds it pushes out to ultimately become a true aneurysm. Patients with severe triple-artery disease rarely develop a typical aneurysm; instead they develop a diffusely dilated ventricle with poor function in all areas. In general the larger the aneurysm the more favorable is the prognosis after surgery. Surgical risk in patients with aneurysms does not relate to the size of the aneurysm except in those areas where its resection constitutes greater than 40 percent of the effective filling volume of the left ventricle. The risk of surgery for patients with aneurysms correlates more positively with the degree of functioning myocardium in the remaining heart. Patients with large aneurysms usually have a good circumflex artery and good myocardium in that area and sometimes good functioning muscle over the inferior surface of the ventricle. Hypo- or akinetic myocardium has not been resected routinely since its function nearly always improves with bypass surgery.

Acute ventricular septal defects continue to be a major disaster. If the patient survives 4 to 6 weeks after the infarct and surgery is performed at that stage, the results are good. The ventricular septal defect is closed and the aneurysm is resected, if present, along with bypass grafts to suitable arteries. However, in patients with massive heart failure who deteriorate rapidly following the ruptured septum, surgery has rarely been successful, although it continues to be performed since the outlook without intervention is hopeless. However, the results have been very disappointing. The intra-aortic balloon pump appears to benefit these patients and may help in getting some through this early high-risk period to a point where the results with surgery are acceptable.

Mitral insufficiency secondary to coronary disease again presents difficult judgment problems at the time of surgery. On occasion ventricular performance has improved markedly and mitral incompetency disappeared completely following effective revascularization. In patients with mitral disease related to coronary insufficiency it has been our policy to do the bypass grafts first and then determine whether or not the patient will be able to come off bypass without insufficiency. If the mitral insufficiency disappears, obviously no examination nor replacement of the valve is indicated. If mitral incompetence continues after the bypass grafts are inserted, the atrium is opened and the valve repaired or replaced.

Secondary Procedures

Patients who have had previous coronary procedures are seen with increasing frequency but to select any one of these for a second or third operation depends on many factors. Those wth recurrent symptoms following another operation usually should be recatheterized. Occasionally, patients are seen in whom bypass grafts are functioning, but the disease has progressed to other arteries. Progression of disease is the determining factor in recurrent symptoms in nearly 20 percent of the cases. These patients generally do well with repeat surgery. More often patients are seen in whom the previous implantation or bypass procedure has failed.

Operative reports examined from the initial procedure should contain such pertinent information as (a) the condition of the coronary arteries, (b) the flow through the bypass graft at the initial operation, and (c) the condition of the myocardium with respect to scar, hypertrophy, or dilatation. If the flows through an initial bypass graft are only 20 to 30 ml/min into a diffusely diseased coronary vessel supplying an area of scarafied myocardium, it would be quite inadvisable to attempt to reoperate on this condition. Conversely, if the flow were large, it would heavily favor repeat surgery. For this reason alone, flow measurements at the time of surgery have been useful and continue to be taken routinely. The coronary vessels can usually be identified at a second procedure, although frequently it is difficult to identify branches of the circumflex artery. In the rare patient who has had a previous poudrage procedure, the decision for repeat surgery is extremely difficult to reach. With poudrage, the anterior descending and circumflex arteries are encased in the fibrous sheath, frequently beyond recognition, and hence it is unlikely that any effective graft can be inserted into the left coronary system. Most patients reoperated with this condition require only a right bypass graft. In patients in whom the heart has been covered with omentum, little difficulty has been encountered in localizing the left coronary system. One is particularly conservative in doing secondary operative procedures on patients with severely compromised ventricular function, or on those with previous operative findings of gross ventricular hypertrophy, low graft flows, or unusually diffuse disease.

Intra-Aortic Balloon Pump

In patients with very low ejection fractions, aortograms are taken routinely prior to surgery. The aortogram indicates whether the iliac and lower aortic areas are suitable for the insertion of the balloon catheter. In patients in whom this has been done preoperatively, there have been no complications. However there have been instances in which one iliac artery was narrowed and the other normal and it helped to know this before the balloon catheter was inserted.

In some patients with extremely poor ventricular performance the balloon catheter is inserted at the beginning of the operative procedure. The balloon pump assists with pulsatile flow, is run automatically during the bypass procedure, and provides a high degree of pulsatile pressure for the patient. As the patient is weaned off bypass, it is synchronized with heart function. Usually the balloon is left in for 1 to 3 days after surgery. Its use has been equally successful in patients who fail to regain adequate heart function following the bypass grafts. The heart usually continues to improve after the balloon is used, and the balloon can be removed within a few days.

The balloon catheter also has markedly reduced mortality associated with surgery for patients with poor ventricular function. Eighty-five percent of patients in whom the balloon was used to assist them through surgery recovered and survived. Most of these patients would not have made it through the operative procedure if the balloon catheter had not been used. The balloon proved to be such a valuable asset in assisting patients through surgery that in the authors' opinion, almost no cardiac surgery should be done unless this assist device is available.

Impending Infarct

For 6 years it has been our philosophy that the more severe the angina the more urgently surgery is indicated. This continues to be the policy at this Center. Once again, this brings us to the problem of the patient with impending infarct. Despite numerous reports in the literature, it is still not possible to agree on a single definition of impending myocardial infarction or preinfarction angina. In terms of risk for surgery, these patients appear to be at very little risk above the ordinary elective patient. Even in patients with symptoms of impending infarction, the risk of surgery relates much more closely to the degree of ventricular function than it does to the degree of symptoms or diffuseness of coronary disease. While symptoms do not correlate with surgical risk, they clearly relate to the urgency for surgery. In patients with constant and progressive angina plus severe threatening coronary disease, surgery is indicated at a very early date.

For the acute infarct, surgery must still be considered experimental. Patients with acute infarction, plus a failing left ventricle occasionally can be handled under ideal circumstances. Even under these circumstances, with catheterization studies and the patient in the hospital, risk and mortality are heightened with acute infarction, and each service must define its own philosophy with regard to these patients.

Summary

The definition of indications for coronary artery surgery requires a close look at the natural history of coronary artery disease patterns. Left main coronary artery stenosis, high left anterior descending stenosis, and three-vessel disease have qualified as anatomic patterns associated with early death. Crescendo anginal pain associated with the above is indication for urgent surgery.

Age, obesity, smoking, and associated disease states, such as diabetes mellitus, hypertension, and chronic organ failure are considered relative factors in planning coronary artery surgery. Significant carotid stenosis or ulcerating plaque may require concomitant surgery. Threatening aortic aneurysms should be removed at the same time, although other peripheral vascular surgical problems may usually be corrected as a secondary procedure.

Single nondominant-vessel disease is not associated with early death and often is treated successfully with medical management. As the amount of coronary artery involvement increases, the risk of death also increases. The most significant determinants of graft patency to the coronary arteries appears to be vein graft flow, use of the internal mammary artery, and the individual surgical team.

Patients with poor ventricular function are candidates for surgery only when severe life-threatening coronary artery disease is also present. Complications of myocardial infarction, which may be indications for surgery, include ventricular aneurysm, ventricular septal defect, and mitral valve regurgitation. Patients are accepted for reoperation if there is some assurance of reasonable ventricular function, with bypassable arteries in which reasonable flows were demonstrated at the first procedure. The intra-aortic balloon pump continues to be a boom in management of patients with ventricular compromise.

Coronary artery surgery has evolved significantly during the past several years with the definition of certain coronary artery disease patterns associated with early death and which comprise the leading indications for coronary artery surgery.

References

1. Bernhard, V. M., Johnson, W. D. and Peterson, J. J. Carotid artery stenosis. Arch. Surg., 105:837, 1972.
2. Bruschke, A. V. G., Proudfit, W. L. and Sones, F. M. Jr. Clinical course of patients with normal, and slightly or moderately abnormal coronary arteriograms. Circulation, 47:936, 1973.

3. Bruschke, A. V. G., Proudfit, W. L. and Sones, F. M. Jr. Progress study of 590 consecutive non-surgical cases of coronary disease followed 5–9 years. I. Arterographic correlations. Circulation, 47:1147, 1973.
4. Brymer, J. F., Buter, T. H., Walton, J. A. Jr. and Willis, P. W. A natural history study of the prognostic role of coronary arteriography. Am. Heart J., 88:139, 1974.
5. Johnson, W. D. Surgical techniques of myocardial revascularization: An overview. Bull. N.Y. Acad. Med., 48:1146, 1972.
6. Johnson, W. D. and Kayser, K. L. An expanded indication for coronary surgery. Ann. Thorac. Surg., 16:1, 1973.

Chapter 13 Cardiomyopathy Diagnostic Criteria and Classification

GEORGE E. BURCH, M.D. and THOMAS GILES, M.D.

General Considerations

The history of cardiomyopathy from 1800 to 1965 was briefly reviewed by Mattingly (49). It is evident from this review that serious interest in diseases of the myocardium developed only during the present century. In recent years considerable knowledge has been gained concerning the ultrastructure and function of the normal and diseased myocardium. However, it seems that progress in clinical application of accumulating knowledge has possibly been retarded because of differences of opinion and confusion regarding criteria for diagnosis and classification of the cardiomyopathies.

Many investigators and clinicians have reserved the term *cardiomyopathy* for noncoronary diseases of the myocardium of unknown etiology (6). Other investigators have accepted essentially the same definition, except that they also include diseases of the endocardium and even the pericardium among the cardiomyopathies (35). However, with such definitions the term *cardiomyopathy* excludes myocardial disease of known cause. Yet, every disease has a cause, and in time the causes of all diseases will become known. We are of the opinion that most definitions of cardiomyopathy are too restrictive and of little value to the clinician. For practical clinical reasons, as indicated below, we introduced a more extensive classification and definition of the cardiomyopathies.

Cardiomyopathy literally means heart muscle pathology. Therefore, we are of the opinion that a broad definition and broad classification of heart muscle pathology are necessary for proper diagnosis and management of all patients with heart muscle disease. After all, it is the muscle of the heart that does the work and pumps the blood. Application of the term cardiomyopathy only to the heart of patients who have no evidence of coronary artery disease, valvular disease, systemic arterial hypertension, congenital defects, or other known diseases (33, 36, 43) may omit the major aspect of the patient's cardiac disease, the state of health of the myocardium. Cardiomyopathy (pathology of the myocardium) can certainly exist alone or in combination with any other type of heart disease. Cardiomyopathy (cardiac muscle pathology) may be produced by any agent or circumstance, both known and unknown, capable of damaging myocytes. The physician, therefore, should search extensively for the cause of cardiomyopathy and manage it early and completely. Only when such an extensive search fails to reveal the cause must the physician tentatively classify the cardiac muscle disease as primary (idiopathic or unknown), even though he continues to search for a cause.

We consider it unnecessary for diagnosis to insist that patients with cardiomyopathy have clinically detectable cardiomegaly or any other specific cardiovascular manifestation or combination of manifestations. The criteria for *early* diagnosis must be extremely finite, so that early subtle clinical manifestations are noted for proper care. Rigid criteria limited to manifestations of the late stages of cardiomyopathy would cause physicians to ignore extremely early stages of the disease at which time very little cardiac pathology is present and a cure is more likely. Certainly, rigid criteria exhibited by extensive disease of the myocardium would severely hamper preventive management and cure of the various types of cardiomyopathy.

The term *primary cardiomyopathy* has caused some difficulty in communication among physicians and has even affected their management of patients with cardiomyopathy. Some physicians insist that the term primary cardiomyopathy should be used to indicate that only the muscle of the heart is involved in the disease, with the cause usually being unknown or the disease idiopathic (33, 50). It should be abundantly clear, however, that any classification that divides the cardiomyopathies into *primary*, i.e., only the myocardium is diseased, and *secondary*, i.e., the myocardium is involved secondary to or as a part of a major systemic illness, is purely arbitrary. Some physicians use the term primary synonymously with idiopathic. The thoroughness with which the clinician takes a history and performs a physical examination is the main factor in the determination of the etiologic, pathologic, and/or clinical categories for a given cardiomyopathy. For example, idiopathic cardiomyopathy may be due to several inter-related factors, e.g., excessive alcohol ingestion, malnutrition, and viral infection. When other classifications of cardiomyopathy are accepted, infections and/or coronary artery disease may be found to be associated with alcoholism in the production of cardiomyopathy. Thus, labeling a particular patient's cardiomyopathy as primary or idiopathic should follow the exclusion of all known causes of heart muscle disease. Since all diseases have a cause, it is the physician's responsibility to search for the cause of the disease of the myocardium and to consider it idiopathic or, preferably, of unknown cause only after an exhaustive search has failed to establish the etiology of the disease.

Classification of Cardiomyopathy

The classification of cardiomyopathy that we have suggested is shown in Table 13-1 (12). This classification is based upon the attitude discussed above. We have found this classification extremely useful in prevention, early care, and management of even late stages of cardiomyopathy.

The discussion that follows will be concerned with selected types of cardiomyopathies, which do not cause obstruction to left ventricular outflow or are not associated with asymmetric septal hypertrophy. It should be noted that idiopathic hypertrophic subaortic stenosis is considered to be genetically transmitted as an autosomal dominant and can produce obstruction to the outflow tract of the left and/or right ventricles (30). A characteristic feature of the disease is a disproportionate hypertrophy of the interventricular septum near the base of the heart.

It is suggested that endomyocardial fibrosis may be secondary to an infectious agent (27)—a concept that, if established, would place endomyocardial fibrosis in the category of secondary heart muscle disease. The remainder of the patients

Table 13-1. Classification of Heart Muscle Disease

I. Primary heart muscle disease
- A. Familial cardiomyopathy
  - 1. With ventricular outflow tract obstruction
  - 2. Without ventricular outflow tract obstruction
- B. Nonfamilial idiopathic cardiomyopathy
  - 1. With ventricular outflow tract obstruction
  - 2. Without ventricular outflow tract obstruction
- C. Endomyocardial fibrosis

II. Secondary heart muscle disease
- A. Infectious myocarditis
  - 1. Viral
  - 2. Bacterial
  - 3. Rickettsial
  - 4. Protozoal
  - 5. Metazoal
- B. Alcoholic cardiomyopathy
- C. Puerperal (postpartal) cardiomyopathy
- D. Metabolic cardiomyopathy
  - 1. Hyperthyroidism
  - 2. Hypothyroidism
  - 3. Amyloidosis
    - a. Secondary amyloidosis
    - b. Primary systemic amyloidosis
    - c. Primary cardiac amyloidosis
  - 4. Glycogen storage disease
    - a. Pompe's disease
    - b. Forbe's disease
  - 5. Nutritional deficiency
    - a. Thiamine deficiency (beriberi)
    - b. Protein deficiency
    - c. Avitaminosis
- E. Allergy-related cardiomyopathy
  - 1. Postvaccinal
  - 2. Serum sickness
  - 3. Urticaria
- F. Cardiomyopathy associated with systemic disease of unknown etiology
  - 1. Rheumatoid arthritis
  - 2. Autoimmune disease (?)
  - 3. Collagen vascular disease
- G. Toxic cardiomyopathy
  - 1. Drugs (emetine, arsenic, isoproterenol)
  - 2. Anesthetic gases
  - 3. Poisons
  - 4. Foods
  - 5. Heavy metals (cobalt, cadmium, etc.)
- H. Infiltrative cardiomyopathy
  - 1. Carcinomatosis (lung, thyroid)
  - 2. Leukemia
  - 3. Hemochromatosis
  - 4. Sarcoidosis
- I. Cardiomyopathy due to physical agents
  - 1. Nonpenetrating chest injury
  - 2. Heat sickness
  - 3. Ionizing radiation
  - 4. Electric shock
  - 5. Solar radiation
- J. Cardiomyopathy associated with neuromuscular disorders
  - 1. Progressive muscular dystrophy
    - a. Duchene dystrophy
    - b. Limb girdle dystrophy (Erb)
    - c. Fascioscapulohumeral dystrophy (Landouzy-Dejerine)
    - d. Dystrophia myotonia
  - 2. Friedrich's ataxia
- K. Primary tumors of the myocardium
- L. Senile cardiomyopathy
- M. Ischemic cardiomyopathy

From Burch, G. E. and DePasquale, N. P. Recognition and prevention of cardiomyopathy. Circulation, 42:A-47, 1970.

classified as having primary heart muscle disease would be those in whom no acceptable etiology for the cardiomyopathy is known. When all patients with heart muscle disease in the United States are considered, very few with cardiomyopathy fail to reveal the cause of their illness, i.e., relatively few have idiopathic cardiomyopathy.

The *secondary* cardiomyopathies are those in which the etiology of the heart muscle disease is reasonably well established and the etiologic agent or circumstance is known. However, it is not logical to limit the term cardiomyopathy, even when secondary, to situations in which only the myocardial pathology dominates the clinical picture. For reasons discussed below, we included postpartal and alcoholic cardiomyopathy in the secondary category rather than consider them idiopathic, as proposed by others (60).

The classification of cardiomyopathies into congestive, obstructive, and restrictive (constrictive) types (36) limits the physician in his diagnosis to only the late and usually terminal and irreversible stages of myocardial disease. This classification clearly indicates the physiologic state of the late or terminal stages of the cardiomyopathy; however, when this form of classification is employed, the cardiologist is usually consulted when it is too late to cure the patient or to employ preventive measures. Moreover, it is abundantly clear that there is a great overlap among these forms of cardiomyopathy and none is necessarily specific for any particular etiologic type of heart disease. Certainly, by the time the disease has progressed to one of these categories of myocardial disease, there is relatively little to be offered therapeutically to effect a cure. Thus, this particular classification is of little value to the clinician and even less to his patients, except in diagnosis and understanding of the hemodynamic state at the time. Finally, the general practitioner and internist are the physicians who will see patients with cardiomyopathy early and will be the ones who will have the opportunities for prevention, early care, and cures. Early detection of active etiologic agents is necessary for prevention, and early diagnosis is necessary for cure.

Most of the diseases listed in the secondary category of the cardiomyopathies are noncontroversial. However, some of those listed are not accepted by all physicians (vide infra). Only some of the specific cardiomyopathies are discussed, but the general principles of clinical care indicated for these selected cardiomyopathies apply to all cardiomyopathies.

Alcoholic Cardiomyopathy

Cardiomyopathy caused by excessive alcohol ingestion is becoming firmly accepted by physicians (13). The term *alcoholic cardiomyopathy* implies that alcohol alone may produce myocardial disease and that, although alcohol may produce and may also contribute to the production of heart muscle disease, associated nutritional disturbances, or toxins in alcohol, or both may be necessarily associated etiologic or conditioning factors or both. Clinicians have placed great emphasis on the nutritional aspects of alcoholic heart muscle disease (13) and have even frequently modified the criteria for beriberi heart disease to include patients with alcoholic cardiomyopathy (13). However, many chronic alcoholics with cardiomyopathy do not have the clinical features of nutritional heart disease nor do they respond to therapy with appropriate vitamins or other nutritional substances (6, 26, 29, 31). Furthermore, an adequate diet is consumed by many patients with alcoholism and cardiomyopathy. These data, however, do not preclude, in an individual patient, the possibility that other toxic substances, malnutrition, and other agents, such as cobalt (53), can contribute to the pathogenesis of the myocardial disease and that alcohol may act as a conditioning factor for toxins and other noxious agents, such as viruses (15).

Some investigators still doubt that alcohol alone can produce cardiomyopathy (36). Lack of differences between the drinking habits of patients with and without cardiomyopathy is cited as one reason for this doubt. Yet, all patients who drink do not develop cirrhosis of the liver, but the whole spectrum of cirrhosis has now been produced by alcohol in subhuman primates (63). That there is variation in individual sensitivity to alcohol is well known. Some people are extremely sensitive to alcohol. This is readily detectable for the central nervous system. Whereas improvement in the cardiomyopathy following abstinence from alcohol has not been noted by some observers (36), we and others have noted dramatic results (16, 59). Again, the response to therapy is certainly related to the extent of the damage, i.e., whether or not the disease is in the early or late stage.

Twenty-one percent of 97 patients with a history of considerable alcohol intake had pathologic evidence of congestive heart failure when examined at necropsy (68). Moreover, 108 of 240 hearts from patients with Laennec's cirrhosis weighed greater than 400 g, with 42 exceeding 500 g (52). Some reports indicate an incidence of 60 percent (48) to 83 percent (1) of instances of cardiomyopathy being due to alcohol.

Observations in man and experimental animals indicate that alcohol alone may act as a myocardial toxin, as well as a toxin for other tissues throughout the body (19). Animal experiments have shown metabolic disturbances (45, 55, 58) as well as structural damage (10, 22) following the ingestion of alcohol. Physiologic studies in animals also revealed depression of myocardial function following ingestion of alcohol (47, 70).

Acute administration of alcohol to normal man has been shown to reduce mechanical efficiency of the heart (51), and even one alcoholic drink will alter the electrocardiogram of some people with heart disease (37). Chronic ingestion of ethanol induces leakage of cardiac enzymes into the coronary sinus blood, even in the absence of clinical evidence of heart disease, or metabolic disturbances (73, 74). Thus, important metabolic and physiologic myocardial changes are produced by ingestion of alcohol.

The histopathology and electron microscopic changes of alcoholic cardiomyopathy are not specific (7). This is not surprising since the heart, as well as other organs, is limited in the manner in which it can react to noxious stimuli. However, the pathology of alcoholic cardiomyopathy differs greatly from that of coronary heart disease in that the coronary arteries are usually widely patent in patients with alcoholic cardiomyopathy and usually remarkably free from arteriosclerotic plaques.

Fully developed alcoholic cardiomyopathy is characterized by a large, pale, flabby, hypertrophied heart with diffuse areas of myocardial degeneration, fibrosis, and occasional endocardial thickening. Although no gross or light microscopic changes may be seen in early stages of the disease, electron microscopy may reveal extensive ultrastructural degeneration (42). Because of its ability to detect early and subtle ultrastructural change, the electron microscope has been most valuable in helping to establish alcohol as a myocardial toxin. Swollen mitochondria with fragmented cristae, swollen sarcoplasmic reticulum and disrupted myofibrils, mitochondrial inclusions, increased number of lysosomes, and lipofuscin granules are ultrastructural changes seen in hearts obtained at necropsy from patients with clinical alcoholic cardiomyopathy (42) and have also been noted in needlebiopsies from living patients (2). It is important to note that similar electron microscopic changes can be produced in adequately fed mice that consume large quantities of a variety of alcoholic beverages, including pure ethyl alcohol (10, 22).

The clinical course of alcoholic cardiomyopathy is partially distinctive. The disease usually has its onset in the second to sixth decades of life, a slightly younger age than one usually anticipates for arteriosclerotic heart disease and ischemic cardiomyopathy. The initial symptoms may be so mild as to suggest anxiety, tension, or smoking as the cause rather than excessive ethanol intake. Such symptoms as mild dyspnea on exertion and palpitation frequently represent the disturbances in cardiac rhythm.

As will be discussed below, the physical examination during the early stages of alcoholic cardiomyopathy may reveal very little. Later, signs and symptoms of congestive heart failure common to all cardiomyopathies will be present. The physical findings may be different from those produced by thiamine deficiency, such as wide pulse pressure.

Viral Cardiomyopathy

Viral cardiomyopathy deserves special attention because increasing evidence implicates viruses in the cardiomyopathy (15). Many patients with viral cardiomyopathy are, no doubt, frequently considered to have idiopathic cardiomyopathy. The exact incidence of viral cardiomyopathy and, indeed, of viral diseases in general, remains unknown primarily because of lack of adequate clinical diagnostic facilities in general hospitals and diagnostic laboratories. It is well established that viruses cause heart disease in man (15, 46, 56). They may produce disease by direct invasion of the myocytes, involvement of the central nervous system with secondary myocardial damage, disturbance of myocardial metabolism, disturbance of vascular supply to the myocardium, and possible elaboration of toxins locally. The role of cellular and humoral immune reactions, so-called *allergic* or *immune* phenomena, have attracted recent interest as mechanisms that may also be responsible for myocardial damage (15). The immunity state may be a response to fragmented tissue released by the viral damage. The precise mechanisms whereby viruses cause acute or chronic cardiomyopathy are not known. The initial loss and partial destruction of functioning myocytes with subsequent healing with scar formation may account for chronic myocardial disease.

It is clear that viral cardiomyopathy was ignored for many years and that premortem diagnosis was not made frequently enough (66, 67). It has been suggested that some instances of chronic idiopathic cardiomyopathy may represent the residual state of acute viral myocarditis (65). Presently, only a few viruses are known to be highly cardiotropic for man. Studies of these viruses will stimulate interest in searching for other cardiotropic viruses yet unknown.

One group of cardiotropic viruses are the picornaviruses. The Coxsackieviruses are prevalent infective agents of man, especially of infants and children. These viruses may serve as a prototype for other cardiotropic viruses, some yet to be discovered. As many as 39 percent of patients with unexplained myocarditis and pericarditis have evidence of Coxsackie B viral infection (39). In one report, 33 percent of patients infected with Coxsackie B viruses were found to develop some form of myocardial disease (40). In another report, 3 of 42 adult patients with clinical evidence of Coxsackie virus B myocarditis developed chronic cardiomegaly (69). Another study of 22 similar patients revealed 5 who had evidence of permanent myocardial damage following viral myocarditis (64). An episode of active myocarditis developed in 7 of these 22 patients.

It is possible that in some instances toxic agents, such as alcohol, may serve as conditioning factors for viral infections of the myocardium. For example, virus-like particles were found in the heart of a patient with alcoholic cardiomyopathy who died a few days after an influenza-like illness (41). Since many viruses are known to produce acute myocarditis, it is likely that more and more cardiomyopathies will be found to be due to viral infections. Conditioning factors such as steroids, radiation, fatigue, physical trauma, malnutrition, toxic agents (chemicals, insect sprays, fumes, and so forth), thermal stress, catecholamines, and drugs may play an important role in the development of viral infections of the myocardium.

That Coxsackie viral infections of the myocardium are common was evidenced by 30 percent of routine postmortem specimens of myocardium which showed the presence of Coxsackie viral antigen by immunofluorescent antibody staining technique (25). Slightly over 50 percent of unselected hearts of infants and children examined at routine necropsy revealed interstitial myocarditis, and slightly over 50 percent of these were associated with the presence of Coxsackie B viral antigen detected by the immunofluorescent staining method (24). These findings in man are supported by a large number of laboratory studies in experimental animals (15).

The clinical manifestations of viral heart disease may be sufficiently characteristic to permit one to suspect the diagnosis clinically in patients. It is now evident that many patients with acute viral illnesses will manifest evidence of myocardial disease, at least as indicated by changes in the electrocardiogram. In one study of 18 patients admitted to hospital with proved viral or mycoplasma infections, 6 showed electrocardiographic evidence of myocardial disease (44).

The diagnosis of viral heart disease is usually indirect during the acute illness (11). However, in most instances, the episode of myocarditis will follow a febrile illness, usually upper respiratory, after a latent period of several days during which time the patient is asymptomatic. However, the patient may not inform his physician of the previous viral infection, so that the clinician does not associate the infection with the myocarditis or cardiomyopathy. The more general criteria for the diganosis of early and late cardiomyopathy will be discussed below.

It is possible that any infectious agent could produce cardiomyopathy. However, the exact role of viruses in the production of cardiomyopathy will never be appreciated until adequate facilities for routine clinical diagnosis and study of viral infections are as available as those that now exist for bacteriologic diseases.

Postpartal Cardiomyopathy

Postpartal cardiomyopathy is a clearly defined clinical entity when restricted to women who develop signs and symptoms of heart disease between the second and twelfth weeks following delivery and in whom the presence of a normal cardiovascular system can be documented during the entire period of gestation (54, 72). Of course, no other recognizable cause for the heart disease should be present. Those clinicians who do not accept postpartal cardiomyopathy as a distinct diagnostic entity usually attribute the heart disease to poor nutrition, toxemia of pregnancy, previous hypertension, a specific myocarditis, or possible drug reactions (3, 5). The disease is often termed *peripartal* cardiomyopathy. This term, of course, means the cardiac disease can develop prior to delivery. However, by our criteria, this is not postpartal heart disease. More recently, it has been argued that hypertension plays a significant role in the development of postpartal cardiomyopathy (8). This is not true from our own experience and rigid diagnostic criteria. Furthermore, many of the patients do not have hypertension.

None of the above suggestions as to etiology explains the clinical picture of patients who satisfy the strict criteria we suggested for postpartal heart disease. It must be remembered that patients with postpartal heart disease may be well nourished (21). Patients with typical postpartal heart disease are not hypertensive (21, 62). The recent suggestion that viruses may play a role in the pathogenesis of postpartal cardiomyopathy (15, 64) is interesting. It fits with experimental evidence showing the pregnant state to be a conditioning factor for viral infections (32). The production of antimyocardial antibodies by the fetus has been suggested as a pathogenetic mechanism (4), but sufficient supporting evidence is lacking.

Although, as discussed above, the complete pathophysiology of postpartal cardiomyopathy is not known, it is still important to recognize the association of cardiomyopathy with pregnancy so that proper treatment of and advice to the patients are possible. Thus, we place postpartal cardiomyopathy in the secondary rather than the idiopathic category of cardiomyopathies. The incidence of postpartal cardiomyopathy varies with different reports from approximately once per 1,300 live births to once per 3,000 to 4,000 confinements (21). The peak incidence of the disease occurs during the second and third decades of life (childbearing years), and a large percentage of the reported patients are black (18).

Ischemic Cardiomyopathy

Ischemic cardiomyopathy is the most common type of cardiomyopathy in the United States, and the etiology is almost always coronary arteriosclerosis. Yet, this common form of cardiomyopathy due to ischemic heart disease was ignored for many years (17, 20). This was due primarily to two reasons: (a) Many physicians considered obstructive lesions of the coronary arteries to produce disease in an all-or-none fashion, i.e., they considered myocardial ischemia that was not severe enough to produce necrosis to be unimportant, and (b) the term cardiomyopathy, by definition, excluded hearts with myocardial diseases of known cause, especially when significant coronary artery disease was present (33, 36, 43).

Myocardial ischemia that is not sufficiently marked to produce large areas of myocardial necrosis can still produce cellular damage (38). When extra work is required of the myocardium in the presence of partial coronary arterial obstruction, then significant ischemia occurs. When the rate of coronary blood flow is only adequate to meet the needs of the patient at rest, it is easy to understand why virtually all cells of the hearts of patients with advanced ischemic cardiomyopathy develop disease during the stresses of living (17). The morphologic changes noted at necropsy are not always visible grossly or even detectable with light microscopy. Electron microscopy usually reveals the ultrastructural damage (17).

The process of ischemic cardiomyopathy actually begins during the very early phases of the coronary disease (17). Electrocardiographic or hemodynamic evidence of ischemic cardiomyopathy may be present prior to the development of x-ray evidence of cardiac enlargement or to the development of symptoms of severe congestive heart failure (75). The incidence and severity of ischemic cardiomyopathy parallel the incidence, severity, and duration of coronary arteriosclerosis. Ischemic cardiomyopathy, therefore, is primarily a disease of older people. Although the clinical course is usually characterized by angina pectoris and myocardial infarction terminating at times with congestive heart failure, the course can be atypical and quite variable (17, 57).

Senile Cardiomyopathy

Senile cardiomyopathy is heart muscle disease related to the ageing process itself (14). Myocardial function declines over the years (9), although the precise mechanisms remain unclear (9, 14, 28). Characteristic changes in the myocardium of Drosophila (23) and rats (71) are associated with ageing. Predictable changes are also observed in the hearts of senescent man (9).

Older patients may, of course, have more than one disease affecting the heart (9). However, in one study, no explanation could be found for one-third of the cases of heart failure occurring in older patients (61). Usually, such heart failure becomes apparent only when the heart is stressed, e.g., as with fever, infections, anemia, thyroid disturbances, physical exertion, or psychic stress.

Diagnostic Criteria for Cardiomyopathy

Once the clinician understands the scope of cardiomyopathy, recognition and treatment become easier. Although the development of cardiomyopathy is a continuous spectrum, we present below three general stages of development to assist the clinician in diagnosis and treatment of his patients.

Potential Cardiomyopathy

Potential cardiomyopathy exists when circumstances and etiologic factors are present which might be expected to produce myocardial damage, but no myocardial disease is clinically detectable. If physicians expect to practice preventive cardiology, this stage of development of cardiomyopathy must be recognized and constantly kept in mind.

For example, a man chronically consuming large quantities of alcohol is in danger of developing heart muscle disease. In one study (59) abnormal cardiac physiology was demonstrated in alcoholic patients when they were stressed even though they had no clinically detectable heart disease at rest. Surely, a stage of heart disease must exist prior even to that which can be brought out by stress with methods presently available for evaluation.

Patients with any acute viral or other infections should be considered to have potential heart muscle disease. Obviously, infection with a known cardiotropic virus increases the likelihood of myocardial damage by the virus. It is known that, during acute febrile illnesses, electrocardiographic evidence of myocardial involvement is often present (15, 44). These changes may be reflected only by slight alterations in the ST segments and T waves. However, there must be a critical number of diseased myocytes to change the electrocardiogram in a detectable fashion. Nevertheless, myocardial disease surely must exist prior to the time that the repolarization process becomes abnormal.

A patient with diabetes mellitus should be regarded as having potential ischemic and/or diabetic (metabolic) cardiomyopathy. Likewise, a patient with thyrotoxicosis will develop cardiac muscle pathology unless the thyroid disease is cured early. Once the concept of potential cardiomyopathy is recognized, the physician can apply the same concept to all of the diseases listed in the diagnostic classification shown in Table 1. This concept is obviously applicable to other organ systems. The therapeutic and preventive implications of recognizing the etiologic agent are clear.

Early Cardiomyopathy

At the stage of early cardiomyopathy, the disease is barely detectable clinically, although the clinical manifestations may be extremely subtle and may be limited to changes noted on history taking, physical examination or routine laboratory tests (ECG, chest x-ray, ECHO, and so forth). The electrocardiogram is most likely to reveal earliest myocardial disease. The value of the ECG cannot be overemphasized. Such an early stage of cardiomyopathy obviously precludes classification of the disease as congestive, obstructive, or restrictive. When very early, the disease has not yet produced such late and terminal stages of myocardial damage. It is at the *early* stages of cardiomyopathy that the *etiology* may be most apparent!

History-taking is an important aspect of the examination of the patient with early cardiomyopathy (16). For example, previous viral infections (flu, coryza, URI, and so on), exposure to toxic agents, poor dietary habits, alcohol ingestion, hypertension and other problems can usually only be evaluated properly from the history. In taking the history from a patient with suspected early cardiomyopathy, every aspect of the patient's life, occupation, past medical records (insurance examination, Army physicals, pre-employment examinations, and the like), patent medicine habits, exposure to toxic agents, and so forth should be carefully explored. This tedious task often supplies the clue to the etiology of the heart disease and, in turn, results in proper care of the patient.

Gradual onset of mild exertional dyspnea and palpitation are frequent symptoms of early cardiomyopathy. Palpitation is often the result of premature contractions or other cardiac arrhythmias associated with myocardial damage. Atrial fibrillation occurring with no apparent cause may frequently be the first indication of cardiomegaly.

The physical examination in early cardiomyopathy may reveal minimal evidence of heart disease. However, inappropriate tachycardia, minimal cardiomegaly, abnormally loud fourth heart sound, or an arrhythmia may be present early.

The electrocardiograph is the most sensitive instrument for the detection of very early cardiomyopathy. Early changes are usually seen in the T waves. Several types of T waves ("spinous," "dimpled," or "cloven") have been described for early alcoholic cardiomyopathy (31). Such changes may be present in the ECG recorded from patients with other causes of myocardial disease. As mentioned above, various types of cardiac arrhythmias may also occur early. Electrocardiographic evidence of ventricular hypertrophy may be seen early. In early ischemic cardiomyopathy "ischemic T waves" may be present, and often only following exercise.

The chest x-ray of the patient with early cardiomyopathy may reveal only minimal cardiac enlargement, if any at all. The distinction of such enlargement from pericardial effusion can be made by echocardiography (ECHO) or carboangiography. The ECHO may reveal, in addition to minimal cardiomegaly, other evidence of cardiac dysfunction (34). In the case of asymmetric septal hypertrophy and/or idiopathic hypertrophic subaortic stenosis, the ECHO can be extremely useful.

Valuable negative information is also obtainable from the history, physical examination, and routine laboratory procedures. When this negative information is combined with positive information, cardiac catheterization is seldom, if ever, needed to make a diagnosis.

Late Cardiomyopathy

The late stage of cardiomyopathy is characterized by signs and symptoms of left and right ventricular congestive heart failure. Routine laboratory studies (chest x-ray, ECG, ECHO, and the like) will show evidence of diffuse myocardial disease. Cardiac catheterization is never needed by the experienced and master cardiologist for diagnosis or management of cardiomyopathy.

Comments

As indicated above, the most important aspects of the management of cardiomyopathy are prevention and early diagnosis. To prevent cardiomyopathy it behooves the physician to recognize the presence or potential presence of etiologic agents that can produce cardiomyopathy. These etiologic factors should be removed immediately or avoided. For example, the stopping of alcohol consumption will prevent people from developing alcoholic cardiomyopathy. A person who never drinks alcoholic beverages cannot develop alcoholic cardiomyopathy. This concept is well exemplified with the prevention of cobalt cardiomyopathy. Since cobalt is no longer added to beer, cobalt damage to the myocardium from beer has been eliminated. Such principles in prevention can be applied to other forms of cardiomyopathy.

We are of the opinion that patients who develop febrile illnesses from viral infections should remain at bed rest for two days after the fever has disappeared and should avoid physical stress and fatigue until they have fully recovered from the viral infections in order to prevent viral cardiomyopathy. To be even more thorough, an ECG should be recorded during viral infections and if the ECG is abnormal the patient should remain at bed rest and under highly restricted physical activity until the tracing returns to normal. As with all diseases, it is important for the physician to recognize the potential situation for the production of cardiomyopathy and manage that situation promptly.

Early diagnosis is essential for a high incidence of cure of cardiomyopathy. When the late stages of the disease develop, an irreversible state exists. The prognosis for the late stages is extremely poor. It is unfortunate that some clinicians equate cardiomyopathy with the late stages and depend upon the manifestations of the late stages for diagnosis and even for classification. All disease states have a beginning, and it is at the beginning and before irreversible structural and functional damage occurs that the physician has the best opportunity to offer the most to his patient. Success in arriving at an early diagnosis depends upon a thorough knowledge and understanding of heart muscle disease. If the potential and possible cardiomyopathetic illnesses are kept in mind when a patient is seen, an early diagnosis is readily and correctly reached. Then, proper therapy must be vigorously instituted.

Heart muscle disease is common—much more common than physicians realize. For example, an abnormal electrocardiogram is pathognomonic evidence of heart muscle disease. The physician is obligated to follow up with a complete investigation and diagnosis, and to establish a prognosis and vigorous management. The muscle of the heart performs the work of the heart. And, the heart must work even when it is sick.

Summary

A broad definition of cardiomyopathy is necessary to prepare for the best care of the patient. It should therefore include all diseases of the myocardium, even those due to myocardial ischemia and senescence. An etiologic classification is useful and can be conveniently divided into primary (idiopathic) and secondary (etiology known) categories. Present evidence indicates that alcoholic and postpartal cardiomyopathies should be considered as secondary types. The role of viruses in the production of heart disease is probably large, and intensive efforts should be directed towards establishing the true incidence of viral cardiomyopathy and the specific types of viruses involved. Ischemic cardiomyopathy is the most common form of cardiomyopathy and is a true form of heart muscle disease.

Cardiomyopathy may be considered clinically as existing in three stages: *potential*, without clinical evidence of heart disease but with circumstances present which can produce cardiomyopathy; *early*, without advanced heart disease but with early, subtle clinical abnormalities, often manifested only in the ECG; and *late*, characterized by congestive heart failure and its complications.

Prevention and early diagnosis with early vigorous treatment cannot be overemphasized when considering cardiomyopathy.

Acknowledgment

This study was supported by Grant HL-14789 from the National Heart and Lung Institute of the U.S. Public Health Service, the Rudolph Matas Memorial Fund for the Kate Prewitt Hess Laboratory, the Rowell A. Billups Fund for Research in Heart Disease and the Feazel Laboratory.

References

1. Alexander, C. S. Idiopathic heart disease. I. Analysis of 100 cases, with special reference to chronic alcoholism. Am. J. Med., 41:213, 1966.
2. —— Electron microscopic observations in alcoholic heart disease. Br. Heart J., 29:200, 1967.

3. Bashour, F. and Winchell, P. "Postpartal" heart disease—A syndrome? Ann. Intern. Med., 40:803, 1954.
4. Becker, F. F. and Taube, H. Myocarditis of obscure etiology associated with pregnancy. N. Engl. J. Med., 266:62, 1962.
5. Benchimol, A. B., Carneiro, R. D., and Schlesinger, P. Post-partum heart disease. Br. Heart J., 21:89, 1959.
6. Brigden, W. Uncommon myocardial diseases; the non-coronary cardiomyopathies. Lancet, 2:1179, 1243, 1957.
7. —— Alcoholic cardiomyopathy. *In* Brest, A., ed., Burch, G., guest ed. Cardiovascular Clinics: Cardiomyopathy. Philadelphia, F. A. Davis Co., 1972, Vol. 4, No. 1, pp. 187–201.
8. Brockington, I. F. Postpartum hypertensive heart failure. Am. J. Cardiol., 27:650, 1971.
9. Burch, G. E. Interesting aspects of geriatric cardiology. Am. Heart J., 89:99, 1975.
10. Burch, G. E., Colcolough, H. L., Harb, J. M., and Tsui, C. Y. The effect of ingestion of ethyl alcohol, wine and beer on the myocardium of mice. Am. J. Cardiol., 27:522, 1971.
11. —— and DePasquale, N. P. Viral myocarditis. *In* Wolstenholme, G. E. W. and O'Connor, M., ed. Ciba Foundation Symposium on Cardiomyopathies. London, J. and A. Churchill, Ltd., 1964, pp. 376–407.
12. —— and DePasquale, N. P. Recognition and prevention of cardiomyopathy. Circulation, 42:A-47, 1970.
13. —— and Giles, T. D. Alcoholic cardiomyopathy: Concept of the disease and its treatment. Am. J. Med., 50:141, 1971.
14. —— and Giles, T. D. Senile cardiomyopathy. J. Chron. Dis., 24:1, 1971.
15. —— and Giles, T. D. The role of viruses in the production of heart disease. Am. J. Cardiol., 29:231, 1972.
16. —— and Giles, T. D. Diagnosis and treatment of cardiomyopathy. *In* Changing Concepts in Cardiovascular Disease. Proceedings of the American College of Cardiology. Baltimore, The Williams and Wilkins Co., 1972, pp. 80–95.
17. —— and Giles, T. D. Ischemic cardiomyopathy: Diagnostic, pathophysiologic and therapeutic considerations. *In* Brest, A., ed., Burch, G., guest ed. Cardiovascular Clinics: Cardiomyopathy. Philadelphia, F. A. Davis Co., 1972, Vol. 4, No. 1, pp. 203–220.
18. —— and Giles, T. D. Incidence of cardiomyopathy. *In* Bajusz, E., and Rona, G., ed., with Brink, A. J. and Lochner, A. Recent Advances in Cardiac Structure and Metabolism: Cardiomyopathies. Baltimore, University Park Press, 1973, Vol. 2, pp. 59–76.
19. —— and Giles, T. D. Alcoholic cardiomyopathy. *In* Kissin, B., and Begleiter, H., ed. The Biology of Alcoholism: Clinical Pathology. New York, Plenum Press, 1974, Vol. 3, pp. 435–460.
20. —— Giles, T. D., and Colcolough, H. L. Ischemic cardiomyopathy. Am. Heart J., 79:291, 1970.
21. —— Giles, T. D., and Tsui, C. Y. Postpartal cardiomyopathy. *In* Brest, A., ed., Burch, G., guest ed. Cardiovascular Clinics: Cardiomyopathy. Philadelphia, F. A. Davis Co., 1972, Vol. 4, No. 1, pp. 269–282.
22. —— Harb, J. M., Colcolough, H. L., and Tsui, C. Y. The effect of prolonged consumption of beer, wine and ethanol on the myocardium of the mouse. The Johns Hopkins Med. J., 129:130, 1971.
23. —— Sohal, R., and Fairbanks, L. D. Ultrastructural changes in Drosophila heart with age. Arch. Pathol., 89:128, 1970.
24. —— Sun, S. C., Chu, K. C., Sohal, R. S., and Colcolough, H. L. Interstitial and Coxsackie virus B myocarditis in infants and children. J.A.M.A., 203:1, 1968.
25. —— Sun, S. C., Colcolough, H. L., Sohal, R. S., and DePasquale, N. P. Coxsackie virus valvulitis and myocarditis observed at routine autopsy. Experientia, 23:1041, 1967.
26. —— and Walsh, J. J. Cardiac insufficiency in chronic alcoholism. Am. J. Cardiol., 6:864, 1960.
27. Davies, J. N. P. African endomyocardial fibrosis. *In* Brest, A., ed, Burch, G., guest ed. Cardiovascular Clinics: Cardiomyopathy. Philadelphia, F. A. Davis Co., 1972, Vol. 4, No. 1, pp. 345–359.
28. Dock, W. Cardiomyopathies of the senescent and senile. *In* Brest, A., ed., Burch, G., guest ed. Cardiovascular Clinics: Cardiomyopathy. Philadelphia, F. A. Davis Co., 1972, Vol. 4, No. 1, pp. 361–373.
29. Eliaser, M. Jr. and Giansiracusa, F. J. The heart and alcohol. Calif. Med., 84:234, 1956.
30. Epstein, S. E., Henry, W. L., Clark, C. E., Roberts, W. C., Maron, B. J., Ferrans, V. J., Redwood, D. R., and Morrow, A. G. NIH Conference: Asymmetric septal hypertrophy. Ann. Intern. Med., 81:650, 1974.
31. Evans, W. Alcoholic cardiomyopathy. Am. Heart J., 61:556, 1961.

32. Faber, P. A. and Glasgow, L. A. Viral myocarditis during pregnancy: Encephalomyocarditis virus infection in mice. Am. Heart J., 80:96, 1970.
33. Fejfar, Z. Definition and classification of the cardiomyopathies. Pathol. Microbiol., 35:17, 1970.
34. Giles, T. D., Burch, G. E., and Martinez, E. C. An echocardiographic study of cardiomyopathy. To be published.
35. Goodwin, J. F., Gordon, H., Hollman, A., and Bishop, M. B. Clinical aspects of cardiomyopathy. Brit. Med. J., 1:69, 1961.
36. —— and Oakley, C. M. The cardiomyopathies. Br. Heart J., 34:545, 1972.
37. Gould, L., Reddy, C. V. R., Patel, N., and Gomprecht, R. F. Effects of a cocktail on the human conduction system. Clin. Res., 22:277A, 1974 (abstr.).
38. Gould, S. E. and Ioannides, G. Ischemic heart disease. *In* Gould, S. E., ed. Pathology of the Heart and Blood Vessels. Springfield, Ill., Charles C. Thomas, 1968, pp. 601–648.
39. Grist, N. R. and Bell, E. J. Coxsackie viruses and the heart (Editorial). Am. Heart J., 77:295, 1969.
40. Helin, M., Savola, J., and Lapinleimu, K. Cardiac manifestations during a Coxsackie B_5 epidemic. Br. Med. J., 3:97, 1968.
41. Hibbs, R. G., Ferrans, V. J., Black, W. C., Walsh, J. J., and Burch, G. E. Virus-like particles in the heart of a patient with cardiomyopathy: An electron microscopic and histochemical study. Am. Heart J., 69:327, 1965.
42. Hibbs, R. G., Ferrans, V. J., Black, W. C., Weilbaecher, D. G., Walsh, J. J., and Burch, G. E. Alcoholic cardiomyopathy: An electron microscopic study. Am. Heart J., 69:766, 1965.
43. Hudson, R. E. B. The cardiomyopathies: Order from chaos. Am. J. Cardiol., 25:70, 1970.
44. Lewes, D., Rainford, D. J., and Lane, W. F. Symptomless myocarditis and myalgia in viral and *Mycoplasma pneumoniae* infections. Br. Heart J., 36:924, 1974.
45. Lieber, C. S., Spritz, N., and DeCarli, L. M. Accumulation of triglycerides in heart and kidney after alcohol ingestion. J. Clin. Invest., 45:1041, 1966 (abstr.).
46. Lyon, E. Virus Diseases and the Cardiovascular System. New York, Grune and Stratton, 1956.
47. Maines, J. E. III and Aldinger, E. E. Myocardial depression accompanying chronic consumption of alcohol. Am. Heart J., 73:55, 1967.
48. Massumi, R. A., Rios, J. C., Gooch, A. S., Nutter, D., DeVita, V. T., and Datlow, D. W. Primary myocardial disease: Report of fifty cases and review of the subject. Circulation, 31:19, 1965.
49. Mattingly, T. W. Changing concepts of myocardial diseases. J.A.M.A., 191:33, 1965.
50. Mattingly, T. W. The clinical concept of primary myocardial disease: A classification and a few notes on management and prognosis. Circulation, 32:845, 1965.
51. Mitchell, J. H. and Cohen, L. S. Alcohol and the heart. Mod. Concepts Cardiovasc. Dis., 39:109, 1970.
52. Morgan, R. R. Heart disease and alcoholism. Circulation, 24:1001, 1961.
53. Morin, Y. and Daniel, P. Quebec beer drinkers' cardiomyopathy: Etiological considerations. Can. Med. Assoc. J., 97:926, 1967.
54. Musser, J. H., Sodeman, W. A., and Turner, R. H. Heart failure or acute nephritis with onset about 3 weeks after delivery. Ann. Intern. Med., 12:739, 1938.
55. Opie, L. H. Metabolism of the heart in health and disease. Part III. Am. Heart J., 77:383, 1969.
56. Pankey, G. A. Effect of viruses on the cardiovascular system. Am. J. Med. Sci., 250:103, 1965.
57. Raftery, E. B., Banks, D. C., and Oram, S. Occlusive disease of the coronary arteries presenting as primary congestive cardiomyopathy. Lancet, 2:1146, 1969.
58. Regan, T. J., Koroxenidis, G., Moschos, C. B., Oldewurtel, H. A., Lehan, P. H., and Hellems, H. K. The acute metabolic and hemodynamic responses of the left ventricle to ethanol. J. Clin. Invest., 45:270, 1966.
59. Regan, T. J., Levinson, G. E., Oldewurtel, H. A., Frank, M. J., Weisse, A. B., and Moschos, C. B. Ventricular function in noncardiacs with alcoholic fatty liver: Role of ethanol in the production of cardiomyopathy. J. Clin. Invest., 48:397, 1969.
60. Roberts, W. C. and Ferrans, V. J. Morphologic observations in the cardiomyopathies. *In* Fowler, N. O., ed. Myocardial Diseases. New York, Grune and Stratton, 1973, pp. 59–115.
61. Rose, G. A. and Wilson, R. R. Unexplained heart failure in the aged. Br. Heart J., 21:511, 1959.
62. Rosen, S. M. Puerperal cardiomyopathy. Br. Med. J., 2:5, 1959.
63. Rubin, E. and Lieber, C. S. Fatty liver, alcoholic hepatitis and cirrhosis produced by alcohol in primates. N. Engl. J. Med., 290:128, 1974.
64. Sainani, G. S., Krompotic, E., and Slodki, S. J. Adult heart disease due to the Coxsackie virus B infection. Medicine, 47:133, 1968.

65. Sanders, V. Idiopathic diseases of myocardium: A prospective study. Arch. Intern. Med., 112:661, 1963.
66. Saphir, O. Myocarditis: A general review with analysis of 240 cases. Arch. Pathol., 32:1000, 1941.
67. —— Myocarditis: A general review with analysis of 240 cases. Arch. Pathol., 33:88, 1942.
68. Schenk, E. A. and Cohen, J. The heart in chronic alcoholism: Clinical and pathological findings. Pathol. Microbiol., 35:96, 1970.
69. Smith, W. G. Coxsackie B myopericarditis in adults. Am. Heart J., 80:34, 1970.
70. Spann, J. F. Jr., Mason, D. T., Beiser, G. D., and Gold, H. K. Actions of ethanol on the contractile state of the normal and failing cat papillary muscle. Clin. Res., 16:249, 1968 (abstr.).
71. Sulkin, N. M. Senescence as reflection of cellular changes. Triangle, 8:304, 1968.
72. Walsh, J. J. and Burch, G. E. Postpartal heart disease. Arch. Intern. Med., 108:817, 1961.
73. Wendt, V. E., Wu, C., Balcon, R., Doty, G., and Bing, R. J. Hemodynamic and metabolic effects of chronic alcoholism in man. Am. J. Cardiol., 15:175, 1965.
74. —— Ajluni, R., and Bruce, T. A. Acute effects of alcohol on the human myocardium. Am. J. Cardiol., 17:804, 1966.
75. Yatteau, R. F., Peter, R. H., Behar, V. S., Bartel, A. G., Rosati, R. A., and Kong, Y. Ischemic cardiomyopathy: The myopathy of coronary artery disease. Natural history and results of medical versus surgical treatment. Am. J. Cardiol., 34:520, 1974.

Chapter 14 Therapeutic Approach to Idiopathic Hypertrophic Subaortic Stenosis

RONALD S. GOTTLIEB, M.D. and EDWARD K. CHUNG, M.D.

General Considerations

An understanding of the pathophysiology of idiopathic hypertrophic subaortic stenosis (IHSS) began in the late 1950s and early 1960s. Investigative studies by Brock and Braunwald *et al.* have contributed significantly for better understanding of IHSS (4, 5). Unlike valvular, subvalvular, and supravalvular fixed stenosis, the degree of outflow tract obstruction in IHSS varies from beat to beat. The participation of contracting myocardium in the formation of the obstruction renders surgical approach more difficult and, at the same time, provides a unique susceptibility to pharmacologic therapy.

Surgical therapeutic approaches were developed before beta-blocking agents became available for clinical use. Surgical approaches included myotomy, or myectomy, or both, of hypertrophied muscle to relieve obstruction. More recently, various other surgical procedures have been proposed.

To evaluate therapeutic maneuvers appropriately, the natural history of this entity must be well documented. Ideally, the natural history should be uniform but, unfortunately, in IHSS it is extremely variable. Therefore, the therapeutic approach in IHSS is further complicated and results in significant controversy.

In general, disorders in which good objective data can be obtained are easier to evaluate therapeutically since it is relatively easy to compare experimental results. Hemodynamic evaluation by cardiac catheterization is an excellent objective method for evaluating idiopathic hypertrophic subaortic stenosis. Nevertheless the information obtained during evaluation remains open to question because of the dynamic nature of the lesion, resulting in moment-to-moment changes in hemodynamic characteristics. Hence, data obtained at different occasions are not easily compared. The situation is somewhat improved by the judicious application of physiologic and pharmacologic maneuvers to increase the gradient, but comparison nevertheless remains difficult.

Significant controversy in the therapeutic approach to idiopathic hypertrophic subaortic stenosis cannot be avoided because of variable natural history, frequently changing hemodynamic characteristics, and relatively low incidence in addition to many available therapeutic methods. The purpose of this Chapter is to review the data that created the controversy and attempt to place it in perspective. A few representative and recent references have been chosen in an attempt to present a fair overview. No effort has been made to provide an encyclopedic or definitive bibliography. Hopefully, the reader will find this Chapter useful in choosing a therapeutic approach for his or her patient.

Clinical Data

At the present time there are three basic therapeutic approaches to idiopathic hypertrophic subaortic stenosis. These are (a) the pharmacologic approach with beta blocking agents, (b) the surgical approach using ventriculomyotomy with or without resection, and (c) replacement of the mitral valve with a low profile prosthesis. Although several different operative methods for myotomy and myectomy, with approach through the left ventricle, right ventricle, left atrium and aorta, have been devised, the information presently available seems to warrant considering these under a single category.

Pharmacologic Therapy

Beta-blocking agents are effective in the treatment of idiopathic hypertrophic subaortic stenosis because of the physiology of the normal ventricular myocardium and the pathophysiology of the ventricular septum. It is well documented that obstruction of the left ventricular outflow tract becomes worse when beta-adrenergic stimulating agents or digitalis preparations are used because the contractile force of the left ventricular myocardium is increased (3). The contractile force of normal myocardium is decreased by beta-blockade (13).

Using the physiologic data, Cohen *et al.* (7) and Cherian *et al.* (6) demonstrated for the first time that beta-blockade was a feasible approach to therapy. Since then evidence for the beneficial effect of beta-blockade on idiopathic hypertrophic subaortic stenosis has continued to accumulate. Sloman (26) studied 5 patients with proved muscular subaortic stenosis treated with propanolol. Four patients from his study improved symptomatically, although the improvement appears to have been mainly effected by a reduction in heart rate. Therapy had to be discontinued in the fifth patient because of fluid retention (26).

Flamm *et al.* (12) studied the efficacy of intravenous propanolol administration in 11 patients with idiopathic hypertrophic subaortic stenosis by cardiac catheterization. A variety of stimulating maneuvers were used to either produce or enhance an intraventricular gradient. They differentiated between latent, labile, and fixed obstruction and demonstrated that propanolol was of value in reducing spontaneous variations in the gradient, the increase in postexercise gradient, and the increase induced by isoproterenol. In one patient with fixed obstruction, symptoms became worse with propanolol. All patients with latent or labile gradients benefited symptomatically, and the authors considered propanolol the drug of choice in those groups.

Kristinsson (15) utilized exercise testing in the evaluation of both propanolol and practolol in the treatment of idiopathic hypertrophic subaortic stenosis. He demonstrated that myocardial oxygen consumption was reduced. Webb-Poplow (29) provided some insight into the mechanism of improvement by beta-blockade when he documented increased left ventricular compliance in those patients on the drug.

It should be noted that all beta-blocking agents are, however, not equally effective. Matlof and Harrison (17), using cardiac catheterization, demonstrated that intravenous propanolol was more effective than practolol. Hubner *et al.* (14) reached

Table 14-1. Beta-Blockade Therapy of Idiopathic Hypertrophic Subaortic Stenosis

Authors	No. of patients	Clinical improvement		Hemodynamic improvement	
		No. of patients	Percent	No. of patients	Percent
Cherian *et al.* (6)	13	10	77	3	23
Sloman (26)	5	4	80	—	—
Flamm *et al.* (12)	11	9	82	11	100
Kristinsson (15)	2	2	100	2	100
Webb-Peploe (29)	9	—	—	9	100
Hubner *et al.* (14)	16	16	100[a]	—	—
Stenson *et al.* (22)	13[b]	10	77	9	100
Powell *et al.* (28)	26	12	46	—	—

[a] Studied as a group. Only mean values presented.
[b] Only 9 of the 13 were evaluated hemodynamically.

the same conclusion in a double-blind study of 16 patients on oral propanolol and practolol therapy.

More recently long-term follow-up study of larger numbers of patients treated with beta-blockade has been carried out. Stenson *et al.* (28) studied 13 patients for an average of 17 months and 9 underwent follow-up catheterization. Most patients had a favourable response initially. However, the long-term clinical response tended to correlate best with the results of the second catheterization. They concluded that propanolol had a favorable effect on the patients' symptoms but did not appear to change the course of the underlying process of idiopathic hypertrophic subaortic stenosis. The nature of the gradient (i.e., latent, labile, or fixed) was not helpful in the prognosis.

Powell *et al.* (22) studied 29 patients in a fashion similar to that of Stenson *et al* (28). They were also able to demonstrate a beneficial symptomatic effect in most patients but stressed the difficulty of predicting which patients would stabilize or improve on oral drug therapy.

Table 14-1 summarizes some representative data from the literature showing the efficacy of beta-blocking agents on idiopathic hypertrophic subaortic stenosis. It is evident from these data that a great many patients can be symptomatically and hemodynamically improved by such treatment. However, it is less clear whether or not classifying the patients into latent, labile, or fixed categories is valuable in deciding who should be treated medically.

Ventriculomyotomy and Myectomy

Shortly after idiopathic hypertrophic subaortic stenosis was recognized as a distinct entity, various surgical procedures were developed rapidly to reduce or abolish left ventricular outflow obstruction. Namely, various surgical approaches included different types and locations of incisions and the presence and extent to which muscle was excised. Various surgical approaches will be discussed under a single therapeutic category because of their basic anatomic and physiologic similarity.

Morrow (19) pioneered much of the early work in this area, describing his first 2 cases with Brockenbrough in 1961. An excellent report of the operative procedure, with illustrations, can be found in a later publication in which results in their first 10 patients are described (21). Morrow (20) continued to perform this procedure and has periodically reported his results.

The most recent results report 68 patients operated since 1960 (10). This report, however, is in editorial form and does not describe the results in as detailed a fashion as was done in an earlier but recent, review (18). The results of the two reports are similar, and for that reason the earlier work showing 56 patients operated from 1960 to 1972 will be cited. All patients operated had rather severe clinical manifestations (angina, presyncope, syncope and/or congestive heart failure) of the disease and had not responded adequately to propanolol therapy.

Of 56 patients operated, 48 are still living, 6 died during the hospitalization for surgery, and 2 died at a later time of causes unrelated to idiopathic hypertrophic subaortic stenosis. Forty-five of the surviving patients have been followed for 1 year or more. All of these patients, except 1, have improved at least one functional class, according to the New York Heart Association criteria. The 1 patient that did not improve, has not become worse.

Forty-five of the postoperative patients were studied hemodynamically; the peak systolic gradient at rest was reduced in all. No patient has had a recurrence of the gradient during the postoperative period. The left ventricular end diastolic pressure was abnormal in 31 patients preoperatively; it improved in 28 of those postoperatively.

Mitral regurgitation is, of course, a common finding in patients with idiopathic hypertrophic subaortic stenosis. Morrow reported it in 36 of 46 patients who had adequate contrast studies. Fourteen of the 36 had postoperative contrast studies which demonstrated that 8 were free of mitral regurgitation and 6 retained it in a mild form.

Complications of the operative procedure included the production of complete AV block in 2 patients and left bundle branch block in approximately one-third of those operated. In addition, 3 patients developed ventricular septal defects secondary to the procedure. They have not been symptomatic and have not required treatment.

Table 14-2 summarizes Morrow's presently reported work. From these data it appears that this operative procedure offers an opportunity for significant improvement, at an acceptable risk, to those patients who have been treated with propanolol but have not had an adequate response. Other groups have obtained similar results using a comparable surgical procedure (1, 2).

Table 14-2. Morrow's Operative Results Using Ventriculomyotomy and Myectomy

No. of patients	56	No. of patients	56
Living		Clinically improved	
Number	48	Number	43
Percent	86	Percent	98[b]
Dead		Hemodynamically improved	
Number	8[a]	Number	45
Percent	14	Percent	100[c]

[a] Two late deaths unrelated to idiopathic hypertrophic subaortic stenosis.
[b] Only 44 patients followed for 1 or more years.
[c] Only 45 patients had follow-up catheterization.

Mitral Prosthesis

The importance of the mitral valve apparatus in the pathophysiology of idiopathic hypertrophic subaortic stenosis has been clearly demonstrated (11, 30). An attractive hypothesis has been advanced to explain this association (23, 25). Echocardiography in patients with idiopathic hypertrophic subaortic stenosis who have mitral regurgitation has shown that the anterior leaflet returns to the open position during systole. It is postulated that this occurs because the hypertrophied anterolateral papillary muscle is maloriented and contracts excessively so that the leaflet returns to the open position.

Having noted the importance of the mitral apparatus in idiopathic hypertrophic subaortic stenosis, Cooley *et al.* (8) reported the treatment of 4 patients by mitral valve replacement in 1971. Two are alive and 2 died, 1 from extension of an old dissecting aortic aneurysm and the other from a cerebral embolism following placement of the prosthetic valve. By 1973, the number of reported patients had been extended to 9, with the 2 deaths continuing to constitute the only mortality (9). All survivors have undergone hemodynamic studies and have had either complete abolition or marked reduction of the gradient. The operative result is listed as excellent in all surviving cases, although detailed analysis of the symptomatic changes is not presented.

Of the three modes of therapy discussed, the least objective data, by far, is available for evaluation of mitral valve replacement. Only one group of investigators has published their results and these include a total of only 9 patients. It does appear, however, that the outflow obstruction of idiopathic hypertrophic subaortic stenosis can be treated successfully by this method and that marked improvement results clinically in the survivors.

Discussion

The efficacy of beta-blockade in the treatment of idiopathic hypertrophic subaortic stenosis is well documented in many cases. Proponents of the various surgical procedures uniformly select patients to be operated from those who have not improved adequately on medical therapy. It is therefore apparent that symptomatic patients with idiopathic hypertrophic subaortic stenosis should have a trial of therapy with beta-blocking agents before any surgical procedure is considered.

Asymptomatic patients, investigated because they had heart murmurs, present a different problem. Obviously no symptoms exist to be improved or abolished. Therefore, should such patients be treated at all? If so, how can they be followed? If the patient is not asthmatic or diabetic, does not have pulmonary disease, and has never been in congestive heart failure, the risk of beta-blocking agents, even in very large doses, is quite small. If one of the above contraindications exists, then the risk will have to be weighed against the potential benefit.

But what is the potential benefit to the asymptomatic patient? Even though the symptoms are not present, a gradient must either exist or be demonstrable with appropriate stimulation. If that were not so, the diagnosis could not be established. That being the case, a gradient is very likely produced with some daily activities, especially during physical or emotional exertion where increased beta-stimulation exists. It is not definitely known whether the presence of a gradient leads to progression of the disease. It is likely that the gradient leads to at least some additional left ventricular hypertrophy. This in turn leads to further outflow tract obstruction and a "vicious cycle" of hypertrophy and obstruction is produced. In addition, the added hypertrophy reduces ventricular compliance and increases both the left atrial pressure and the likelihood of angina pectoris. On this basis it would appear worthwhile to treat the asymptomatic patient with beta-blocking agents, provided no contraindication to such therapy exists in sufficient degree to be dangerous.

The great majority of patients have a good response to beta-blocking therapy and no further intervention is necessary. Approximately 10 percent, however, do not respond adequately. In this group surgical intervention must be considered. The problem lies in choosing the surgical procedure. It should be kept in mind that the etiology of the hypertrophy is unknown and no medical or surgical approach cures the underlying pathology. The best that can be expected is relief of symptoms at the same time that the gradient is abolished. It may be that the intrinsic disease process causes no harm unless a gradient is present at some time, but not enough information is presently available to evaluate that point.

Of the two surgical procedures available, there is much more objective evidence available for evaluation of myotomy and septectomy. That evidence, discussed previously in detail, is impressive. Mortality and morbidity seem to be acceptable when dealing with individuals who are refractory to medical therapy. Hemodynamic and clinical results are excellent in the immediate postoperative period and Morrow has not been able to demonstrate the reappearance of a ventricular gradient in any operated patient. Clinical improvement has been almost universal.

Disability following surgery is minimal. There is no risk of thrombus formation or systemic embolization, hence no requirement for anticoagulation. Thus the long-term outlook is improved. No prosthesis is required and therefore complications such as malfunction, displacement, infection, hemolytic anemia, and periprosthetic leaks are avoided.

A note of caution should be added. Idiopathic hypertrophic subaortic stenosis is an unusual disease and as a result only a few cardiovascular surgeons are likely to acquire a large experience with ventriculomyotomy and myectomy. In the hands of surgeons less experienced with the procedure, the results may not be as impressive.

Much less objective evidence is available for the newer procedure of mitral valve replacement with a low profile prosthesis. The initial mortality would appear to be at least as high, if not higher, than myotomy and septectomy, although the numbers are very small. The gradient is abolished, however, and the survivors have an excellent clinical result. If this alone were the evidence upon which a choice had to be made, it would be a difficult choice indeed.

The price the patient must pay for improvement must also weigh heavily in the decision. It has been pointed out by Roberts (24) that "prosthetic cardiac valve" is indeed a disease in itself. The evidence for this view is provided by the work of Levine *et al.* (16) who demonstrate a higher mortality for mitral valve replacement than may be expected from symptomatic idiopathic hypertrophic subaortic stenosis. A cardinal point of the good practice of cardiology and one about which a great deal of information has been gathered, is to avoid prosthetic mitral valve replacement in rheumatic mitral valvular disease until the "appropriate time." The "appropriate time" is that moment when the risk of acquiring the prosthetic valve and living with it is less than the risk of persisting with the diseased valve. If that criteria were applied to idiopathic hypertrophic subaortic stenosis, very few mitral valves would be replaced.

Dwight Harkin (27), in defending his position as a reviewer of Cooley's paper (9), states that "... a surgical technique is safe enough to use when it is safer than the condition that it is designed to correct and is the best available." The very application of that principle, using existing knowledge and data, would raise very serious questions as to the use of the low profile prosthetic mitral valve as treatment for idiopathic hypertrophic subaortic stenosis.

On the basis of the above information it would appear reasonable to conclude that propanolol should be the first therapeutic approach to idiopathic hypertrophic subaortic stenosis. An adequate trial, both in terms of duration and dosage, should be carried out before deciding the response has not been adequate. Once an inadequate response to propanolol has been documented, surgical intervention must be considered. Myotomy and septectomy, along the lines of Morrow's prototype, seem to be the surgical procedure of choice at present. It is at least as safe as mitral valve replacement and has far fewer postoperative complications and potential hazards.

There may well be situations where myotomy and septectomy are tried without a good result. If such a patient should have persistent and severe symptoms, it would appear justified to consider replacing the mitral valve. Otherwise the later procedure should probably be restricted to use in a research protocol, under special circumstances, until more data are available for its evaluation and comparison to myotomy and septectomy.

Summary

Controversies exist in the treatment of idiopathic hypertrophic subaortic stenosis, but it is reasonable to conclude that all symptomatic patients should have a trial of beta-blocking agents and be maintained on such therapy if an adequate response is obtained. The asymptomatic patient should be placed on a regimen of drugs that could be expected to substantially reduce, or abolish, left ventricular outflow tract gradient. Only those patients who prove to be refractory to such medical therapy should be considered for surgical intervention. At present the great majority of documented evidence favors the choice of ventriculomyotomy and myectomy over mitral valve replacement with a low profile prosthesis. The results are at least as good and there are fewer postoperative complications.

References

1. Adelman, A. G., Wigle, E. D., Ranganathan, N., Webb, G. D., Kidd, B. S. L., Bigelow, W. A., and Silver, M. D. The clinical course in muscular subaortic stenosis. A retrospective and prospective study of 60 hemodynamically proved cases. Ann. Intern. Med., 77:515, 1972.
2. Barratt-Boyes, B. G. and O'Brien, K. P. Surgical treatment of idiopathic hypertrophic subaortic stenosis using a combined left ventricular-aortic approach. In Wolstenholme, G. E. W. and O'Conner, M. eds. Hypertrophic Obstructive Cardiomyopathy, Ciba Foundation Study Group. London, J. and A. Churchill, 1971, pp. 150–159.
3. Braunwald, E. and Ebert, P. A. Hemodynamic alterations in idiopathic hypertrophic subaortic stenosis induced by sympathomimetic drugs. Am. J. Cardiol., 10:489, 1962.

4. —— Morrow, A. G., Cornell, W. P., Aygen, M. M., and Hilbish, T. F. Idiopathic hypertrophic subaortic stenosis. Clinical, hemodynamic and angiographic manifestations. Am. J. Med., 29:924, 1960.
5. Brock, R. Functional obstruction of the left ventricle (Acquired aortic subvalvular stenosis). Guy's Hosp. Rep., 106:221, 1957.
6. Cherian, G., Brockington, I. F., Shah, P. M., Oakley, C. M., and Goodwin, J. F. Beta-adrenergic blockade in hypertrophic obstructive cardiomyopathy. Br. Med. J., 1:895, 1966.
7. Cohen, J., Effat, H., Goodwin, J. F., Oakley, C. M., and Steiner, R. E. Hypertrophic obstructive cardiomyopathy. Br. Heart J., 26:16, 1964.
8. Cooley, D. A., Leachman, R. D., Hallman, G. L., Gerami, S., and Hall, R. J. Idiopathic hypertrophic subaortic stenosis. Surgical treatment including mitral valve replacement. Arch. Surg., 103:606, 1971.
9. —— —— Wukosch, D. C. Diffuse muscular subaortic stenosis: Surgical treatment. Am. J. Cardiol., 31:1, 1973.
10. Epstein, S. E., Morrow, A. G., Henry, W. L., and Clark, C. E. The role of operative treatment in patients with idiopathic hypertrophic subaortic stenosis. Circulation, 48:677, 1973.
11. Fix, P., Moberg, A., Sodesberg, H., and Kornell, J. Muscular subvalvular aortic stenosis: Abnormal anterior mitral leaflet possibly the primary factor. Acta Radiol. Diagn., 2:177, 1964.
12. Flamm, M. D., Harrison, D. C., and Hancock, E. W. Muscular subaortic stenosis—Prevention of outflow obstruction with propanolol. Circulation, 38:846, 1968.
13. Harrison, D. C., Braunwald, E., Glick, G., Mason, D. T., Chidsey, C. A., and Ross, J. Jr. Effects of beta-adrenergic blockade on the circulation, with particular reference to observations in patients with hypertrophic subaortic stenosis. Circulation, 29:84, 1964.
14. Hubner, P. J. B., Ziady, G. M., Lane, G. K., Hardarson, T., Scales, B., Oakley, C. M., and Goodwin, J. F. Double-blind trial of propanolol and protocol in hypertrophic cardiomyopathy. Br. Heart J., 35:1116, 1973.
15. Kristinsson, A. Beta-adrenergic blockade in hypertrophic cardiomyopathy with emphasis on exercise studies. In Wolstenholme, G. E. W. and O'Conner, M. eds. Hypertrophic Obstructive Cardiomyopathy, Ciba Foundation Study Group. London, J. and A. Churchill, 1971, pp. 113–123.
16. Levine, F. H., Copeland, J. G., and Morrow, A. G. Prosthetic replacement of the mitral valve: Continuing assessments of the 100 patients operated upon during 1961–1965. Circulation, 47:518, 1973.
17. Matlof, H. J. and Harrison, D. C. Acute hemodynamic effects of practolol in patients with idiopathic hypertrophic subaortic stenosis. Br. Heart J., 35:152, 1973.
18. Morrow, A. G. Operative treatment in idiopathic hypertrophic subaortic stenosis. In Sharma, D., Newby, D., and Hegyeli, R. J., eds. Proceedings USA–USSR Joint Symposium on Congenital Heart Disease. Bethesda, National Heart and Lung Institute, 1973, pp. 113–127.
19. —— Brockenbrough, E. C. Surgical treatment of idiopathic hypertrophic subaortic stenosis: Technic and hemodynamic results of subaortic ventriculomyotomy. Ann. Surg., 154:181, 1961.
20. —— Fogarty, T. J., Hannah, H., and Braunwald, E. Operative treatment in idiopathic hypertrophic subaortic stenosis—Technique and the results of preoperative and postoperative clinical and hemodynamic assessments. Circulation, 37:589, 1968.
21. —— Lambrew, C. T., and Braunwald, E. Idiopathic hypertrophic subaortic stenosis: II. Operative treatment and the results of pre- and postoperative hemodynamic evaluations. Circulation, 30:Suppl. 4:120, 1964.
22. Powell, W. J., Whiting, R. B., Dunsmore, R. E., and Sanders, C. A. Symptomatic prognosis in patients with idiopathic hypertrophic subaortic stenosis. Am. J. Med., 55:15, 1973.
23. Pridie, R. B. and Oakley, C. Mitral valve movement in hypertrophic obstructive cardiomyopathy. Br. Heart J., 31:390, 1969.
24. Roberts, W. C. Operative treatment of hypertrophic obstructive cardiomyopathy. The case against mitral valve replacement. Am. J. Cardiol., 32:377, 1973.
25. Simon, A. L., Ross, J. Jr., and Gault, J. H. Angiographic anatomy of the left ventricle and mitral valve in idiopathic hypertrophic subaortic stenosis. Circulation, 36:852, 1967.
26. Sloman, G. Propanolol in management of muscular subaortic stenosis. Br. Heart J., 29:783, 1967.
27. Spodick, D. H., Cooley, D. A., Leachman, R. D., and Harkin, D. E. Operative treatment of hypertrophic obstructive cardiomyopathy. Am. J. Cardiol., 34:117, 1974.
28. Stenson, R. E., Flavin, M. D., Harrison, D. C., and Hancock, E. W. Hypertrophic subaortic stenosis—clinical and hemodynamic effects of long-term propanolol therapy. Am. J. Cardiol., 31:763, 1973.

29. Webb-Poploe, M. Management of hypertrophic obstructive cardiomyopathy by beta-blockade. In Wolstenholme, G. E. W. and O'Conner, M. eds. Hypertrophic Obstructive Cardiomyopathy, Ciba Foundation Study Group. London, J. and A. Churchill, 1971, pp. 103–112.
30. Wigle, E. D., Adelman, A. G., and Silver, M. D. Pathophysiologic considerations in muscular subaortic stenosis. In Wolstenholme, G. E. W. and O'Conner, M. eds. Hypertrophic Obstructive Cardiomyopathy, Ciba Foundation Study Group. London, J. and A. Churchill, 1971, pp. 63–76.

Chapter 15 Current Concepts of Hemiblocks

Calvin L. Weisberger, M.D. and Edward K. Chung, M.D.

General Considerations

For many years the intraventricular conduction system had been considered as only two branches consisting of right and left bundle branches. Right bundle branch block and left bundle branch block have been known as distinct electrocardiographic entities for decades. Various investigators recognized and described other forms of intraventricular conduction block and coined various names for them (12). There were, however, no clearcut anatomic, physiologic, and electrocardiographic descriptions of these various electrocardiographic entities. They, therefore, existed as curiosities without implying useful information for the clinician. In 1967, Rosenbaum and colleagues published their text *Los Hemibloqueos*, which clearly documented, described and demonstrated significance for electrocardiographic patterns signifying blocks in subdivision of the left bundle branch system. These included and superseded to a great extent many of the previously described, partial intraventricular conduction blocks. Since their publication the term, *hemiblocks* has become a unique and popular electrocardiographic term. There still exists a debate over (a) the real anatomic nature of the intraventricular conduction system and (b) over the true clinical implications of the various forms of hemiblocks. In this Chapter, the purpose is to explore what is known about hemiblocks and what implications this knowledge holds for the clinicians.

The Cardiac Conduction System

Anatomic Considerations

Within the human heart the major components of the cardiac conduction system (Figure 15-1) include:

1. The sinus node
2. The atrial preferential pathways
3. The atrioventricular (AV) node
4. The His bundle
5. The right and left bundle branches
6. The Purkinje network

The sinus node is the primary pacemaker of the heart, it is generally located near the junction of the superior vena cava and the right atrium. Its blood supply is the sinus nodal artery, which arises from the proximal right coronary artery in 60 per-

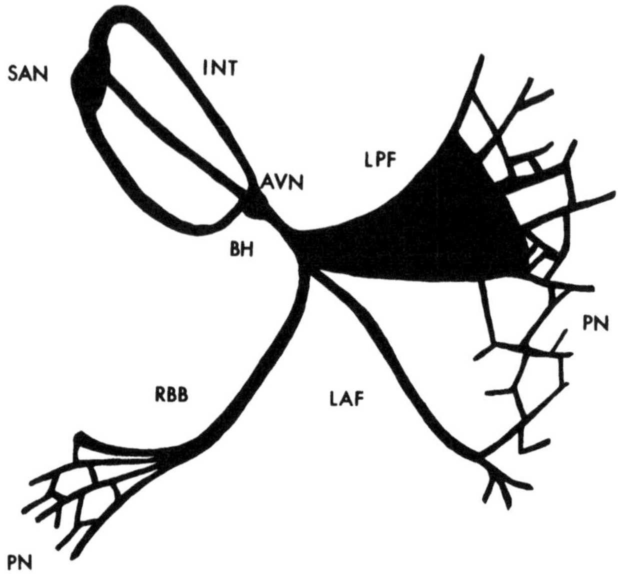

Fig. 15-1. Schematic drawing of the intracardiac conduction system. SAN = sinus node, INT = internodal pathways, AVN = atrioventricular node, BH = bundle of His, RBB = right bundle branch, LAF = left anterior fascicle, LPF = left posterior fascicle, PN = Purkinje network.

cent and from the proximal left circumflex coronary artery in 40 percent of cases. The sinus node receives both sympathetic and parasympathetic innervation (2).

The atrial preferential pathways are bands of specialized myocardium, which run between the sinus and AV nodes. James (7) and Truex (15) reported their anatomic existence. It is still a matter of controversy as to whether these tracts truly function electrophysiologically to conduct the sinus impulse to the atrioventricular node or whether they simply exist as an anatomic structure.

The AV node is located in the inferior portion of the right side of the interatrial septum. It is bounded by the ostium of the coronary sinus, the inferior vena cava, and the base of the septal leaflet of the tricuspid valve (2). The blood supply to the AV node is the AV nodal artery, which is usually the first branch of the posterior descending coronary artery. In 90 percent of cases it is a branch of the right coronary artery, in the other 10 percent from the left circumflex artery. The nerve supply to the AV node includes both sympathetic and parasympathetic fibers.

The Bundle of His is the direct continuation of the AV node. It is a thin bundle oriented anteriorly and inferiorly and extending for a distance of 1 to 2 cm from the AV node. Initially it runs within the central fibrous body and then close to the membranous septum (14). At the level of the noncoronary cusp of the aortic valve, the His bundle leaves the central fibrous body and branches of the left bundle branch begin to be given off. The His bundle blood supply is predominantly from the AV node artery with some contribution from the first septal perforating branch of the left anterior descending coronary artery.

The right bundle branch is the continuation of the His bundle after the left bundle branch fibers have been given off. The right bundle branch averages 45 to 50 mm in length and 1 to 2 mm in diameter. It runs along the membranous septum in the subendocardium, through the muscular septum and then down the right side of the septum to the anterior papillary muscle of the tricuspid valve (14). Proximally its blood supply is the AV node artery, within the muscular septum it receives branches

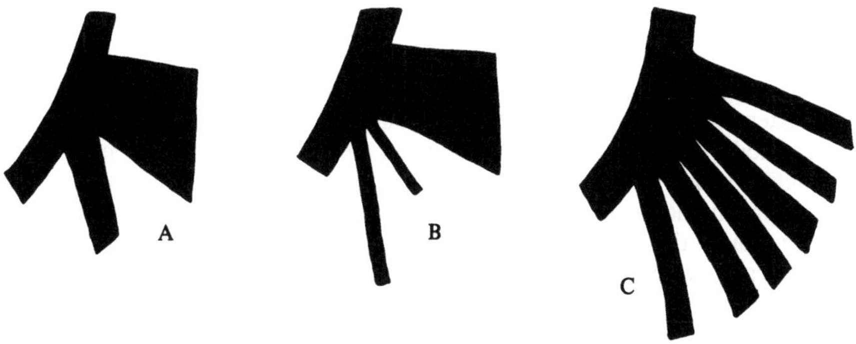

Fig. 15-2. Variations in described anatomy of left bundle branch divisions: A = bifascicular, B = trifascicular, and C = fan distribution (multifascicular).

from septal perforating arteries from the left anterior descending. The right bundle branch does not divide until it reaches its terminus at the anterior papillary muscle of the right ventricle.

The left bundle branch is, at present, the most controversial component of the intraventricular conduction system. Fibers to the left ventricle begin separating from the His bundle at the level of the noncoronary aortic cusp. The radiation from the bundle of His encompasses a length of 4 to 6 mm. The actual form of the left bundle branch is at debate. Rosenbaum and his colleagues (14) found that, in most of their dissections, there existed a main left bundle branch which was located along the membranous septum just below the aortic valve. After a short distance it was found to divide with the anterior one-third moving across the left ventricular outflow tract and terminating in the base of the anterior papillary muscle. The posterior two-thirds turns posteriorly and inferiorly and terminates at the base of the posterior papillary muscle. Other investigators have reported the absence of a main left bundle branch and instead a fan-like radiation extending from the His bundle out along the septum to the bases of the papillary muscles (3). Other dissections have shown three main branches of the left bundle branch system: the anterior and posterior division described by Rosenbaum and also a midseptal fascicle (3) (Figure 15-2).

The blood supply to the left bundle branch system includes branches from both the left and right coronary arterial systems. Those fibers located near the AV node and His bundle or found in the posterior area of the septum receive blood supply from the AV node artery and branches of the posterior descending coronary artery (usually right coronary branches), those fibers located anteriorly in the septum receive branches from the septal perforating branches of the left anterior descending coronary artery.

After the fibers of the bundle branch systems reach their destinations they seem to ramify into what has been called the Purkinje network. This is an interconnected series of differentiated myocardial fibers which extend subendocardially over essentially entire ventricles. The fibers branch inward perpendicularly from the endocardium to the epicardium.

The human cardiac conduction system then is still not incontrovertibly delineated from the anatomic viewpoint. The existence of sinus node, AV node, His bundle and main bundle branches is well accepted. The ramifications of these structures remains still in question.

Physiologic Considerations

The electrophysiology of the cardiac conduction system is rather complicated, and an extensive discussion thereof is beyond the scope of this chapter. Basically the sinus node is the primary pacemaker of the heart and the action potential of this structure shows a steeper rise to phase 4 than that of any other normal anatomical structure in the heart. For this reason, the sinus node reaches threshold potential more rapidly than the other structures and discharges at a rate in excess of them in the normal state. Many other components of the conduction system possess the property of automaticity. That is, they have a spontaneous rise to phase 4 and thus can discharge themselves if not depolarized earlier by an impulse coming from elsewhere in the heart. There are variations in the action potential waveform between various parts of the conduction system which affect conduction velocity and refractory periods at different levels of the conduction pathways. The property of decremental conduction also exists within parts of the AV conduction system, especially the AV node (2). This is the property whereby the conductive fiber changes so that the action potential becomes progressively less effective as a stimulus to more distal unexcited portions of the fiber. When an action potential is produced in the sinus node, it traverses the sinoatrial junction, passes through either the atrial muscle or atrial preferential pathways, and arrives at the AV node. After traversing the AV node, the impulse goes through the His bundle and its branches. The first detectable activation of the ventricular myocardium takes place within the left ventricular endocardium. Three areas are simultaneously activated:

1. High on the anterior paraseptal wall just below the attachment of the mitral valve
2. Left central portion of intraventricular septum
3. Posterior paraseptal wall about one-third the distance from the apex to the base (5).

Activation spreads from these three areas, rapidly encompassing the endocardium and spreading outward to the epicardium. The net resultant vectors of this process produce the surface potentials recorded as the electrocardiogram or vectorcardiogram. This consists of an initial vector to the right, representing depolarization of the left septum with respect to the right and then leftward, and posterior forces representing greater total mass of depolarized muscle on the left with respect to the right ventricle, the gradient being endocardial to epicardial.

If one considers the anatomic structure of the conduction system correlates with the normal ventricular activation process, the following factors can be considered. If the left-sided conduction system is functionally or anatomically composed of two fascicles, why are there three discrete areas of initial left ventricular activation? The data reported by Durrer (5) certainly supports the idea of a trifascicular left bundle branch system either anatomically or functionally. One could, of course, argue that the series of human hearts studied by him was small and so may be biased. Recent studies of Lazzara *et al.* (9) in dog hearts show rather rapid subendocardial conduction throughout the left ventricle. There were only minor differences in time to reach end-fiber destination, except for the fibers at the edges of the left bundle radiations, *border fibers*. They were unable to produce any of the characteristic hemiblock patterns except by interrupting the border fibers. Lesions located in that portion of the left bundle branch medial to the border fibers produced no change in surface ECG. This explains the absence of a third divisional block pattern and also explains the existence of left anterior and posterior hemiblocks, even if such discrete fascicles are not present in all cases. Functionally then, while the anatomic controversy of the left bundle divisions continues, we may think of the conduction system as behaving as if it were bifascicular.

Diagnostic Criteria of Hemiblocks

The diagnostic criteria of right bundle branch block are well described in standard texts of electrocardiography, as are criteria for left bundle branch block (1). If we recall the areas of earliest activation of left ventricular endocardium, we can forecast the appearance of left anterior and posterior hemiblocks. A block of normal activation of the anterior paraseptal wall would mean that the spread of depolarization would start in the posterior and inferior portion of the left ventricle with normal septal activation and the wave of depolarization would then sweep superiorly and to the left (Figure 15-3). If the fibers to the posterior paraseptal wall were blocked, the

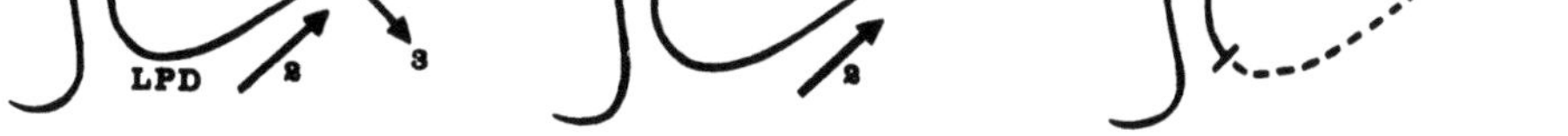

Fig. 15-3. Hemiblocks. When both anterior and posterior divisions of left bundle branch system are intact (diagram A), the left ventricle is activated via both divisions (vectors 1 and 2) so that the resultant forces of vectors 1 and 2 will produce vector 3. When one of two divisions of the left bundle branch system is blocked, however, the impulses must travel through the intact division only. That is, in anterior hemiblock (diagram B) vector 1 is no longer present as a result the left ventricule is activated via intact posterior division (vector 2). In this case the electrical axis shifts to the left and superiorly (marked left axis deviation). For the same reason, posterior hemiblock (diagram C) produces right axis deviation because the left ventricle is activated via intact anterior division (vector 1). RB = right bundle branch, AVN = AV node, LAD = left anterior division, LPD = left posterior division.

wave of depolarization through the septum would again be normal, but the spread of activation would be from the anterior paraseptal wall inferiorly to the right (Figure 15-3). These would then be the correlates of anterior and posterior hemiblock. Delay in activation of the central septum would either produce only an absence of initial septal forces or no noticeable change in the ECG.

Left Anterior Hemiblock

The ECG pattern of left anterior hemiblock is usually related to the diseased left ventricle. The ECG criteria for left anterior hemiblock have been defined by Rosenbaum *et al.* (14) and have not been seriously challenged.

The diagnostic criteria for left anterior hemiblock (1, 14) are as follows (Figures 15-3 and 15-4):

1. Marked left axis deviation (–45° to –90°.)
2. Small q wave in lead I and small r wave in lead III.
3. Little or no prolongation of QRS interval (usually 0.10 second or less).
4. No evidence of other factors responsible for left axis deviation.

It should be noted that certain clinical conditions and ECG entities may produce similar ECG findings. Chronic obstructive lung disease may produce left axis deviation as may diaphragmatic myocardial infarction and cardiomyopathy (6). There are other causes for left axis deviation as well, but we believe that understanding ventricular activation and possible variants to it from different causes are the simplest means of identifying left anterior hemiblock in the presence of other processes or ruling out its presence despite leftward axis. For example, diaphragmatic myocardial infarction commonly causes QS or QR complexes in leads II, III, and aVF. These may persist from the time of acute myocardial infarc-

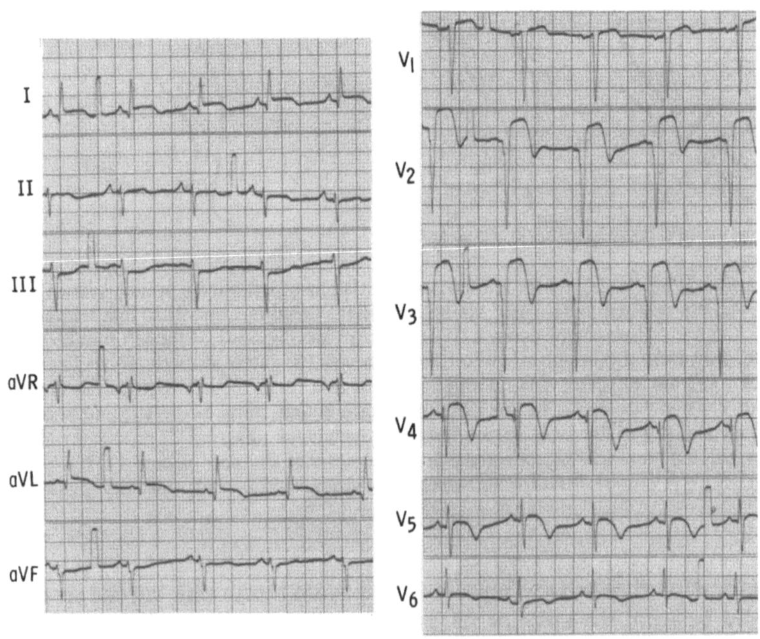

Fig. 15-4. Acute extensive anterior myocardial infarction associated with left anterior hemiblock (QRS axis: –45°). The rhythm is sinus with a rate of 76 beats per minute.

tion. The terminal forces in left anterior hemiblock are superiorly directed; the presence of inferiorly directed terminal forces would weigh against left anterior hemiblock. One should also consider in these patients the magnitude of the superiorly directed forces in these leads. The diaphragmatic infarction without left anterior hemiblock (and in the absence of other myocardial disease or infarction) has its QS complex formed with the presence of intact wavefronts from left anterior and left posterior divisions. Therefore the summation of these usually results in low voltage QS in leads II and III, whereas in left anterior hemiblock, the wavefront from the anterior division is missing so the terminal forces would produce relatively large S waves in leads II, III, and aVF. Using reasoning in this manner, one can make it less difficult to decide whether an ECG tracing that shows left axis deviation in the frontal plane really indicates left anterior hemiblock (Figure 15-4).

Left Posterior Hemiblock

Diagnostic criteria for left posterior hemiblock (1, 14) are (Figures 15-3 and 15-5):

1. Marked right axis deviation (plus 105° to plus 108°)
2. Small r wave in lead I and small q wave in lead III
3. Little or no prolongation of QRS interval (usually 0.10 second or less)
4. No evidence of other factors responsible for right axis deviation.

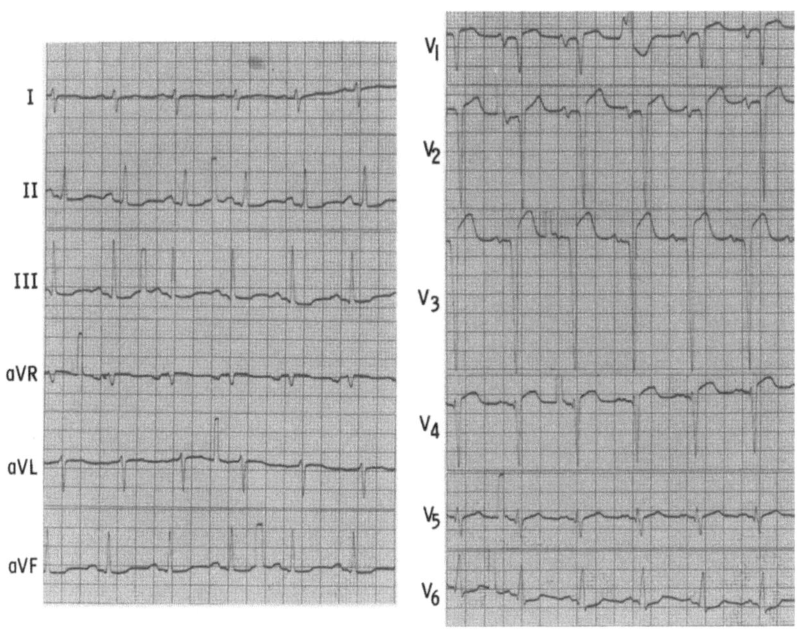

Fig. 15-5. Acute extensive anterior myocardial infarction associated with left posterior hemiblock (QRS axis: +105°). Note a ventricular premature contraction in lead V_1, and evidence of left atrial hypertrophy. The rhythm is sinus with a rate of 90 beats per minute.

Other factors responsible for right axis deviation may include right ventricular hypertrophy, vertical heart, chest deformity, and lateral myocardial infarction. Among them, the most common causes of right axis deviation simulating left posterior hemiblock are right ventricular hypertrophy and lateral wall myocardial infarction. Lateral wall infarction is unlikely to have Q_3, as the net of initial forces is the result of intact anterior and posterior pathways, the summated vector of which is plus 30° to plus 150° in general. When left posterior hemiblock is present, the unopposed forces sweeping around the left ventricular free wall produce the Q_3 seen on the surface ECG.

Right Bundle Branch Block with Left Anterior Hemiblock or Left Posterior Hemiblock

Hemiblock (either anterior or posterior) is often associated with right bundle branch block, the presence of which alters the recognition of hemiblocks. The S waves in leads V_{4-6}, which are responsible for the terminal forces, are usually slurred by the late depolarization of the right ventricle. In general, however, the same diagnostic criteria apply for left anterior and left posterior hemiblock in the presence of right bundle branch block. Initial septal forces are not altered by hemiblock or right bundle branch block. The marked left or right axis deviation is *not* characteristic of a pure right bundle branch block. Therefore, the marked left and right axis deviation in the presence of right bundle branch block represents left anterior and left posterior hemiblock, respectively (Figures 15-6 and 15-7) (1).

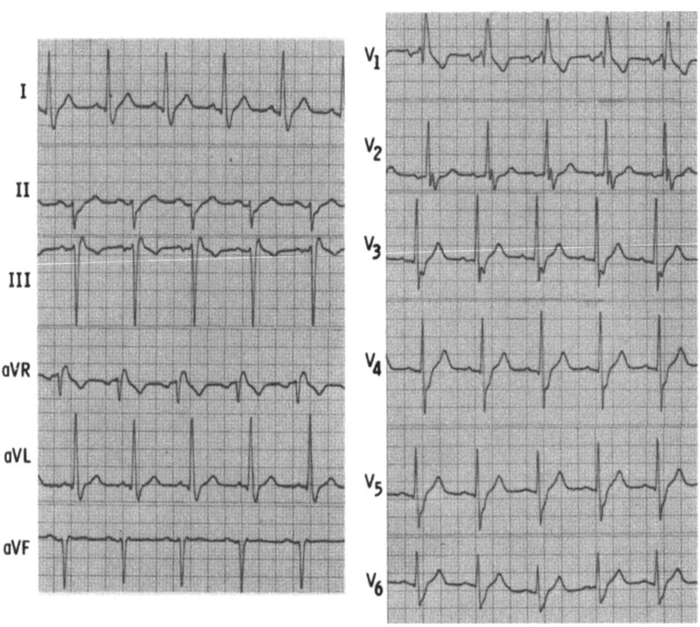

Fig. 15-6. Bifascicular block consisting of right bundle branch block associated with left anterior hemiblock (QRS axis: −50°). The rhythm is sinus with a rate of 86 beats per minute.

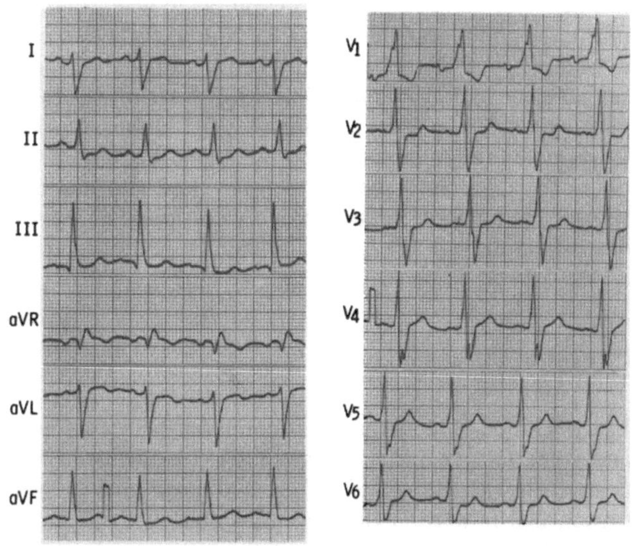

Fig. 15-7. Bifascicular block consisting of right bundle branch block associated with left posterior hemiblock (QRS axis: + 120°). The rhythm is sinus with a rate of 79 beats per minute.

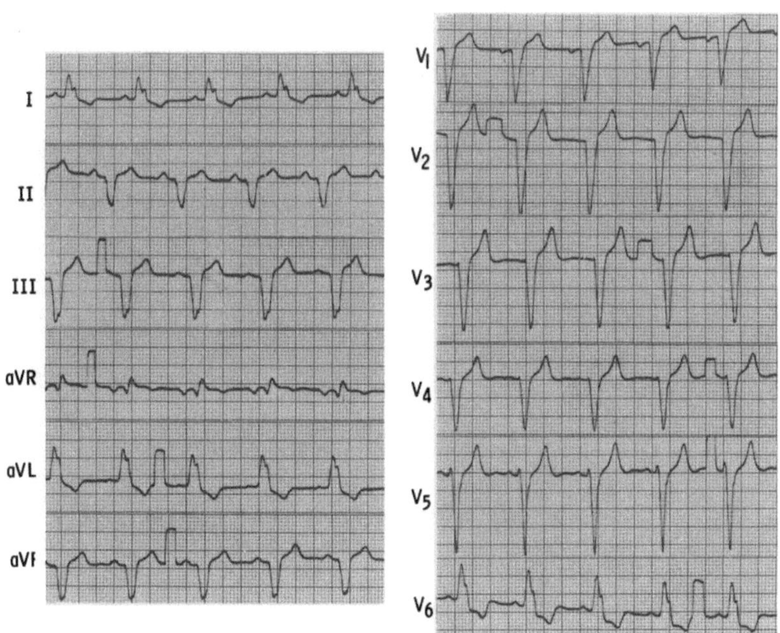

Fig. 15-8. Left bundle branch block. The rhythm is sinus with a rate of 76 beats per minute.

There is a moot debate, at present, as to whether the hemiblocks can occur as part of a left bundle branch block. Certainly if there is a conduction delay (partial block) in one division of the left bundle and complete block in another division, we might see an electrical axis compatible with the hemiblocks in the presence of a markedly prolonged QRS interval (Figure 15-8). However, this ECG finding should be read as left bundle branch block, as it would denote extensive disease in the entire left bundle branch system. In a recent study, by Lev and associates (10) 10 autopsied hearts showing left bundle branch block were found to have proximal bundle branch disease where the left-sided fibers branch from the His bundle.

Causes of Hemiblocks

In the United States, the most common causes of hemiblocks are coronary artery and hypertensive heart disease (13). In particular, hemiblock (either anterior or posterior) with an acute onset is almost always associated with acute anterior myocardial infarction (Figures 15-4 and 15-5). Because the left anterior division is supplied mainly by branches of the left anterior descending, and occasionally by branches of the right coronary artery, disease of these vessels both in theory and in fact is associated with left anterior hemiblock (18). The right bundle branch has a similar blood supply, and frequently a vascular lesion sufficient to cause left anterior hemiblock is also sufficient to cause right bundle branch block (Figure 15-6). Left

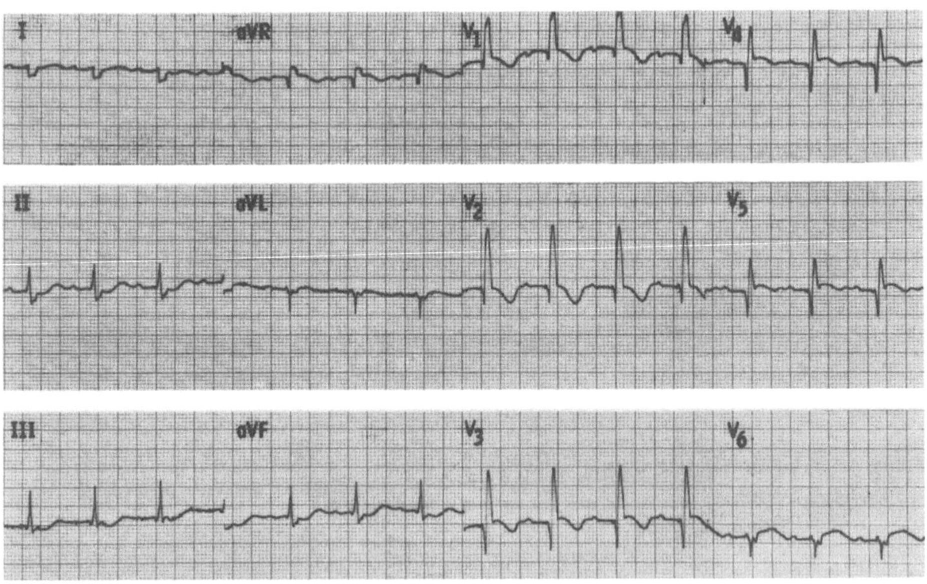

Fig. 15-9. Figures 15-9 and 15-10 were taken on the same patient with acute extensive anterior myocardial infarction on different occasions (few days apart). Figure 15-9 shows bifascicular block consisting of right bundle branch block and left posterior hemiblock (QRS axis: +125°). The rhythm is sinus with a rate of 93 beats per minute.

posterior hemiblock is seen very infrequently with coronary artery disease because the posterior radiation is more extensive and its blood supply is from both the right and left coronary artery systems. At times, left anterior hemiblock is observed on one occasion and left posterior hemiblock on another occasion in the presence of right bundle branch block associated with acute myocardial infarction (Figures 15-9 and 15-10). The hemiblocks presumably are produced by ischemia in coronary artery disease. In the case of hypertension, cardiomyopathy, Lev's disease, and Lenegre's disease the etiology differs (13). Because the left anterior fibers run along the aortic outflow tract, they are exposed to increased mechanical stress in any condition that causes increased impedance to left ventricular ejection. This factor may cause changes in the fibers sufficient to cause the conduction block on an anatomic basis alone. In cardiomyopathy, or extensive anterior myocardial infarction, it cannot, at present, be ruled out that some hemiblocks may be due to unresponsive muscle at the terminus of normal fascicles. That is, if a normal left anterior division terminates in electrically silent muscle, the ECG recorded might well look the same as if the conduction tract itself were blocked. Delay in conduction along a fascicle, caused by anatomic stretch or hypertrophy of its terminal muscle mass, has been shown to produce right bundle branch block patterns in dogs in the absence of anatomic lesion within the right bundle branch. We may say then that the hemiblocks or bundle branch blocks represent either anatomic or effective physiologic delay of activation of specific areas of ventricular musculature. The exact etiology of any given hemiblock may be unclear, but the presence of a hemiblock in a previously normal ECG implies an abnormal ventricle.

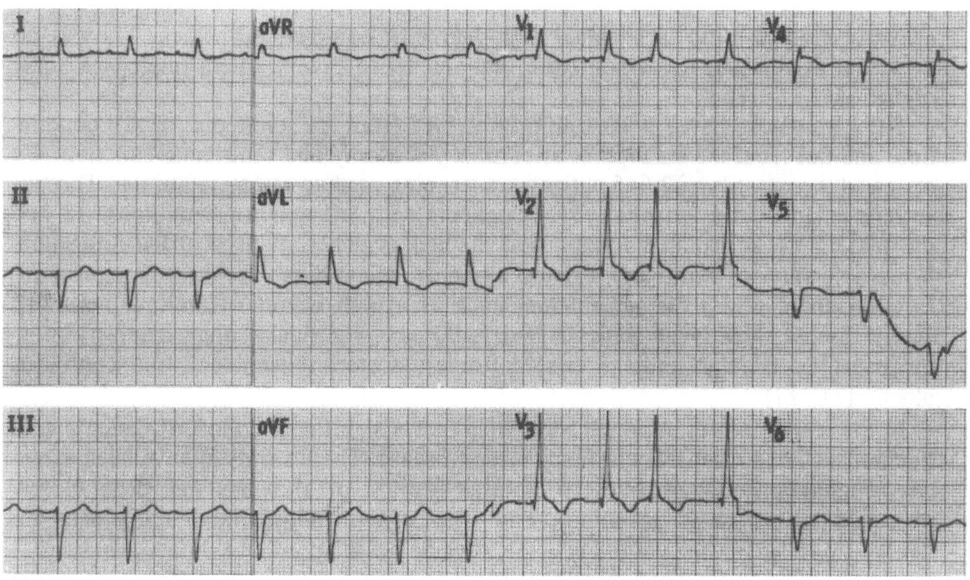

Fig. 15-10. Bifascicular block consisting of right bundle branch block and left anterior hemiblock (QRS axis: −75°). The rhythm is sinus with a rate of 88 beats per minute. Note one atrial premature beat.

Clinical Significance of Hemiblocks

The presence of hemiblock is generally accepted as evidence of AV conduction system disease. There appears to be no evidence to show that isolated right bundle branch block or isolated left hemiblocks not associated with acute myocardial infarction precedes advanced AV block.

When a combined lesion of the right bundle branch block and left anterior hemiblock was associated with acute myocardial infarction in 32 patients, 16 of the group developed either a high degree or complete AV block (4). Mortality in this group was three times that of a control group in the coronary care unit. In a group of patients with right bundle branch block and left anterior hemiblock not associated with acute myocardial infarction, there was no increased incidence of a high degree or complete AV block compared with control groups. All patients with right bundle branch block and left anterior hemiblock had advanced myocardial disease frequently associated with congestive heart failure.

In a series of 12 patients with right bundle branch block and left posterior hemiblock, no patients followed for up to 3 years showed complete AV block. Other studies have shown a 10 to 15 percent incidence of complete AV block in this lesion over a period of approximatley 10 years. Patients with right bundle branch block associated with left posterior hemiblock were, in general, older than 60 years and about 45 percent were found to have coronary artery disease (16).

His bundle recordings were used to predict the possible development of complete AV block in patients with right bundle branch block and either left anterior or left posterior hemiblock. A prospective study is now underway to determine whether the prolonged His to ventricle conduction time in patients with bifascicular block is an accurate prediction of an eventual high degree or complete AV block. There is no evidence, at present, to demonstrate that this is so except where related to acute myocardial infarction.

The hemiblocks have, in general, been viewed from the standpoint of AV conduction, and not from the standpoint of coronary anatomy and ventricular function. We reviewed the records of 2,645 patients undergoing cardiac catheterization at Thomas Jefferson University Hospital. Of 48 patients with left anterior hemiblock, 18 had the pattern as an isolated finding and 30 had evidence of myocardial infarction. When left anterior hemiblock existed alone or in combination with myocardial infarction, there was a 50 percent incidence of a high degree of multiple coronary artery disease. Nearly all patients had significant ventricular angiographic abnormalities (18). Similar findings existed for left posterior hemiblock and combined blocks (11, 17).

In the United States, it would seem then that a significant cohort of patients with hemiblocks have extensive coronary artery disease. There seems to have been extensive conduction disease but the natural history of this has not been clearly demonstrated. In those patients in whom single and multiple fascicular blocks are caused by an active myocardial process, such as acute myocardial infarction, there is a good possibility they will develop a high degree or complete AV block. In those cases of chronic asymptomatic hemiblocks, there appears to be no evidence, at present, for eventual progression to complete AV block.

Therapy of Hemiblocks

The hemiblocks alone do not require treatment. There has been controversy over the need for prophylactic pacing of patients with bifascicular block. Nevertheless, it is generally agreed, at present, that in patients with combined blocks (either right bundle branch block with left anterior hemiblock or left posterior hemiblock), associated with acute myocardial infarction an artificial pacemaker should be inserted to prevent complete AV block. This particular intervention has shown no alteration in the high mortality statistics associated with these patients, however. Nevertheless, the concept has been accepted from the standpoint that though the patient may die from cardiogenic shock, he should not die from complete AV block. The recommendation for patients with chronic bifascicular or trifascicular block has been not to pace unless the patient experiences syncope or has documented evidence of advanced or complete AV block on other occasions (8). His bundle electrocardiography to assess the need for cardiac pacing in bifascicular or trifascicular blocks remains to be proven, as previously mentioned.

With respect to coronary artery disease and ventricular abnormality, it would appear that fascicular blocks imply advanced disease with its increased risk of sudden death. Probably these patients should undergo cardiac catheterization so that coronary anatomy can be visualized. In this way, the physician can best determine the course of treatment to recommend for individual patients.

Summary

The anatomy of the AV conduction system has been shown to consist of a well-defined AV node, a well-delineated His bundle, and branches to the right and left ventricles. The anatomic distribution of the left ventricular fibers remains in dispute, but with respect to the electrocardiogram the left bundle branch functions as a bifascicular system. Block in the anterior superior division of the left bundle branch system results in marked left axis deviation (QRS axis: –45° and –90°), small q wave in leads I and aVL and small r wave in lead III, and little or no prolongation of the QRS interval. Left posterior hemiblock results in marked right axis deviation (+105° and +180°), small r wave in lead I and small q wave in lead III, and little or no prolongation of the QRS interval. Hemiblocks may coexist with right bundle branch block or first- or second-degree AV block (bifascicular or trifascicular block), giving evidence for diffuse conduction system disease.

In the United States coronary artery disease, hypertension, cardiomyopathy, Lev's and Lenegre's disease, are common causes of hemiblocks. When correlated with coronary arteriograms in symptomatic patients, left anterior hemiblock is associated with both left anterior descending coronary disease and multiple total coronary artery disease. Hemiblocks, when they occur in the course of acute myocardial infarction, especially as bifascicular block, is associated with a very poor prognosis. Chronic bifascicular block has not been shown to progress to complete AV block in most cases. The treatment of hemiblocks is related to their causes. In general, artificial pacemakers are indicated for acute bifascicular blocks in acute myocardial infarction and for patients with syncope in the presence of chronic bifascicular block. Because of the high incidence of multiple coronary artery lesions in patients with hemiblocks and chest pains or shortness of breath, these patients should be considered candidates for coronary angiography for precise diagnosis and appropriate treatment.

The recognition of fascicular blocks then carries significant diagnostic importance. The recognition of these entities by physicians can be facilitated by a simple understanding of normal ventricular depolarization pathways and the possible alteration thereof by various pathologic states.

References

1. Chung, E. K. Electrocardiography: Practical Applications with Vectorial Principles. Hagerstown, Harper and Row, 1974.
2. —— Principles of Cardiac Arrhythmias. Baltimore, Williams and Wilkins Co., 1971.
3. Demoulin, J. C. and Kulbertus, H. E. Histopathologic examination of concept of left hemiblock. Am. Heart J., 34:807–814, 1972.
4. DePasquale, N. P. and Bruno, M. S. Natural history of combined right bundle branch block and left anterior hemiblock. Am. J. Med., 54:297, 1973.
5. Durrer, D., VanDam, R. T., Freud, G. E., Janse, M. J., Meijler, F. L., and Arzbaecher, R. C. Total excitation of the isolated human heart. Circulation, 41:899, 1970.
6. Grant, R. P. Left axis deviation: an electrocardiographic pathologic correlation study. Circulation, 14:233, 1956.
7. James, T. N. The specialized conducting tissue of the atria. In Dreifus, L. S. and Likoff, W. eds. Mechanism and Therapy of Cardiac Arrhythmias. New York, Grune and Stratton, 1971.
8. Kulbertus, H. E. The magnitude of risk of developing complete heart block in patients with LAD–RBBB. Am. Heart J., 86:278, 1973.
9. Lazzara, R., Yeh, B. K., and Samet, P. Functional anatomy of the canine left bundle branch. Am. J. Cardiol., 33:623, 1974.
10. Lev, M., Unzer, P. N., Rosen, K. M., and Bharate, K. The anatomic substrate of complete left bundle branch block. Circulation, 50:479, 1974.
11. Lie, K. I., Wellens, H. J., Schulenberg, R. M., Becker, A. E., and Durrer, D. Factors influencing prognosis of bundle branch block complicating acute antero-septal infarction. The value of His bundle recordings. Circulation, 50:935, 1974.
12. Pryor, R. and Blount, S. G. The clinical significance of true left axis deviation. Am. Heart J., 72:391, 1966.
13. Rosenbaum, M. B., Elizari, M. V., Lazzari, J. O., Kretz, A., and DaRuos, H. A. The clinical causes and mechanisms of intraventricular conduction disturbances. In Schlant, R. C. and Hurst, J. W. eds. Advances in Electrocardiography. New York, Grune and Stratton, 1972.
14. Rosenbaum, M. B., Elizari, M. V., and Lazzari, J. O. The Hemiblocks, Oldsman, Fla., Tampa Tracings, 1970.
15. Truex, R. C. Comparative anatomy and functional considerations of the cardiac conduction system. In De Carravello, A. P. ed. Specialized Tissues of The Heart. New York, American Elsevier Publishing Co., 1962.
16. Varriale, P. and Kennedy, R. J. Right bundle branch block and left posterior fascicular block. Am. J. Cardiol., 29:459, 1972.
17. Weisberger, C. L. Unpublished data.
18. —— Scariato, A., Kasparian, H., Duca, P., Gottlieb, R., and Brest, A. N. Coronary angiographic significance of left anterior hemiblock. Unpublished data.

Chapter 16 Physical Activity and Coronary Heart Disease

SAMUEL M. FOX, III, M.D.

General Considerations

Physical inactivity, permitted or encouraged by mechanization within this century, is often mentioned as one of the factors contributing to the reported major increase in the morbidity and mortality of coronary heart disease in many developed countries. Although not as extensively investigated as elevated blood pressure, serum lipids and smoking within the prospective population studies that have provided the basis for the concept of a multifactorial etiology for coronary heart disease, there are many reports that suggest that physical inactivity is important and an increase in habitual physical activity will contribute to a preventive approach.

This chapter aims to review the data and present an informed proposal for patient advice. Some authors insist that various proposed preventive or therapeutic programs be categorized as either proved or unproved on a crude binary coding ("zero" or "one") unproved or proved, that suggests we pay no attention to an hypothesis unless it is proved beyond reasonable doubt. Coronary heart disease has yet to have even one risk factor accepted as firmly proved capable of preventive modification. Thus, if such a narrow binary code was accepted nothing might be done at this time until data are wholly convincing to the appropriately skeptical scientific community. Since the Multiple Risk Factor Intervention Trial (MRFIT) is only just starting and 5 or more years are probably required to develop statistically significant data, a policy of such "purist" form would appear unjustified.

Concerning physical activity or inactivity, there are no known *primary* preventive trials under way or in an advanced state of planning. Therefore there is little hope for specific definition in this area in the foreseeable future. Accordingly, interim guidelines are needed so long as the required specific, definitive information is lacking. Spreading levels of acceptance on the following format may permit constructive action while the desired further knowledge is being developed.

Levels of Acceptance of Regimens

Proven—Beyond reasonable doubt.
Prudent Action—Justified by substantial, although incomplete data and acceptably low hazard.
Promising—But more data needed.
Possible—Hypothesis only.

Beneficial effects resulting from an increase in habitual physical activity may be grouped into four general areas. For each, requirements of intensity, frequency, duration, and type of activity may be different:

1. Physiologic improvement
2. Psychologic benefit
3. Socioeconomic rewards
4. Epidemiologic changes (decreased morbidity/mortality)

An extension of life in the eighth decade or later, without regard for its quality, might be a socioeconomic and psychologic calamity, illustrating how values can conflict. Risk factor reduction has often been evaluated by epidemiologic parameters alone, yet, intervention, such as increased physical activity, is likely to influence the other three aspects in important ways.

To attract and maintain the involvement of individuals, a preventive program should include not only the extension of life without disease, but the preservation and enhancement of the quality of that life. Individuals and society may be far more interested in investing time, effort, and resources in activities that improve total human performance throughout life than in those that merely increase the chances for individuals to experience old age.

The idea that man prospers best if he is physically active has been with us at least since the time of Plato. In the *Dialogues*, Timaeus tells Socrates that "... concerning the mode of treatment by which the body and mind are to be preserved ... moderate exercise reduced to order, according to their affinities, the particles and affections which are wandering about the body." More than 2,000 years later, the Intersociety Commission on Heart Disease Resources (ICHD) reports, "Primary prevention of the atherosclerotic diseases" was less definite in its summary:

> Regular exercise, particularly those forms of endurance exercise which enhance cardiovascular fitness, may have a role to play in the prevention of atherosclerotic diseases. It is important to emphasize, however, that exercise is not free of danger both to the musculoskeletal and the cardiovascular systems. This is particularly true for middle-aged individuals—especially coronary-prone persons—who suddenly take up vigorous exercise after years of minimal physical activity. Physicians and other professionals need aid in guiding a concerned public to avoid these problems. Research on the role and programming of exercise for the prevention of atherosclerotic diseases must be pursued vigorously to obtain more definitive information (37).

Although the ICHD report on preventing atherosclerotic diseases indicates physical inactivity, or sedentary living, is important as a possible risk factor, it was classed as a "minor" risk factor secondary to the "major" factors of diet and elevated serum lipid levels, cigarette smoking and hypertension. Among the risk factor modifications most frequently proposed, an increase in habitual physical activity and the reduction of psychosocial tensions may have the greatest potential for improving the quality of life and enhancing human performance in addition to contributing to preventive efforts. For these reasons it appears urgent that an accelerated effort be made in investigating the effects of increases in physical activity and the modification of psychosocial tensions as part of the effort to produce a vigorous and creative society as well as to reduce the cost of medical care and disability.

This chapter will review major population studies on the risk factor status of physical inactivity and also discuss mechanisms by which an increase in habitual physical activity may produce beneficial effects.

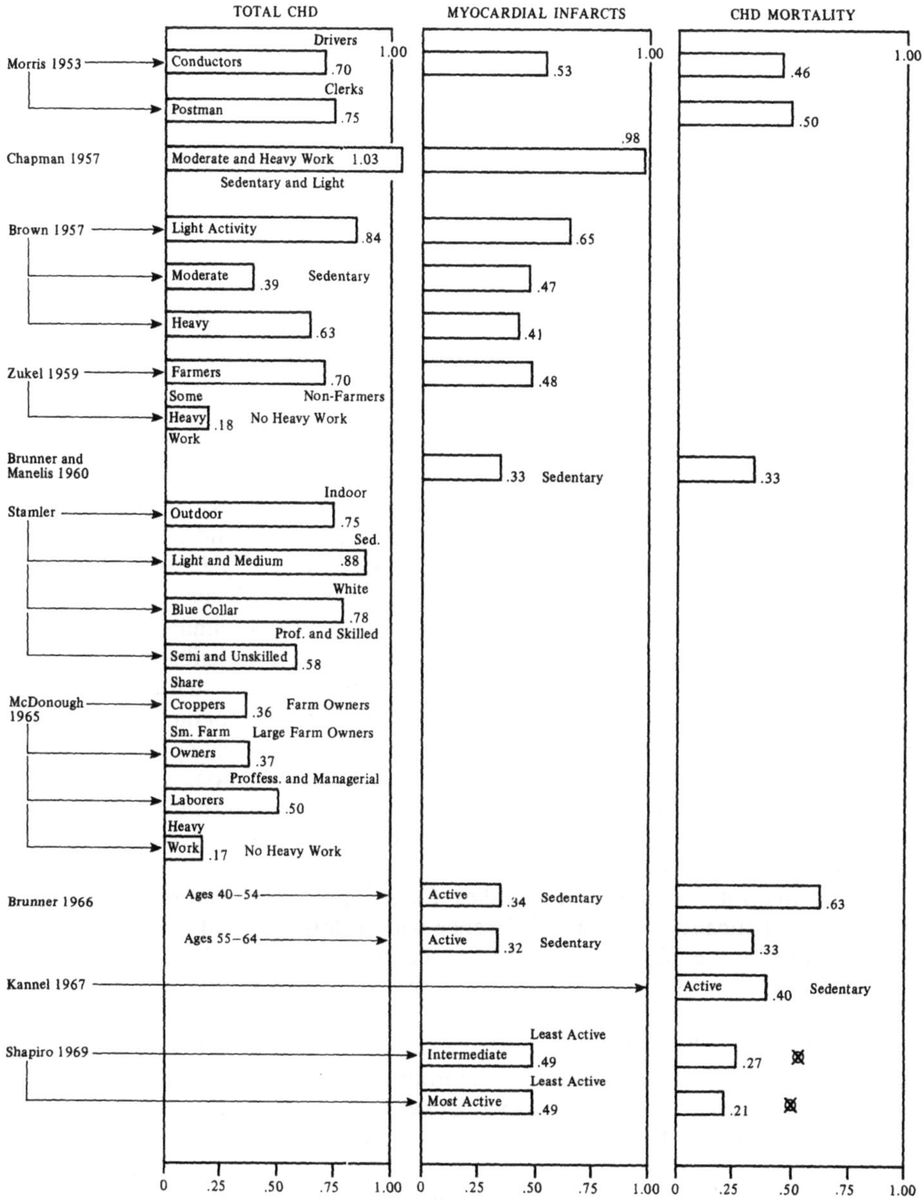

Figure 16-1. Data from many observational studies comparing groups of differing habitual physical activity relative to total coronary heart disease (CHD) manifestations, myocardial infarction and mortality. The horizontal bars, and the number near their ends, represent the relative occurrence of a manifestation in those of presumed or measured *greater* physical activity as compared to their more sedentary colleagues. A bar representing the experience of the more sedentary group would, in each study, extend exactly to the line labeled 1.00. Except for Chapman's data there is a lesser occurrence of coronary manifestations in those of greater habitual physical activity. Reproduced with permission from Fox, S. M. Relationship of activity habits to coronary heart disease. In Naughton, J. P., Hellerstein, H. K., and Mohler, I. C. eds. Exercise Testing and Exercise Training in Coronary Heart Disease. New York, Academic Press, 1973, p. 5.

Evidence Supporting the Physical Activity Hypothesis

The first important evidence in support of a statistically significant relationship between physical activity and coronary heart disease was reported by J. N. Morris and his colleagues in 1953 (49). Figure 16-1 indicates that among London bus conductors, presumably more active than the drivers since they moved around while collecting tickets, there was but 70 percent of the age-corrected incidence of all manifestations of coronary heart disease found among the drivers. The psychologic stress and strain of driving and ticket collection were not evaluated. Another study by the same authors compared London postmen and postal clerks and reported a similar reduced incidence of coronary manifestation in the more physically active postmen. It is significant and encouraging that the postmen did not have to climb many flights of stairs, nor were they required to be strenuously active for more than a usual 5 hours in making their rounds.

We must recognize, as Morris and his colleagues did, that the data reported from these and other population studies indicate an *association of less coronary heart disease with more physical activity* and not necessarily a cause and effect relationship. In a subsequent article with the intriguing title *The Physique of London Busmen; the Epidemiology of Uniforms* Morris and his colleagues indicated that factors of perhaps personal and also system selection, such as a height limitation for the conductor applicants, might have influenced the distribution and eligibility of individuals for their respective job categories (48). The authors also noted that newly employed drivers had a greater average girth for a given height than do conductors. In 1966 the same group reported that serum lipid and blood pressure levels appear to make the greatest contribution to the observed differences in manifestations of coronary heart disease among transport workers, but they considered it impossible to determine if an increase in physical activity had contributed to the lesser levels of both blood pressure and cholesterol (50).

In the majority of the many studies following Morris' pioneer work there is usually a statistically significant difference with a definite trend toward an association between more physical activity in occupation and total life pattern and a decrease in the incidence, prevalence, severity and/or mortality of coronary heart disease (Figures 16-1 and 16-2).

Zukel and his colleagues (75) reported a striking difference in the incidence of coronary heart disease between persons performing heavy work and those doing almost no physical labor. Later analysis (21) of Zukel's data revealed that people engaged in from 1 to 2 hours of heavy physical activity per day had less than one-sixth the incidence of coronary events as those whose usual life pattern included no heavy work. Unfortunately, the data did not permit an analysis relative to heavy physical activity lasting less than 1 hour per day. Data on lesser periods of physical activity is of

---

▷

Fig. 16-2. Data concerning coronary mortality relative to previous levels of physical activity from many, but not all relevant observaitonal studies. This graph includes some of the data from Figure 16-1 and has the same design. Reproduced with permission from Fox, S. M. Relationship of activity habits to coronary heart disease. *In* Naughton, J. P., Hellerstein, H. K., and Mohler, I. C. Exercise Testing and Exercise Training in Coronary Heart Disease. New York, Academic Press, 1973.

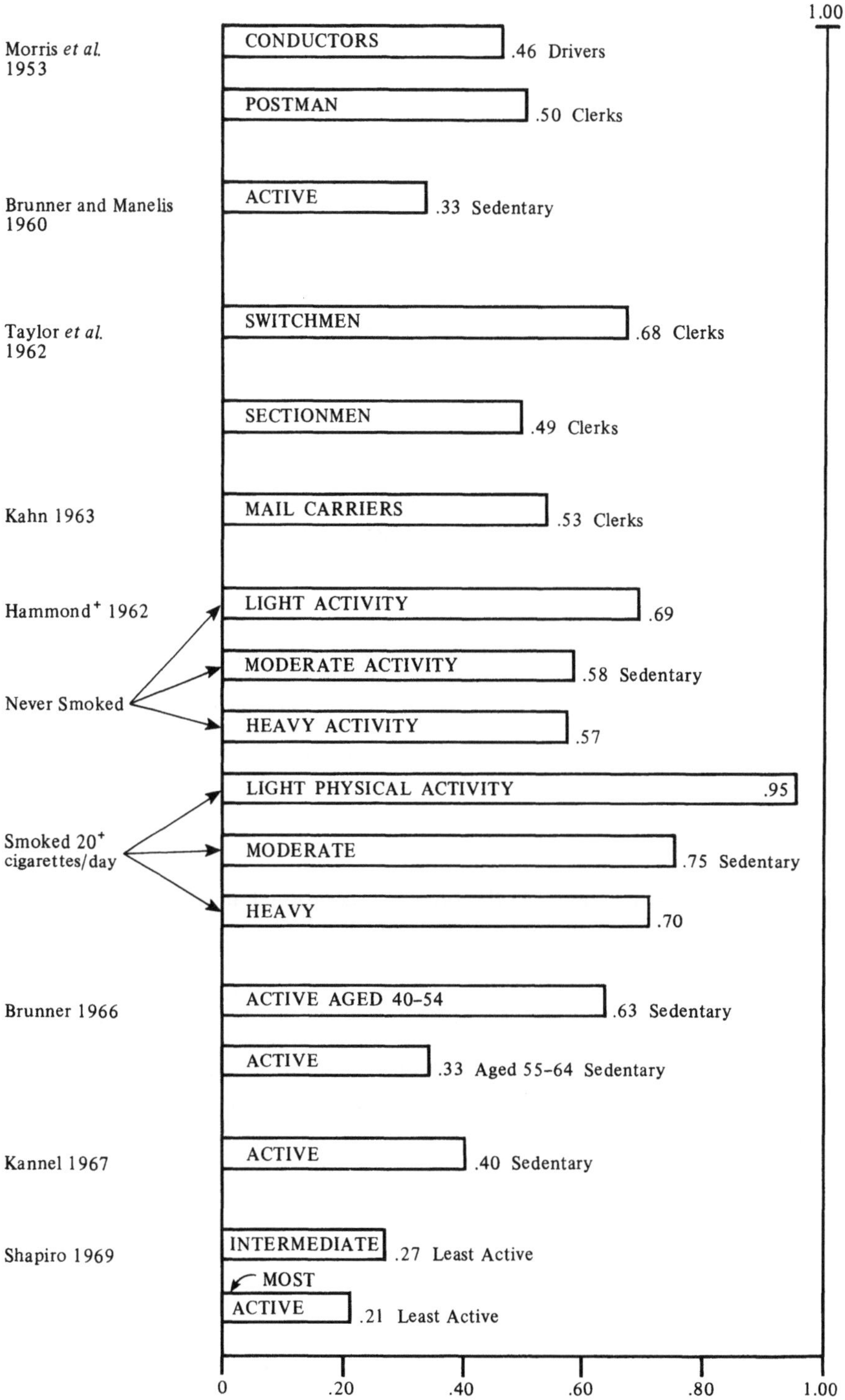
1.00
Morris et al. 1953
CONDUCTORS
.46 Drivers
POSTMAN
.50 Clerks
Brunner and Manelis 1960
ACTIVE
.33 Sedentary
Taylor et al. 1962
SWITCHMEN
.68 Clerks
SECTIONMEN
.49 Clerks
Kahn 1963
MAIL CARRIERS
.53 Clerks
Hammond+ 1962
LIGHT ACTIVITY
.69
Never Smoked
MODERATE ACTIVITY
.58 Sedentary
HEAVY ACTIVITY
.57
LIGHT PHYSICAL ACTIVITY
.95
Smoked 20+ cigarettes/day
MODERATE
.75 Sedentary
HEAVY
.70
Brunner 1966
ACTIVE AGED 40-54
.63 Sedentary
ACTIVE
.33 Aged 55-64 Sedentary
Kannel 1967
ACTIVE
.40 Sedentary
Shapiro 1969
INTERMEDIATE
.27 Least Active
MOST
ACTIVE
.21 Least Active
0
.20
.40
.60
.80
1.00

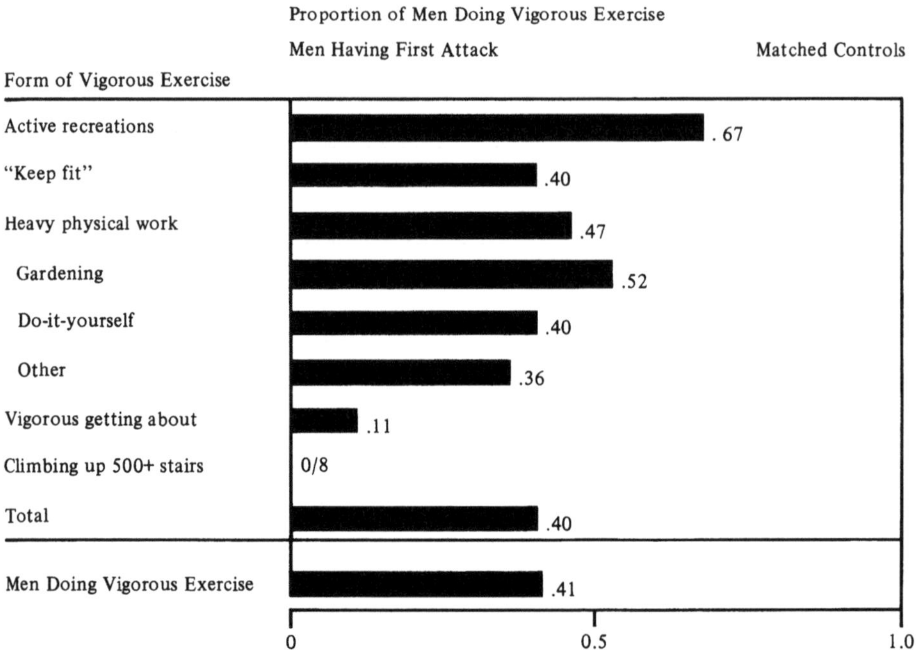

Fig. 16-3. Graphic representation of the recent report of Morris, *et al.* It can be seen that those men who suffered a first attack of coronary heart disease had previously reported less involvement in "Active Recreations" (0.67). "Keep Fit" activity (0.40) etc. with an average or total involvement of 0.40 (40 percent as frequently reported) as the matched controls who did not develop a coronary. It was considered unlikely that this lesser involvement was due to unadmitted coronary symptoms which supports the inference of lesser activity predisposing to more coronary manifestations.

particular interest relative to the type of recreational activity, either games, jogging, bicycling, or swimming, and so forth, which might stimulate meaningful changes, if indeed this is possible.

The study by Chapman and his colleagues (12) of Los Angeles Civil Servants, is often mentioned as one of the striking indications that physical activity appears to have no protective effect, as there was no difference in the total manifestations of coronary heart disease or myocardial infarctions among individuals classified as being more or less involved in physical activity. No data were presented on nonoccupational physical activities, which might have compensated for sedentary occupations. Sociologically there is reason to believe that those who are physically active during working hours tend to be inactive in their free time in comparison to the opposite trend among those who have sedentary occupations—at least to some extent.

Another study that is often spoken of as having shown no difference between occupational levels of physical activity and the incidence of coronary heart disease is that of Dr. Oglesby Paul undertaken in the Western Electric Company in Chicago. Although no overall differences in coronary events were observed Paul (24) states, "after 8 years the more active men in Code 4 indeed showed fewer coronary deaths than those in the less active Code 2 but unfortunately, also relatively more infarctions with survival." Certainly it is of importance that individuals have nonlethal episodes (as compared to those with a fatal outcome), although clearly a change in severity is less than the optimum desired. Also from Chicago is the report by Stamler and his associates (69), in which no statistically significant differences were found, perhaps due to the small population studied. The trends were all in a favorable direction, however, in that those individuals with actual or presumed greater physical activity at work, had a lesser incidence of coronary events even though in each category this did not reach high statistical significance.

As previously mentioned, relative to the difference between bus drivers and bus conductors and between mail carriers and clerical personnel in Britain, the choices made by individuals were perhaps influenced by circumstances of employment within the American scene and are of considerable significance in relation to the background of causation of increased coronary disease.

Most of the authors were cognizant of the problems that would result if those persons with symptoms or signs of coronary disease were categorized in the less active group and thus would bias the less active group toward a more rapid collection of morbidity and mortality statistics. There is no way that these investigators could guarantee that some of their population were not influenced by some subtle forms of less than adequate health that may have had a background in coronary insufficiency.

Even in later years the trend continues with fewer coronary manifestations being found in those of lifetime physically more active habits. Brown and his colleagues (6) in a study of males over age 65 on the rolls of the National Health Service in Birmingham, England, found the prevalence of abnormalities associated with coronary disease less in individuals whose life-time activity patterns placed them in the relatively more active group as compared to their more sedentary colleagues. Unfortunately the circumstances of this study did not permit evaluation as to whether these individuals were less of a burden on the social welfare system in Britain after their retirement or whether they were able to pursue more retirement activities of personal or community benefit. While the aforementioned study suggested a persisting effect running on beyond the years of occupational differences in physical activity, Kahn's review (38) of postal workers in Washington, D.C., suggested that the difference in the incidence of coronary heart disease became indistinguishable within 5 years after an individual left the more physically active occupational status. He states that "There is a suggestion here that physical activity of 5, 10, 15 years ago may not be associated with change in current mortality risks."

The above-mentioned studies were all undertaken in populations in which physical activity may have differed, but there were also available differences in diet and other characteristics of individual life-styles that may have played a very important role in coronary risk effects. One of the studies mentioned as being perhaps least influenced by factors of diet and other circumstances, is that of Brunner and Manelis (9), who evaluated differences in coronary heart disease in Kibbutz workers in Israel and reported lower rates among the more physically active. The diet in these communal settlements provided a standard meat ration for workers of both physically active and sedentary occupations. One must discount the purity of the dietary control, however, because it is probable that those who were physically more active supported their greater caloric needs by additional intake of grains, cereals, vegetables, and fruits, which are generally considered low in atherogenic potential. Thus this interesting social experiment is not truly a situation in which dietary factors were controlled throughout the physical activity range.

Taylor and his associates (72) reported greater death rates from arteriosclerotic heart disease among railroad workers with sedentary jobs compared to their more active colleagues in the categories of "switchmen" and, most particularly, to "section repairmen." It appears unlikely that individuals in the age groups studied with undiagnosed or latent coronary heart disease would have transferred in large numbers to the less active jobs, particularly in view of the traditions of nonmobility from the blue collar field workers into clerical work. There was no way in which the investigators could follow the dropouts from the physically active category into other industries, as the follow-up schedules only permitted evaluation of those retained within the railroads. As the study participants aged, it became apparent that the differences in arteriosclerotic manifestations were reduced between those of lesser and greater occupational job classification (39). It is a reasonable assumption that the more physically active men became less active with seniority as they were in a position to oversee the repair of sections of track and undertake other less physically demanding jobs as they obtained seniority.

Few studies have looked at the differences in both blacks and whites relative to levels of physical activity, but McDonough, Hames, and associates in Evans County, Georgia, were able to do so (42). Striking differences were only evident after adjustments were made for social class differences. Skinner and his colleagues (67) in evaluating the same study population with the addition of exercise stress test facilities, confirmed significantly lower CHD prevalence rates in the more active group, but it is of interest that there were no demonstrable difference between the treadmill elicited work capacity of members of the inactive compared to the physically active group.

Angina Pectoris

The usual finding of the more active groups having less severe disease with fewer fatalities and of less early onset did not appear to prevail relative to the subjective symptom of angina pectoris, at least in the earlier studies. In most studies angina pectoris accounts for only approximately 12 to 18 percent of all reported manifestations of coronary heart disease and as such its total impact may not be very large, but the questions raised by the difference in incidence are important to the understanding of the place, if any, of an increase in habitual physical activity as a preventive measure. The more active groups studied by Morris (49) and by Zukel (75) had almost twice the incidence of angina pectoris as the less active groups, and so far the greater reported incidence of angina pectoris in the more active groups has not been adequately explained. No data demonstrate that the greater exertion of the more active persons elicited symptoms of angina more frequently in that group; neither is there proof for the optimistic hypothesis that members of the more active group are living with a less severe anginal syndrome rather than having suffered myocardial infarction or death, which might have occurred had they not stimulated some protective adaptation by their exercise. Less angina in the physically more active segments of the population has been reported by Brunner (8).

Autopsy Studies

The hopeful hypothesis that the hearts of persons conditioned by high energy expenditures can be shown to develop larger coronary arteries less vulnerable to occlusions by a given amount of atherosclerotic accumulation is not yet supported by any convincing data. However, the extensive autopsy studies led by Morris and Crawford (47) of the hearts of some 3,800 individuals who were considered to have died from noncoronary heart disease causes revealed that there were fewer healed infarcts, fibrous patches, scars, and coronary occulusions in those whose occupations throughout life had been classified as "active" or "heavy" as compared to those with job classifications of "light" physical activity. The relative frequency of accumulation of atherosclerotic material within the major coronary arteries was far less striking, however, which supported the findings of Spain and Bradess (68), who found essentially no difference in the amount of atheromatous material in the coronary arteries of patients of differing physical activity patterns studied through the coroner's office in Westchester County, New York.

Although there are no supporting data in humans at this time, it is important in the future to see if some definition can be provided to support or refute the hypothesis that during the developing years an increase in habitual physical activity will stimulate the formation of larger coronary arteries in relation to the total heart mass, particularly in comparison with coronary arteries of those of less physical activity. If this attractive hypothesis could be substantiated, there would be a lessening of the resistance of those involved with educational and recreational programs to invest in facilities that are attractive and which will sustain the physical activity interests of our school and college-age children.

Participation in Athletic Training

In examining the differences in the incidence of coronary heart disease between those person who participated actively in athletics and a matching group of persons of lesser activity patterns it is difficult to sort out constitutional factors that may play a role in the outcome of such things as coronary heart disease. It is quite possible that those who do succeed athletically have a general or "constitutional" superiority that enhances their survival chances in a manner not now definable, but may contribute to the reputed lesser occurrence of coronary heart disease in some athletically well-trained populations. Differences in life style might also be important since the life-long athlete may be more prudent about smoking, diet, body weight, and exposure to some forms of psychic stress. Until we are better able to quantify the relative effects of different life styles and habits, it is difficult to evaluate their influence on coronary heart disease statistics. The reports of Montoye (45), Paffenbarger *et al*, (54), Pomeroy and White (56) and Pyörälä *et al.* (57), reinforce the argument that habitual physical activity, such as that engaged in by athletes, has a beneficial physical effect extending throughout part of their later less active life. The review and data of Polednak and Damon, however, show no differences between athletes and nonathletes after a long-term follow-up (55).

Amount of Increased Physical Activity

If indeed there is a beneficial influence that can be acquired by the introduction of an increase in habitual physical activity, it is important to try to quantify the required amount relative to the facilities and persuasions that must be provided to attract a previously sedentary person to an altered life style. Many studies suggest that the type, intensity, duration, and frequency of physical activity that may have a preventive value are not so great that a useful effect can not be attainable even in the lives of those time-pressured, striving persons in the modern megapolis.

Skinner and his colleagues (67) calculated that daily caloric expenditure differences of 400 to 500 kcal were associated with a significant difference in the prevalence of coronary heart disease in Evans County, Georgia. Taylor reported a similar figure for the railroad workers (71). Even lesser amounts seemed associated with statistically significant differences in coronary manifestations in the studies of Rose (63) and Shapiro and colleagues (66). Rose reported that walking 20 minutes or more to work was associated with a one-third lower prevalence of "ischemic type electrocardiographic abnormalities." Paffenbarger and associates, however, found only a 25 percent reduction in CHD death rates associated with a 925 kcal per day increase among longshoremen (53).

One of the most important recent studies is that representing Morris' continued interest in the potential preventive aspects of physical activity (46). He and his colleagues compared the later appearance of first attacks of coronary disease in 16,882 British male Executive Grade civil servants free of disease of age 40 to 64 in relation to the amounts of physical activity recorded by them for a previous working Friday and free Saturday.

For each of the 232 men who suffered a first clinical attack, two controls not so affected were chosen on the basis of age and other comparable circumstances. The previously recorded activities were analyzed separately, with vigorous activity defined as that likely to reach energy peaks of 7.5 kcal/min, which corresponds to heavy industrial work or about seven multiples of resting metabolic requirements. Morris and his colleagues reported:

> "During the two sample days, 11 percent of the men who developed coronary disease, compared with 26 of the controls, reported such vigorous activities. In men recording vigorous exercise the relative risk of developing coronary disease was about a third that in comparable men who did not, and in men reporting much of it still less. Lighter exercise, and provisional estimates of overall activity, showed no such advantage. Vigorous exercise apparently protected against rapidly fatal heart attacks and other first clinical attacks of coronary disease alike, throughout middle age. The smoking habits of men engaged in such activity were similar to those of the other men in the study."

Moderately heavy activities, those requiring from 4 to 7 kcal/min of energy expenditure, apparently had no influence and included "the most demanding household chores, polishing the car, endless hours of painting and paperhanging, chiseling and drilling, hoeing the garden and cutting hedges, ballroom dancing." The most energetic of these, such as lawnmowing, walking to work whatever the duration, other walking, or playing golf were distributed similarly between cases and controls or with insignificant differences. Morris and his colleagues believed "there is a time threshold before physical work becomes 'beneficial,' but this proved to be over 30 minutes, not 15, a total of at least an hour of such activity during the Friday-Saturday also appeared to be advantageous . . . ."

When the relative risk of developing coronary heart disease was examined, those who had reported the most vigorous activity had the least likelihood, 0.18; those of lesser vigorous activity 0.55; and those doing no vigorous activity, 1.20 times the population mean.

Postinfarct Training

Numerous reports of studies without random allocation to a more and less active group have suggested that those individuals having suffered a myocardial infarction who undertake vigorous physical activity in a well-structured rehabilitation training program have group mortality rates well below those of most infarct groups not involved in physical retraining (59). Encouraging as these reports are, the question is clearly unanswered as to what selection factors went into definition of the active group, particularly questions related to the possibility that those who succeeded and persisted with the exercise training program were among the least damaged and perhaps the individuals most likely to survive among all those with coronary disease. Early results have been published (65) from a controlled study in Göteborg, Sweden, of postinfarct male patients born in 1913 or later in which randomization was performed in hospital, but actual separation into a training and control program occurred after 3 months. Twenty-five percent were not considered candidates for training, mostly because of cardiac contraindications.

The training program consists of three sessions a week of 30 minutes each, with the intensity regulated by a physiotherapist using heart rate as a guide. In months 6 through 20, there was a difference in deaths in the two groups, with deaths being 8 in the exercising group and 19 in the control group. There were 6 deaths attributed to coronary heart disease in the exercising group and 18 in the control group, which were highly significant by the usual statistical criteria. The high rate of nonadherence of individuals in the study has made its continuation less meaningful. The follow-up over 4 years has allegedly continued to show a greater death-rate in those who were not involved in the exercise training program. More studies of this nature need to be pursued in which more individuals stay within designated activity groups, and thus the influence of physical activity increases can be more validly assessed.

In this section many epidemiologic studies have been mentioned which indicate that most groups of individuals with greater occupational or total life physical activities have fewer heart attacks and such attacks that occur are less severe and less frequently fatal than those occurring among their more sedentary colleagues.

Space limitations will not permit further details of these and other studies but the literature contains both supportive (7, 23, 25, 26) and skeptical (36), reviews.

Physiologic Effects of Physical Training

Many studies have indicated that most "unfit" individuals can improve their cardiovascular performance after a physical training program. Although this is also true for those with established coronary heart disease there are some individuals, perhaps largely those with the most severe limitation of "three-vessel" disease, who are refractory to physical training in so far as they show little if any alterations in the parameters of physical performance. A recent review by Dr. Robert A. Bruce (7) of careful studies in his laboratory indicate the clear-cut ability to increase the oxygen consumption, cardiac output, stroke volume, and arteriovenous oxygen difference in younger individuals and all but the last item in males of average age 47. Improvement has also been found in his experience and that of others with the training of individuals who suffered a myocardial infarction.

Recognizing that many training programs produce a lowering of heart rate, both at rest and specifically at any given work load on a test/retest evaluation and that there is a reduction in systolic blood pressure in many individuals that accompanies moderate exertion, it can be postulated that there is increased efficiency of cardiovascular performance even though Bruce and others quite clearly state this may not be due to any improvement in blood supply to the myocardium. Table 16-1 lists some of the physiologic and psychologic parameters that can be influenced to a greater or a lesser degree by physical training and may contribute to a decreased mortality or severity or a delayed time of onset of coronary heart disease.

Animal studies have shown enlargement of collateral vessels around constrictions imposed by surgical ligatures on major coronary branches. Physical training has apparently stimulated an increase in this coronary collateralization in most, but not all, studies, yet similar results have not been found in sizable numbers of diseased humans before and after an exercise training program, including angiographic definition. As yet there is no controlled study in diseased humans to indicate that there is a progression of atherosclerotic restriction of coronary vessels in those who are not physically active, as compared to the status of the vessels of those exercising on various regiments. Thus, in Currens' and White's autopsy findings (14) of large coronary vessels in the marathon runner Clarence DeMar, the large coronaries reported may only mean that he succeeded with superior endowment rather than that his unusually fine coronary tree resulted from his lifetime of marathon running.

Table 16-1. Mechanisms by which Physical Activity may Reduce the Occurrence or Severity of Coronary Heart Disease

Physical Activity—May: Increase	Physical Activity—May: Decrease
Coronary collateral vascularization	Serum lipid levels
Vessel size	Triglycerides
Myocardial efficiency	Cholesterol
Effectiveness of peripheral blood distribution and return	Blood sugar
	Appetite
Electron transport capacity	Obesity-adiposity
Fibrinolytic capability	Platelet stickiness
Blood oxygen content	Arterial blood pressure
Red blood-cell mass and blood volume	Heart rate
Thyroid function	Heart power requirement for a specific task
Growth hormone production	Vulnerability to dysrhythmias
Tolerance to stress	Neurohormonal over-reaction
Prudent living habits	Chronic catecholamine production
Sleep, rest and relaxation	"Strain" associated with psychic "stress"
"Joie de vivre"	

Even in the lack of clear-cut evidence of a better nutritional supply to the myocardium, there are encouraging studies in animals indicating that physical training may also improve myocardial efficiency by increasing available potassium and cytochrome oxidase supplies and the ability to utilize lactate (28, 31, 58). An increase in myocardial electron transport capacity, as noted by Holloszy in rats after 12 weeks of treadmill training (34) may have an equivalent beneficial response in man, but for understandable reasons the opportunity for this type of study is hard to arrange.

Detry and Bruce (15) also indicated that physical training produces a greater arterial oxygen content and that this is more frequently the mechanism of greater oxygen availability than that accomplished by widening the arteriovenous oxygen extraction in older or diseased patients.

Physical activity of light or moderate intensity (10 to 12 minutes walk at 3 mph) will significantly increase fibrinolytic activity in most persons, although only briefly (11, 44, 64). Data on more strenuous activity (18), especially competitive games, is less consistent, with some investigators indicating increased lytic activity whereas others have observed a decrease (20, 36). Though some of these inconsistencies may have resulted from different methods for evaluating blood clotting mechanisms in the type of exercise performed, the data nevertheless suggest that a moderate increase in habitual activity may have a favorable chronic effect on blood clotting, fibrinolytic mechanisms, or both (29), while unaccustomed strenuous exercise tends to temporarily shorten blood clotting time (17), even though it may also stimulate increased fibrinolytic activity. Hames (30) found a decreased tendency for platelet aggregation with acute moderate exertion, but techniques for this type of evaluation have not been applied with great success in many studies.

A small but possibly beneficial chronic increase in thyroid function has been presented verbally in some reports but this finding has not yet been published. Likewise growth hormone stimulation accompanying physical exertion may have a useful lipid lowering effect, but the complex actions of this hormone needs far more evaluation.

There are many reports of peripheral circulatory improvement in the legs after an exercise program, suggesting that benefit can occur even late in the course of atherosclerotic disease (19).

Although studies of psychologic factors in the genesis of coronary heart disease have been regarded with considerable skepticism because methodology is still being developed, there are numerous investigators who believe that stress modification represents a useful approach to preventive programs. Numerous reports indicate that persons involved in physical activity programs believe they develop an increased tolerance or decreased vulnerability to some psychologic stresses either because the person's self-image is enhanced or the individual has the opportunity to work-off or over-ride anxieties by physical activities. A number of recent reports state an increase in "joie de vivre" and tolerance to stress is appreciated by most of the study's participants in almost direct proportion to the degree to which they adhere to prescribed programs (16, 32, 43).

Although some individuals upon initiating a physically more active life report an increase in demands for rest and sleep, there are data indicating that the opposite effects may occur and that in addition to help in avoiding insomnia, a physically more active life may increase the restfulness of sleep (1).

One of the factors which will make the definitive study of the preventive potential of physical activity a difficult task is the natural tendency of those committing themselves to a program of increased physical activity to modify, in a prudent manner, other habits that may contribute to the background of coronary heart disease. Chief among these might be abstinence from cigarette smoking for which there is some encouraging evidence but not as much as is desired (16, 32).

A voluntary reduction in food intake, particularly animal fat, is another example of associated, presumably beneficial changes in life style that may be prompted by commitment to a more prudent way of life that includes increased physical activity. The person who invests the time, effort, and resources required to enhance his physical condition is also likely to be motivated to avoid unnecessary stress/strain relationships or harassment in his life. By thus reducing some of the factors thought to contribute to atherogenesis or the precipitation of sudden catastrophe (through surges in catecholamines and other factors that contribute to dysrhythmias) or both, prudent habits and actions can be a potent by-product of physical activity programs.

The above section has discussed physiologic and psychologic parameters that appear to be enhanced by an increase of physical activity and thereby may lead to a reduction in the incidence and severity of coronary heart disease. Physical activity can also induce decreases in various factors, which will permit an equivalent amount of work to be done at lesser myocardial metabolic cost or have other benefits of potential value in reducing risk.

The legitimate widespread concern about excess serum cholesterol immediately raises the question of the potential lipid lowering effects of increased habitual physical activity. Although there are many reports (27, 35, 51, 61, 62, 70) indicating that cholesterol levels respond favorably in a downward direction to increased physical activity, most reports also included indications that there was some weight reduction or, if not an absolute weight reduction, a reduction in adiposity. On the other hand, a reduction in triglycerides has been almost uniformly reported as being of significance with an increase in physical activity even though the effect may be transitory. The report by Mann (40) is the chief exception to this reported trend of a decrease in triglycerides among those who undertake a metabolically demanding exercise training program.

Reduction of triglyceride levels after exercise, even if that exercise must be performed every 2 to 3 days to maintain the lower serum level, is encouraging, since hyperlipidemia has been associated with accelerated blood clotting, increased blood viscosity, and greater adhesiveness and aggregation properties of platelets (10, 41, 74). Also, reported have been impaired myocardial oxygen extraction, decreased coronary blood flow, and decreased physical performance capacity as a result of the early onset of anginal symptoms in patients with alimentary hyperlipemia (33, 60).

The lowered cholesterol level reported after physical activity in many studies may have been due to "regression toward the mean," or because some newly activated individuals stimulated to loose body weight change their diets along with the increase in physical activity. Tooshi (73), however, reported that middle-age men who walked, jogged, and ran for 15 minutes a day improved their *fitness*; those exercising 30 minutes a day at the same intensity per minute improved *body composition* as well, i.e., more muscle and less fat per given weight, but the significant *change in cholesterol* was found only in the group exercising at the same intensity for 45 minutes per day 5 days a week. It is also possible that individuals with relatively little body adiposity are more able to influence their serum lipid levels than those with larger lipid stores, but further data need to be obtained on this as well as many other points.

We do not know if the physically active person can better tolerate eating more saturated fat than can the less active or if he or she can indulge in other dietary indiscretions beyond enjoying the extra calories that the activities consume, but it is clear that increased physical activity often serves as a useful adjunct to efforts in dietary modifications or the reduction of adiposity. A recent report (2) even suggests that exercise elevates the plasma concentration of anorexigenic or appetite suppressing substances.

With increased interest in the influence of carbohydrate and sugars on atherosclerosis, it is important that more information be developed about the influence of physical activities on metabolic pathways, including the disturbed metabolism of diabetes mellitus. We know that the patient with diabetes requires less insulin when he exercises and, indeed, one must be cautious in prescribing exercise without glucose being available because of the rapid reduction of serum levels in some individuals. As yet there is no firm evidence that a long-term benefit to the carbohydrate-glucose metabolic pathways is achieved by an increase in habitual physical activity.

Elevated blood pressure as a coronary heart disease risk factor, and its reduction as a preventive approach, is one of the most accepted concepts in current efforts to control coronary heart disease. Some studies report that moderately elevated resting blood pressures of patients have been reduced during a physical conditioning program (52), but this has not been a major feature in most controlled studies. The observed reduction may, again, have resulted from a "regression towards the mean" or the fact that most individuals observed over an extended period of time tend to present a decreasing blood pressure on each subsequent examination. Boyer and Kasch (5) indicate considerable improvement in an encouraging report that is not a controlled study.

Perhaps more important than usually obtained resting blood pressure is an "operational blood pressure" with which we live, work, and love. The results of many exercise stress tests indicate operational pressures may be significantly reduced in many individuals during and after exercise programs (13), but studies of blood pressure response during real-life situations are still needed.

One of the most predictable training effects of an exercise program is heart-rate reduction, both at rest and, more impressively, at various levels of submaximal exertion. The exact mechanism by which this training bradycardia is achieved has not been well defined, but the effect appears to be a reliable indicator of the conditioning effect. The bradycardia and the reduced blood pressure level, and the heart rate-systolic blood pressure product calculated from their multiplication, may be major contributors to the markedly increased tolerance to, and capacity for, exertion after physical training seen in most patients with angina pectoris. As yet the available data are too meager to determine whether the conditioning protects the myocardium against further damage or enhances chances for survival after further insults.

In Blackburn's recent report (4) of a decrease in the frequency of premature ventricular complexes in those who had undertaken and adhered well to an exericise training program, there was not only evidence of a decrease in ectopic ventricular impulses at any given work level, but there was a suggestion, although among very few subjects, of the lesser occurrence of premature ventricular complexes at the same heart rate that was associated with a greater work load achieved after training. A decrease in the vulnerability of the myocardium to dysrhythmias would be a factor of great importance for approximately half of the more than 600,000 coronary deaths in the United States occur outside of hospital, presumably more the result of dysrhythmia than early primary myocardial failure. This is particularly relevant until chronic antidysrhythmic medication is proved of value.

A more appropriate neurohormonal responsiveness to both psychic and physical stress resulting from physical conditioning may contribute to a reduced coronary risk as postulated by the late Wilhelm Raab, but too little data are available in this fascinating area. In the current era of psychosocial and economic stress we might all benefit from an enhanced capability to handle stresses more appropriately.

A review of some of the physiologic mechanisms whereby an increase in habitual physical activity may be salutory indicates a capability to increase physical work performance and some strong evidence of psychologic benefits of significance. Studies have yet to document the socioeconomic and epidemiologic benefits with overwhelming persuasion that activity program investments will return to individuals, industry or government, tangible benefits in excess of the required costs in time, effort, and resources.

Summary

What then is a rational position for a clinician in 1975? Although more data are needed—and appear amenable to development within the capability of research teams now existing—it appears *prudent* to recommend an increase in habitual physical activity for both men and women without compromised or unstable cardiac status. After a "clearance" evaluation, which optimally should include an exercise tolerance test, a person appears well advised to try to find some rewarding activities—preferably those that are fun—in which he can participate three or more times per week. If participation is but twice a week, and preferably not on consecutive days, the duration of involvement should presumably be longer to maintain or enhance physiologic performance—the apparently reciprocal relationships between *frequency, duration*, and *intensity* not being well defined even for physiologic response. Although the needs for, and responses to, the intensity of effort probably vary considerably between individuals, it would appear likely that exertion requiring five or more multiples of resting metabolic rate are necessary to create a difference within a year or so. Thus vigorous walking at more than $3\frac{1}{2}$ mph (6 km/hr), bicycle riding at more than 8 mph, vigorous dancing, badminton, and tennis doubles appear within the lower levels of meaningful activity as are energetic leaf raking, hand mowing, hoeing, garden digging, and splitting or sawing wood (22).

Although the major hypothesis that such activities are capable of postponing or decreasing coronary morbidity and mortality remains unproven, the practitioner can recommend participation on the basis of data indicating almost predictable improvement in performance and feeling states with an acceptably low hazard to those properly screened. The physically more active person will usually become more health-conscious and thus achieve a reduction of general health hazards in a total life style of improved quality.

References

1. Baekeland, F. Exercise deprivation: sleep and psychological reactions. Arch. Gen. Psychiat., 22:365, 1970.
2. Belbeck, L. W. and Critz, J. B. Effect of exercise on the plasma concentration of anorexigenic substance in man. Proc. Soc. Exp. Biol. Med., 142:19, 1973.
3. Blackburn, H. Disadvantages of intensive exercise therapy after myocardial infarction. In ref. 7 pp. 162–172.
4. Blackburn, H., Taylor, H. L., Hamrell, B., Buskirk, E., Nicholas, W. C., and Thorsen, R. D. Premature ventricular complexes induced by stress testing: their frequency and response to physical conditioning. Am. J. Cardiol., 31:441, 1973.
5. Boyer, J. L. and Kasch, F. W. Exercise therapy in hypertensive men. J.A.M.A., 211:1668, 1970.
6. Brown, R. G., Davidson, A. G. McKeown, T., and Whitfield, A. G. W. Coronary artery disease: influences affecting its incidence in males in the seventh decade. Lancet, 2:1073, 1957.
7. Bruce, R. A. The benefits of physical training for patients with coronary heart disease. *In* Ingelfinger, F. J., Ebert, R. V., Finland, M., and Relman, A. S., eds. Controversy in Internal Medicine. Philadelphia, W. B. Saunders Co., 1974, pp. 145–161.
8. Brunner, D. The influence of physical activity on incidence and prognosis of ischemic heart disease. In Raab, W., ed. Prevention of Ischemic Heart Disease: Principles and Practice. Springfield, C. C. Thomas, 1966.
9. Brunner, D. and Manelis, G. Myocardial infarction among members of communal settlements in Israel. Lancet, 2:1049, 1950.
10. Buzina, R. and Keys, A. Blood coagulation after a fat meal. Circulation, 14:854, 1956.
11. Cash, J. D. Effect of moderate exercise on the fibrinolytic system in normal young men and women, Br. Med. J., 2:502, 1966.
12. Chapman, J. M., Goerke, L. S., Dixon, W., Loveland, D. B., and Phillips, E. The clinical status of a population group in Los Angeles under observation for two to three years. Am. J. Public Health, 47:33, 1957.
13. Choquette, G. and Ferguson, R. J. Blood pressure reduction in "borderline" hypertensives following physical training. Can. Med. Assoc. J., 108:699, 1973.
14. Currens, J. H. and White, P. D. Half a century of running. N. Engl. J. Med., 265:988, 1961.
15. Detry, J.-M. R., Rousseau, M., Vandenbroucke, G., Kusumi, F., Brasseur, L. A., and Bruce, R. A. Increased arteriovenous oxygen difference after physical training in coronary heart disease. Circulation, 44:109, 1971.
16. Durbeck, D. C., Heinzelmann, F., Schacter, J., Haskell, W. L., Payne, G., Moxley, R., Nemiroff, M., Limoncelli, D., Arnoldi, L., and Fox, S. M. The NASA-USPHS health evaluation and enhancement program. Am. J. Cardiol., 30:784, 1972.
17. Egeberg, O. The effect of exercise on the blood clotting system. Scand. J. Clin. Lab. Invest., 15:8, 1963.
18. Epstein, S. E., Rosing, D. R., Brakman, P., Redwood, D. R., and Astrup, T. Impaired fibrinolytic response to exercise in patients with type-IV hyperlipoproteinemia. Lancet, 2:631, 1970.
19. Ericsson, B., Haeger, K., and Lindell, S. E. Effect of physical training on intermittent claudication. Angiology, 21:188, 1970.
20. Fearnley, G. R. and Lacker, R. The fibrinolytic activity of normal blood. Br. J. Hematol., 1:189, 1955.
21. Fox, S. M. and Haskell, W. L. Physical activity and health maintenance. J. Rehabil., 32:89, 1966.
22. Fox, S. M., Naughton, J. P., and Gorman, P. A. Physical activity and cardiovascular health. Mod. Concepts. Cardiovasc. Dis., 41:17, 1972.
23. —— —— and Haskell, W. L. Physical activity and the prevention of coronary heart disease. Ann. Clin. Res., 3:404, 1971.
24. —— and Paul, O. Physical activity and coronary heart disease. Am. J. Cardiol., 23:305, 1969.
25. —— and Skinner, J. S. Physical activity and cardiovascular health. Am. J. Cardiol., 14:731, 1964.
26. Froelicher, V. F. and Oberman, A. Analysis of epidemiologic studies of physical inactivity as risk factor for coronary artery disease. Prog. Cardiovasc. Dis., 15:41, 1972.
27. Goode, R. C., Firstbrook, J. B., and Shepard, J. R. Effects of exercise and a cholesterol-free diet on human serum lipids. Can. J. Physiol. Parmacol., 44:575, 1966.
28. Gollnick, P. D. and Hearn, G. H. Lactic dehydrogenase activities of heart and skeletal muscle of exercised rats. Am. J. Physiol., 201:694, 1961.

29. Guest, M. M. and Celander, D. R. Fibrinolytic activity in exercise. Physiologist, 3:69, 1960.
30. Hames, C. G. Personal communication relative to Evans County, Georgia, study.
31. Hearn, G. H. The effects of terminating and detraining on enzyme activities of heart and skeletal muscle of trained rats. Int. Z. Angew. Physiol., 21:190, 1965.
32. Heinzelmann, F. and Bagley, R. W. Response to physical activity programs and their effects on health behavior. Public Health Rep., 85:905, 1970.
33. Hellerstein, H. K., Hornsten, T. R., Baker, R. A., and Hoppes, W. L. Cardiac performance during postprandial lipemia and heparin-induced lipolysis. Am. J. Cardiol., 20:525, 1967.
34. Holloszy, J. Biochemical adaptations in muscle: effects of exercise on mitochondrial oxygen uptake and respiratory enzyme activity in skeletal muscle. J. Biol. Chem., 242:2278, 1967.
35. Holloszy, J. O., Skinner, J. S., Toro, G., and Cureton, T. K. Effects of a six month program of endurance exercise on the serum lipids of middle-aged men. Am. J. Cardiol., 14:753, 1964.
36. Ikkala, E., Myllyla, G., and Sarajas, H. S. Platelet adhesiveness and ADP-induced platelet aggregation in exercise. Ann. Med. Exp. Biol. Fenn., 44:88, 1966.
37. Inter-Society Commission for Heart Disease Resources. Atherosclerosis Study Group and Epidemiology Study Group: Primary prevention of the atherosclerotic diseases. Circulation, 42:A55, 1970.
38. Kahn, H. A. The relationship of reported coronary heart disease mortality to physical activity of work. Am. J. Public Health, 53:1058, 1963.
39. Keys, A. Physical activity and the epidemiology of coronary heart disease. In Brunner, D. and Jokl, E. eds. Medicine and Sport, Physical Activity and Aging. Baltimore, University Park Press, 1970, Vol. 4.
40. Mann, G. V., Garrett, H. L., Farhi, A., Murray, H., Billings, F. T., Shutte, E., and Scharten, S. E. Exercise to prevent coronary heart disease: an experimental study of the effects of training on risk factors for coronary disease in men. Am. J. Med., 46:12, 1969.
41. McDonald, L. and Edgill, M. Coagulability of the blood in ischemic heart disease. Lancet, 2:457, 1957.
42. McDonough, J. R., Hames, C. G., Stulb, S. C., and Garrison, G. E. Coronary heart disease among negroes and whites in Evans County, Georgia. J. Chron. Dis., 18:443, 1965.
43. McPherson, B. D., Pavio, A. U., Yuhasz, M. S., Rechnitzer, P. A., Pickard, H. A, and Lefcoe, N. M. Psychological effects of an exercise program for post-infarct and normal adult men. J. Sports Med. Phys. Fitness, 7:95, 1967.
44. Menon, I. S., Burke, F., and Dewar, H. A. Effect of strenuous and graded exercise on fibrinolytic activity. Lancet, 2:700, 1966.
45. Montoye, H. Summary of research on the relationship of exercise to heart disease. J. Sports Med. Phys. Fitness, 2:35, 1962.
46. Morris, J. N., Chave, S. P. W., Adam, C., Sirey, E., Epstein, L., and Sheehan, D. J. Vigorous exercise in leisure-time and the incidence of coronary heart disease. Lancet, 1:333, 1973.
47. Morris, J. N. and Crawford, M. D. Coronary heart disease and physical activity of work. Br. Med. J., 2:1485, 1958.
48. Morris, J. N., Heady, J. A., and Raffle, P. A. B. Physique of London busmen: epidemiology of uniforms. Lancet, 2:569, 1956.
49. Morris, J. N., Heady, J. A., Raffle, P. A. B., Roberts, C. G., and Parks, J. W. Coronary heart disease and physical activity of work. Lancet, 2:1053, 1953.
50. Morris, J. N., Kagan, A. Pattison, D. C., Gardner, M. J., and Raffle, P. A. B. Incidence and prediction of ischemic heart disease in London busmen. Lancet, 2:553, 1966.
51. Naughton, J. and McCoy, J. F. Observations on the relationship of physical activity to the serum cholesterol concentration of healthy men and cardiac patients. J. Chron. Dis., 19:727, 1966.
52. Naughton, J. P., Shanbour, K., Armstrong, R., McCoy, J., and Lategola, M. Cardiovascular responses to exercise following myocardial infarction. Arch. Intern. Med., 117:541, 1966.
53. Paffenbarger, R. S. Jr., Laughlin, M. E., Gima, A. S., and Black, R. A. Work activity of longshoremen as related to death from coronary heart disease and stroke. N. Engl. J. Med., 282:1109, 1970.
54. Paffenbarger, R. S. Jr., Norkin, J., Krueger, D. E. Wolf, P. A., Thorne, M. O., Lebauer, E. J., and Williams, J. L. Chronic disease in former college students: II. Methods of study and observations on mortality from coronary heart disease. Am. J. Public Health, 56:962, 1966.
55. Polednak, A. P. and Damon, A. College athletics, longevity, and cause of death. Hum. Biol., 42:28, 1970.

56. Pomeroy, W. and White, P. D. Coronary heart disease in former football players. J.A.M.A., 167:711, 1958.
57. Pyörälä, K., Karvonen, M. J., Taskinen, P., Takkunen, J., and Kyronseppa, H. Cardiovascular Studies on Former Endurance Runners. Report 19. Helsinki, Institute of Occupational Health, 1965.
58. Raab, W. The nonvascular metabolic myocardial vulnerability factor in "coronary heart disease." Am. Heart J., 66:685, 1963.
59. Rechnitzer, P. A., Pickard, H. A., Pavio, A. U., Yuhasz, M. S., and Cunningham, D. Long-term follow-up study of survival and recurrence rates following myocardial infarction in exercising and control subjects. Circulation, 45:853, 1972.
60. Regan, T. J., Binak, K., Gordon, S., DeFazio, V., and Hellems, H. K. Myocardial blood flow and oxygen consumption during postprandial lipemia and heparin-induced lipolysis. Circulation, 23:55, 1961.
61. Rochelle, R. Blood plasma cholesterol changes during a physical training program. Res. Q. Am. Assoc. Health, Phys. Educ., 32:538, 1961.
62. Romanova, D. and Barin, P. The influence of physical exercise on the content of serum protein, lipoprotein and total cholesterol in persons of middle and elderly age with symptoms of atherosclerosis. Kardiol. Pol., 1:36, 1961.
63. Rose, G. Physical activity and coronary heart disease. Proc. R. Soc. Med., 62:1183, 1969.
64. Rosing, D. R., Brakman, P., Redwood, D. R., Goldstein, R. E., Beiser, G. D., Astrup, T., and Epstein, S. E. Blood fibrinolytic activity in man: diurnal variation and the response to varying intensities of exercise. Circ. Res., 27:171, 1970.
65. Sanne, H., Elmfeldt, D., and Wilhelmsen, L. Preventive effect of physical training after a myocardial infarction. In Tibblin, G., Keys, A., and Werkö, L. eds. Preventive Cardiology, New York, John Wiley and Sons, 1972.
66. Shapiro, S., Weinblatt, E., Frank, C. W., and Sager, R. V. Incidence of coronary heart disease in a population insured for medical care (HIP). Am. J. Public Health, Suppl. to June 1969.
67. Skinner, J. S., Benson, H., McDonough, J. R., and Hames, C. G. Social status, physical activity, and coronary proneness. J. Chron. Dis., 19:773, 1966.
68. Spain, D. and Bradess, V. Sudden death from coronary atherosclerosis: age, race, sex, physical activity and alcohol. Arch. Intern. Med., 100:228, 1957.
69. Stamler, J., Lindberg, H. A., Berkson, D. M., Shaffer, A., Miller, W., and Poindexter, A. Prevalence and incidence of coronary heart disease in strata of the labor force of a Chicago industrial corporation. J. Chron. Dis., 11:405, 1960.
70. Taylor, H. L. Relationship of physical activity to serum cholesterol concentration. In Rosenbaum, F. F., and Belknap, E. L. (eds.). Work and the Heart. New York, Hoeber, 1953.
71. Taylor, H. L., Blackburn, H., Puchner, T., Vasquez, C. L., Parlin, R. W., and Keys, A. Coronary heart disease in selected occupations of American railroads in relation to physical activity. Circulation, 40:Suppl. 3:202, 1969.
72. Taylor, H. L., Klepetar, E., Keys, A., Parlin, W., Blackburn, H., and Puchner, T. Death rates among physically active and sedentary employees of the railroad industry. Am. J. Public Health, 52:1697, 1962.
73. Tooshi, A. Effects of three different durations of endurance exercises upon serum cholesterol. Med. Sci. in Sports, 1:1, 1971.
74. Williams, A., Higginbotham, A. C., and Knisely, M. T. Increased blood cell agglutination following ingestion of fat, a factor contributing to cardiac ischemia, coronary insufficiency, and anginal pain. Angiology, 8:29, 1957.
75. Zukel, W. J., Lewis, R. H., Enterline, P. E., Painter, R. C., Ralston, L. S., Fawcett, R. M., Meredith, A. P., and Peterson, B. A. short-term community study of the epidemiology of coronary heart disease. Am. J. Public Health, 49:1630, 1959.

Chapter 17 His Bundle Electrocardiography—Its Clinical Value

ROBERT L. DEJOSEPH, M.D. and DOUGLAS P. ZIPES, M.D.

General Considerations

Since the introduction by Scherlag and associates (23) of the catheter technique for recording His bundle activity in man, a voluminous amount of knowledge has been obtained about the physiology of normal and abnormal atrioventricular conduction and of arrhythmias. However, recent editorials consider His bundle electrocardiography of limited value in the clinical management of cardiac patients (3, 9, 10). Nevertheless, as these editorials point out, certain clinical situations exist when His bundle electrocardiography can be of considerable value in arriving at therapeutic decisions. In this paper, we will consider briefly the technique of His bundle recording and the physiologic importance of the measurements obtained. The major portion of our discussion will deal with the clinical findings of and indications for His bundle studies.

Technique of His Bundle Recording

His bundle electrocardiography may be performed on patients in a postabsorbtive, nonsedated state wherever fluoroscopic and recording equipment are available. Before the study is started, a reliable intravenous route is begun and a routine 12-

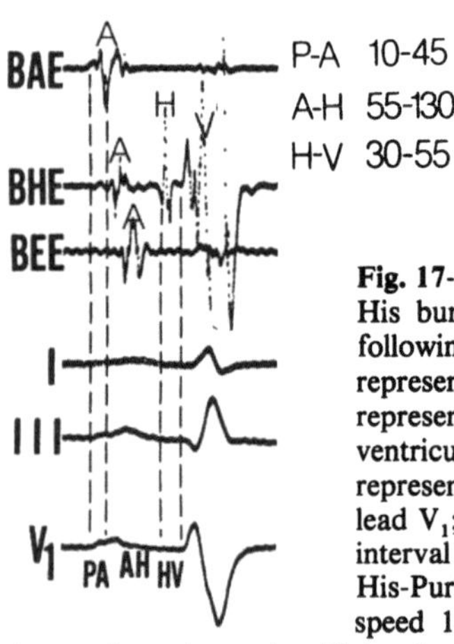

Fig. 17-1. A single cardiac cycle illustrating the intervals measured during His bundle electrocardiography. In this and all subsequent figures, the following abbreviations are used: BAE = bipolar atrial electrogram representing high right atrial activity; BHE = bipolar His electrogram representing low right atrial activity (A), His bundle activity (H) and ventricular septal activity (V); BEE = bipolar esophageal electrogram representing primarily left atrial activity; I, lead 1; II, lead 2; III, lead 3; V_1, lead V_1; P-A, P-A interval representing intra-atrial conduction; A-H, A-H interval representing AV nodal conduction; H-V, H-V interval representing His-Purkinje conduction. All numbers are given in milliseconds. Paper speed 100 mm/sec unless otherwise stated. Interrupted lines demarcate the various intervals. Note the normal sequence of artrial activation recorded with this technique: high right atrial activity precedes low right atrial activity recorded in the BHE lead and this precedes left atrial activity recorded in the BEE lead.

lead electrocardiogram is recorded. Using local anesthesia, a multipolar (usually, a tripolar) catheter electrode is inserted percutaneously into a femoral vein and advanced under fluoroscopic guidance to the right atrium. A quadripolar catheter is also inserted into the right atrium through the femoral vein or an antecubital (basilic) vein. The proximal two electrodes of this catheter are used to record the atrial electrogram and the distal two electrodes are used for atrial pacing. After the catheter is connected to appropriate recording devices, the electrode portion of the His bundle catheter is then advanced across the atrioventricular ring while the electrogram is recorded simultaneously, until the position yielding the optimal His bundle deflection is found (Figure 17-1). In some instances, a right bundle branch deflection also may be recorded (Figure 17-2). The tip of the quadripolar catheter is advanced to the high lateral portion of the right atrium. Once the His and right atrial catheters have been introduced into the vein, it usually takes less than 5 minutes to position them. An esophageal lead may be swallowed, and yield information about left atrial events (30). Additional catheter electrodes may be inserted to record from the coronary sinus, stimulate the ventricle, and so forth, depending on the nature of the study. His bundle recording can also be obtained using an arm or neck vein, or from the aorta.

Complications from His bundle studies are uncommon if the usual precautions observed during cardiac catheterization are performed. One must remember that whenever catheters are introduced into the heart, thus bypassing the high skin resistance, great care must be taken to assure that all equipment is adequately grounded. This may require the help of an experienced electrician or bioengineer. Reported complications involving improperly grounded electrical equipment are not

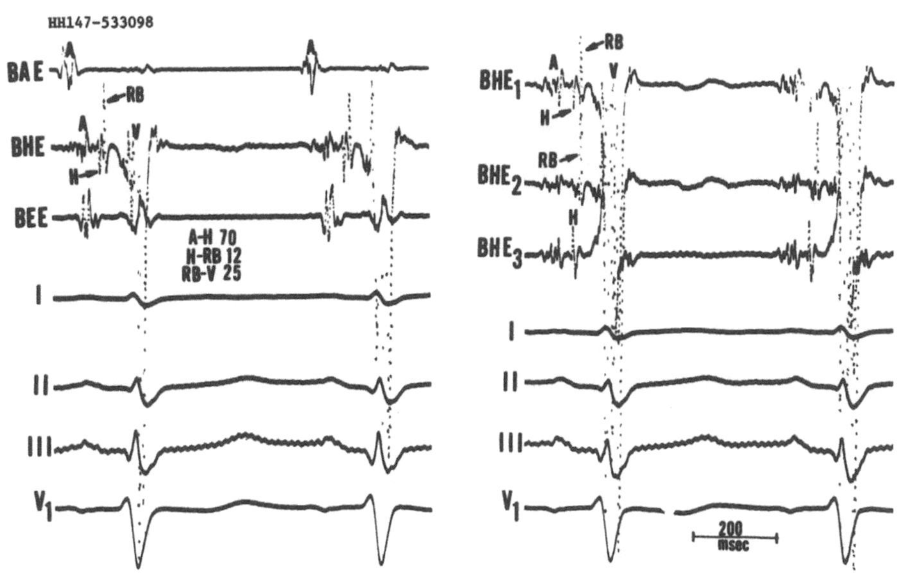

Fig. 17-2. Example illustrating a right bundle branch deflection (RB). In the panel on the right, three His bundle leads recorded simultaneously indicate recordings of both His and right bundle spikes (BHE_1), recording of primarily right bundle spike (BHE_2), and recording primarily a His bundle spike (BHE_3).

common however. The physician must have expertise in at least right heart catheterization techniques, observing the basic principles of sterility, prevention of air emboli, hemostatis, and the like. Hematomas in the femoral area occur but usually resolve uneventfully. Thrombophlebitis happens infrequently, but when it does, one must be concerned about pulmonary emboli and the patient must be anticoagulated. The hazard of inducing arrhythmias during catheter placement or electrical stimulation must be anticipated and appropriate resuscitative equipment, including a direct current cardioverter and airway equipment, must be immediately available.

Conduction Disorders and Block

Significance of Proximal and Distal His Bundle Delay and Block

Pertinent to considering the value of His bundle recordings is a discussion of their electrophysiologic significance and the intervals measured. Three basic measurements are made from the His bundle catheter recording, the P-A, A-H, and H-V intervals (Figures 17-1 to 17-3).

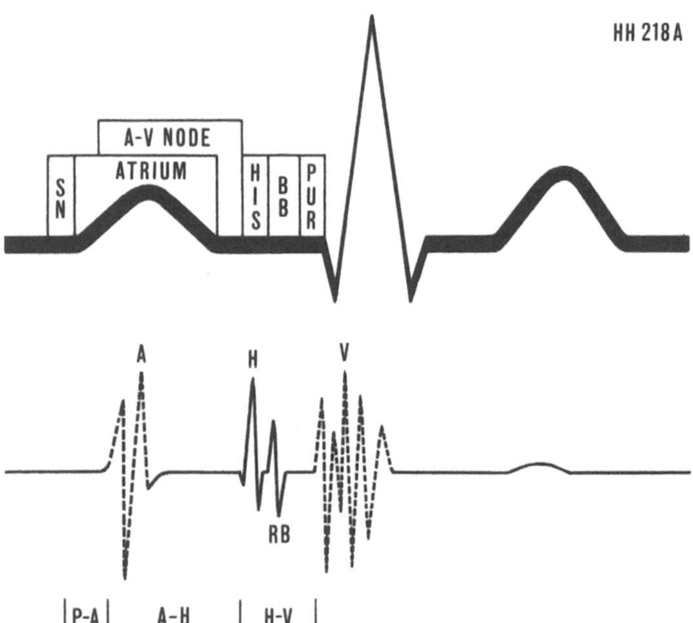

Fig. 17-3. Schematic illustration indicating condition through the various portions of the heart during one cardiac cycle. Note that the impulse has reached the Purkinje fibers prior to the inscription of the QRS complex. It is important to remember that with surface electrocardiography, only atrial depolarization (and sometimes atrial repolarization), ventricular depolarization and ventricular repolarization are recorded. SN = sinus node, BB = bundle branches, Pur = Purkinje fibres. Top portion adapted from Hoffman, B. F. and Singer, D. H. Prog. Cardiovasc. Dis., 7:226, 1964.

The *P-A interval* represents the interval between the onset of the P wave in the surface tracing (which generally coincides with the onset of the high right atrial recording) and the low right atrial deflection recorded in the His bundle lead. This interval reflects intra-atrial conduction and has not proved to be of much clinical value in our experience.

The *A-H interval* is measured from the beginning of the atrial electrogram (A) in the His bundle lead to the beginning of the His (H) deflection. Since the low right atrium and His bundle anatomically delimit the boundaries of the atrioventricular (AV) node, the A-H interval closely approximates AV nodal conduction time. The A-H interval is affected importantly by various interventions (Table 17-1). The normal range for the AH interval in our laboratory is 55 to 130 msec, depending on heart rate and autonomic tone. Some investigators measure the P-H interval from the beginning of the P wave in a simultaneously recorded surface electrocardiogram. This measurement naturally includes intra-atrial conduction time.

The *H-V interval* (H-Q interval) is measured from the beginning of the H deflection to the earliest onset of ventricular depolarization recorded in any lead. This interval represents conduction from the His bundle through the bundle branch-Purkinje system, up to the point of ventricular muscle activation, and is normally between 30 to 55 msec, regardless of heart rate or autonomic tone.

Prolongation of the A-H interval or block before the inscription of the His electrogram indicates delay or block in the AV node. Prolongation of the H-V interval or block after the inscription of His bundle electrogram indicates delay or block distal to the His bundle recording site, in the His-Purkinje system.

Delay or block proximal to the bundle of His must be distinguished from delay or block distal to the bundle of His because the latter generally is of a more serious nature. If an advanced degree of block occurs in the distal His-Purkinje system, pacemaker function for the ventricles must be provided by automatic pacemaker cells in the bundle branch-Purkinje fibers. These cells discharge slowly (approximately 40 beats/min or less), and unreliably, often causing periods of asystole or generating a rate insufficient to maintain cardiac output. The resulting clinical consequences are of a serious nature and may include angina, syncope, or heart failure. However, when block occurs in the AV node, centers in the His bundle or high in the bundle branch fascicles assume pacemaker function and establish reliable, more stable rates usually faster than 40 beats/min (13).

Table 17-1.

	AV nodal conduction time (A–H interval)	His-Purkinje conduction time (H–V interval)
Digitalis	Increase	No effect
Atropine	Decrease	No effect
Isoproterenol	Decrease	No effect/decrease
Propranolol	Increase	No effect
Lidocaine	No effect	No effect
Procainamide	Increase/no effect	Increase
Diphenylhydantoin	Decrease/no effect	No effect
Quinidine	Decrease	Increase
Pacing induced increase in atrial rate	Increase	No change
Exercise induced increase in atrial rate	No change	No change

Considering the etiology of the AV block may provide evidence regarding its site. For example, digitalis-induced AV block virtually always occurs within the AV node, whereas trifascicular block, a common cause of acquired complete heart block (25) generally results within the distal His-Purkinje system and produces distal or intra-His block. In most instances the site of block can be determined from careful analysis of the scalar electrocardiogram, but exceptions do occur (20) and may be detected during His bundle electrocardiography. According to a recent study (15) an important future use of His bundle electrocardiography may be found for patients with bifascicular conduction disturbances, such as right bundle branch block and left anterior hemiblock, or other combinations (22). Although only 5 to 10 percent of these patients develop high degrees of AV block (6), His bundle electrocardiography may be of benefit by selecting, on the basis of significant H-V prolongation, the subset of patients who are prone to developing more advanced forms of AV block. One forseeable problem is that patients with normal H-V times on one occasion, may exhibit high grade AV block at other times (5, 12).

Rapid atrial pacing and premature atrial stimulation using the extrastimulus method can be used to induce proximal and distal His block or demonstrate a prolonged refractory period of the AV node and the His-Purkinje system. These observations must be interpreted with caution, however, because functional block in the His-Purkinje system has been described (4). In some instances, atropine administration may obviate the protective effects of AV nodal conduction and be used to uncover distal His conduction disturbances during premature atrial stimulation. In general, it is difficult to produce distal His block during provocative atrial pacing if the block does not occur spontaneously.

First Degree AV Block

P-R interval prolongation may result owing to conduction delay in the AV node (A-H interval), in the His-Purkinje system (H-V interval), or at both sites, (Figure 17-4) (18). From analysis of the ECG, one may be able to accurately determine the area of conduction delay. If the QRS is normal in contour, the delay is almost always in the AV node; however, if the QRS complex shows a bundle branch block pattern, conduction delay may be within the His-Purkinje system, the AV node, or both. In this instance, His bundle electrocardiography allows localization of the site of conduction delay (Figure 17-5).

Second-Degree AV Block

Second degree heart block is of two types, type I (Wenckebach) and type II. Type I AV block in the surface electrocardiogram (ECG) is characterized by progressive P-R prolongation culminating in a nonconducted P wave. Following the blocked P wave, the P-R interval returns to its previously shortest value and begins the cyclic lengthening anew. Type II AV block is characterized by a constant P-R interval preceding the nonconducted P wave and almost always occurs in the setting of a bundle branch block (19).

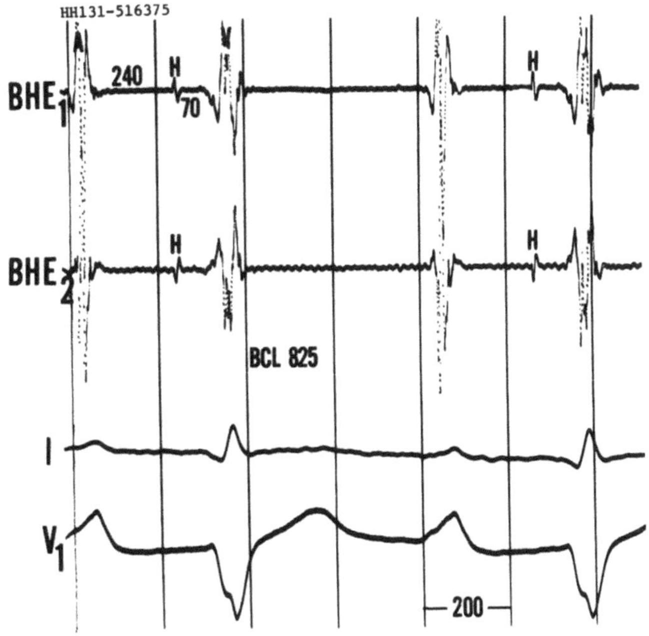

Fig 17-4. P-R prolongation in the surface (360 msec) is due to conduction delay at the level of the AV node (240 msec) as well as in the distal His Purkinje system (70 msec). BCL = basic cycle length during spontaneous discharge.

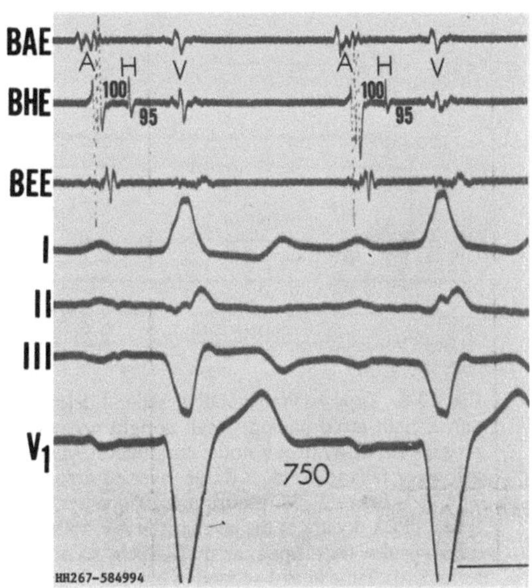

Fig. 17-5. P-R prolongation (230 msec) in the surface tracing during left bundle branch block caused primarily by distal His conduction delay (95 msec).

Type I (Wenckebach) Second Degree AV Block

In the presence of a normal QRS complex, type I (Wenckebach) second degree AV block almost always occurs at the level of the AV node, and is characterized by progressive lengthening of the A-H interval until one atrial deflection is not followed by a His deflection (Figure 17-6). It must be remembered that Wenckebach block is ubiquitous and may result at *any* site in the heart where conduction occurs (17). Type I AV block has been documented within the bundle of His, between an H and H′ deflection (Figure 17-7), as well as distal to the bundle of His, in the bundle branches. Wenckebach block occurs at other levels in the heart and may present between sinus node and atrium, between right and left atria (30), and so forth. In isolated preparations, type I block may take place between two impaled cells in a small piece of tissue. From a clinical point of view, however, in the setting of a *normal* QRS complex, this type of AV block virtually always occurs at the level of the AV node, with only rare exceptions. In general, therefore, unless the patient exhibits

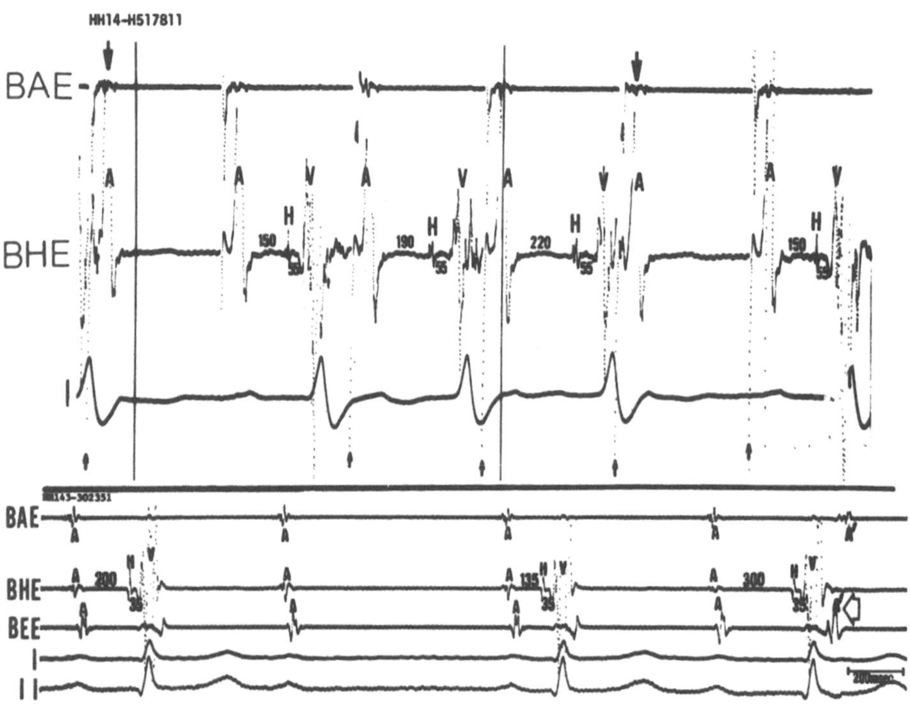

Fig. 17-6. Type I (Wenckebach) second-degree AV block recorded in 2 different patients. In the top panel, right atrial pacing (small upright arrows) in a patient with right bundle branch block results in progressive delay in AV nodal conduction, characterized by a gradual increase in the A-H interval until a P wave fails to conduct (large inverted arrows); following the blocked P wave the cycle begins anew. The H-V interval (55 msec) remains constant. In the lower panel, during spontaneous sinus rhythm, type I block occurs at the level of the AV node. Following the longest A-H interval (300 msec), an atrial echo results (A′, open arrow). Such reentry has been postulated as a cause of Wenckebach periodicity. Time lines 1 second in top panel; horizontal bar 200 msec in bottom panel.

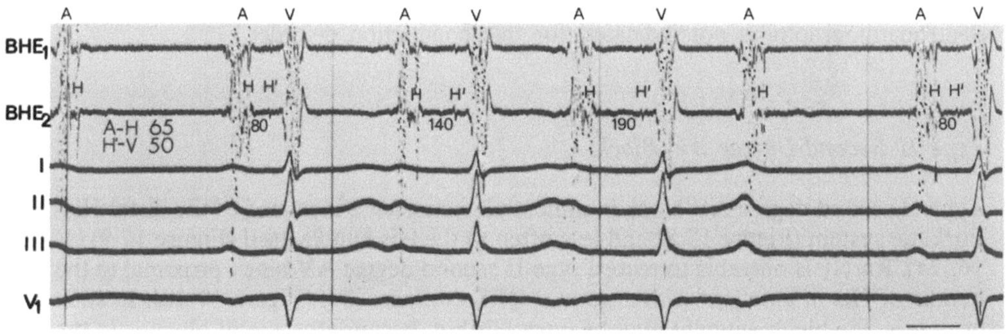

Fig. 17-7. Intra-His type I (Wenckebach) AV block. The A-H interval remains constant (65 msec); the H'V interval also remains constant (50 msec). However, two His bundle spikes can be recorded (H, H') and the interval between them progressively increases until an H is no longer followed by an H'. One cannot entirely rule out that the first deflection labeled H is not really part of the atrial deflection. If this is so, then the example would represent a normal AV nodal Wenckebach block. Time lines in this and other figures are one second. The black bar is 200 msec.

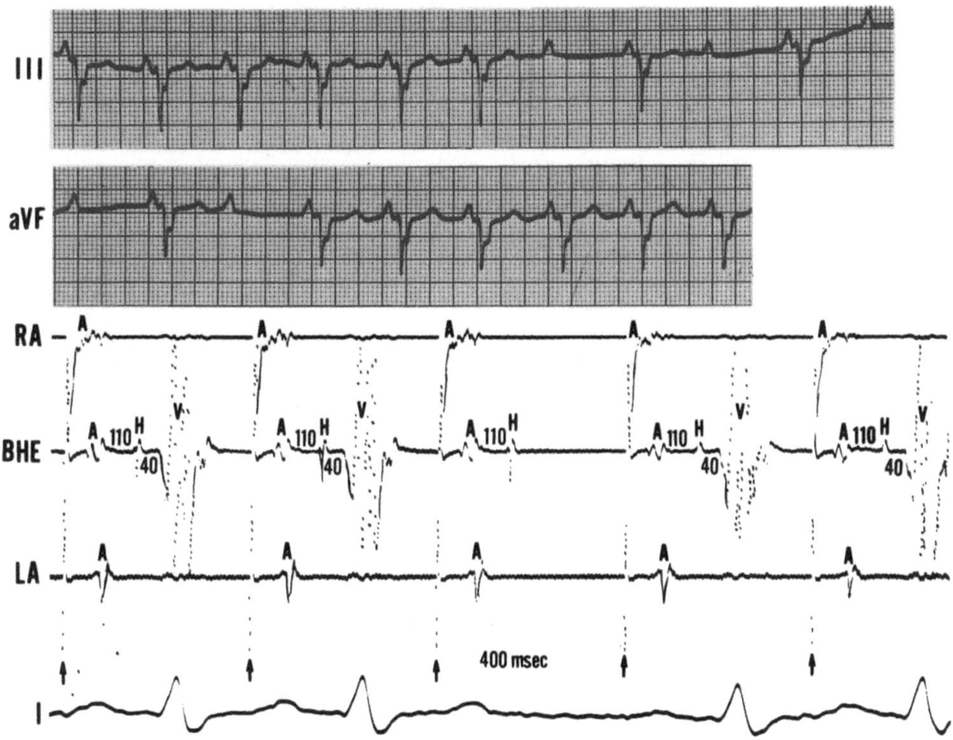

Fig. 17-8. Type II second-degree AV block. The surface electrocardiogram (top) illustrates type II AV block in a patient with right bundle branch block and left anterior hemiblock. During right atrial pacing, at the time of His bundle electrocardiography (lower panel; pacing spikes indicated by small upright arrows), the A-H and H-V intervals remained constant. Sudden failure of conduction occurred distal to the bundle of His following the third P wave.

an unusual type of Wenckebach conduction disturbance (see exceptions), His bundle electrocardiography is not indicated for this conduction disorder.

Type II Second-Degree AV Block

Type II second-degree AV block in almost all instances is localized to the distal His-Purkinje system (Figure 17-8) and less often to the His bundle itself (Figure 17-9) (1, 16, 24). Rarely is one able to record type II second-degree AV block proximal to the bundle of His in a patient with a normal QRS complex (20) (Figure 17-10). In such instances, the block actually may be intra-His but, because the site of block is in the very early portion of the His bundle, an insufficient amount of tissue proximal to the site of block may fail to generate a recordable potential. In virtually all instances of type II AV block, except those occurring within the bundle of His, a bundle branch block also exists. Thus, in the presence of bundle branch block, if nonconducted P waves occur suddenly without antecedent P-R prolongation, one can be fairly certain that this is type II, distal His block (8) and His bundle electrocardiography is generally not necessary. If, however, the P-R interval varies in a patient with a bundle branch block or if the QRS complex is normal during apparent type II AV block, then His bundle electrocardiography may be of value in determining the nature and site of the block.

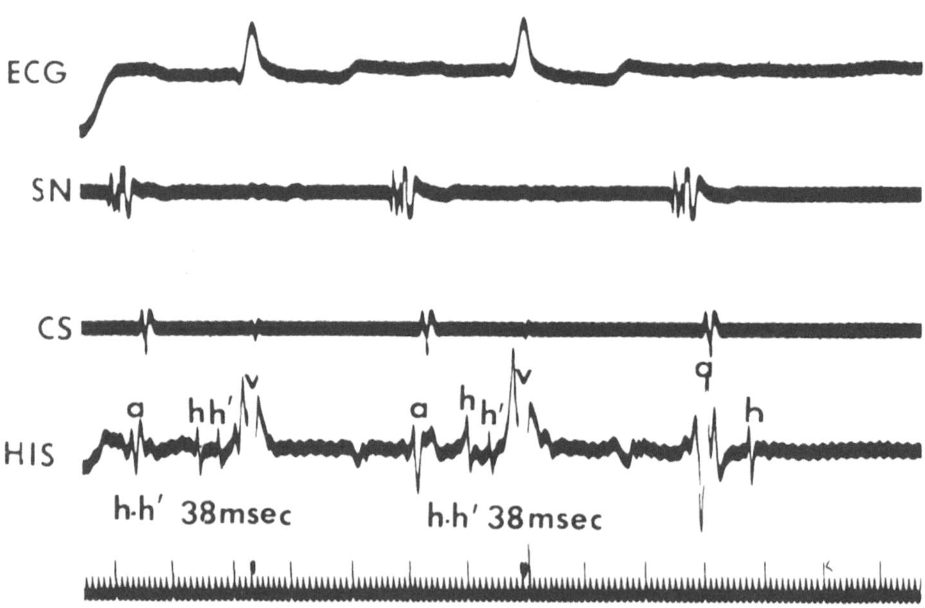

Fig. 17-9. Type II second degree AV block within the bundle of His in a dog. Two His bundle spikes are recorded (H and H'). The interval between them remained constant. Sudden failure of conduction resulted at a site distal to the first H deflection.

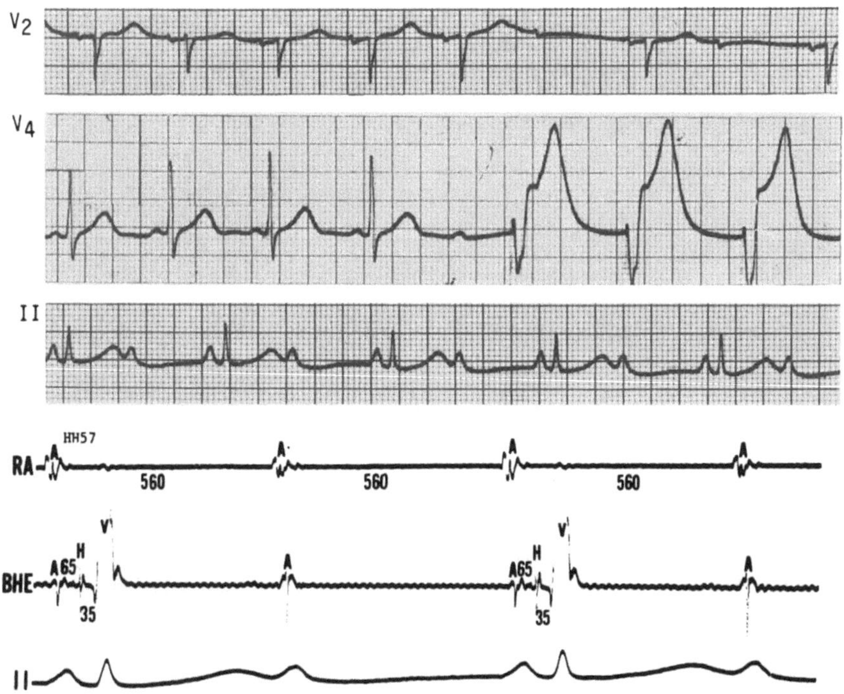

Fig. 17-10. Type II second degree AV block in a patient with a normal QRS complex. Note the constant P-R intervals in V_2, V_4, and lead 2. Sudden failure of AV conduction resulted without antecedent P-R prolongation. In V_4, a demand ventricular pacemaker began discharging. The His bundle recording (bottom panel), reveals that the block occurred proximal to the His bundle recording site; persistent 2:1 conduction occurred during His bundle recording.

Exceptions

Exceptions to these statements must be considered. First, pseudo AV block may occur due to nonconducted premature extrasystoles originating from the bundle of His (21) (Figure 17-11). Concealed retrograde conduction from these His bundle extrasystoles results in block or delay in conduction of the sinus P waves and may simulate first-degree, type I or type II second-degree AV block (Figures 17-11 and 17-12). Second, during Wenckebach AV block, a very high conduction ratio such as 12:11 or 8:7, and so on, or during AV conduction with very prolonged P-R intervals, a P wave may fail to conduct without obvious antecedent P-R prolongation. This may occur because of slight changes in the atrial rate, slight changes in the degree of autonomic tone, or slight P-R interval lengthening, which becomes difficult to measure at the usual paper speeds of 25 mm/sec. It is sometimes helpful to compare the P-R interval of the first beat of the Wenckebach cycle and the last beat preceding the nonconducted P wave. Such comparisons makes the P-R change obvious. Mild exercise, Valsalva maneuver, carotid massage, or atropine may help differentiate the type of AV block and often obviates the need for His bundle electrocardiography. The third exception occurs uncommonly, in patients who have simultaneous prox-

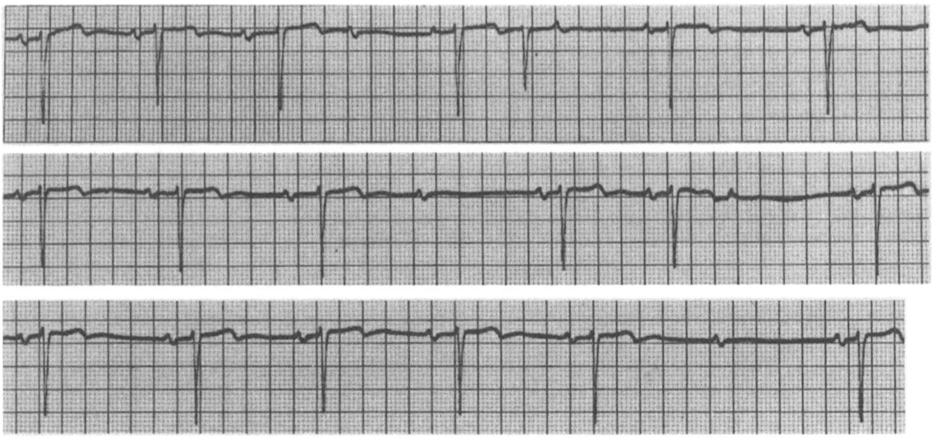

Fig. 17-11. Concealed conduction from blocked bundle of His extrasystoles. Premature His bundle discharge reached the ventricles on one occasion in this example (fifth QRS complex in top tracing). On all other occasions, His bundle discharge failed to activate the ventricles anterogradely, or the atria retrogradely, but did penetrate the AV node to affect subsequent AV conduction. In the top two tracings, concealed His bundle discharge mimicked type I (Wenckebach) AV block, and in the bottom tracing, it mimicked type II AV block. Proof of this explanation can be found during His bundle electrocardiography performed in this patient (Figure 17-12).

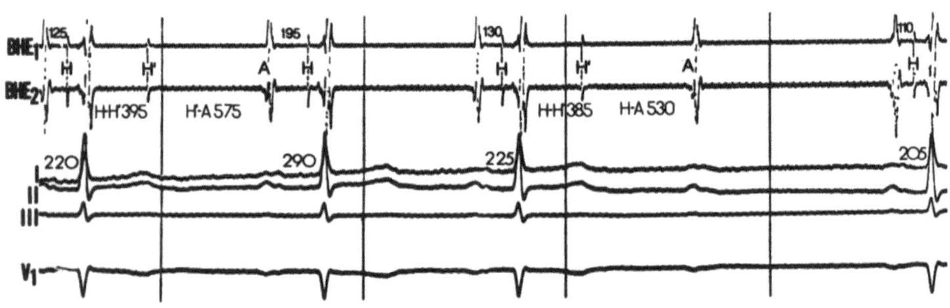

Fig. 17-12. Concealed conduction from blocked bundle of His extrasystoles (same patient as in Figure 17-11). Premature intermittent His bundle discharge (H'), which blocked before reaching the ventricles anterogradely or atria retrogradely, invaded the AV node and made it refractory for a period of time. Depending on the H'A interval, the subsequent P wave conducted with P-R prolongation or was blocked entirely. Thus, concealed bundle of His extrasystoles can mimic first, type I or type II second-degree AV block depending upon their H'A interval.

imal and distal His conduction disturbances (Figure 17-13). In these instances, because the surface electrocardiogram would be clearly inadequate to decipher the nature of the block occurring at two levels, His bundle electrocardiography would be of significant benefit.

2:1 AV Block

The 2:1 AV block may be type I or type II AV block and may therefore occur proximal or distal to the bundle of His (Figure 17-14). In general, when the QRS complex is normal, 2:1 AV block occurs at the level of the AV node. In the presence of a

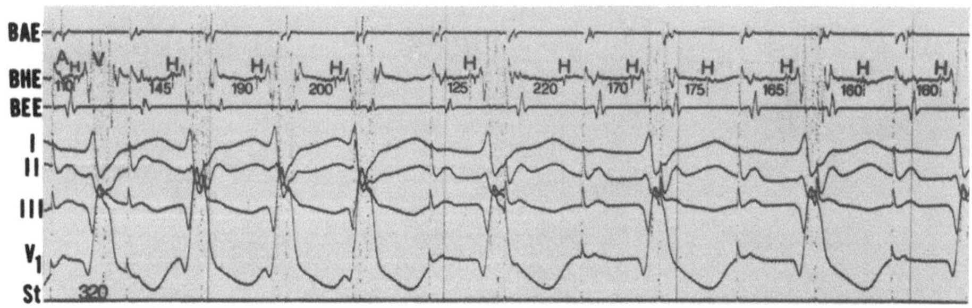

Fig. 17-13. Simultaneous block above and below the bundle of His. During rapid atrial pacing in a patient with intermittent distal His block, the A-H interval progressively lengthened until one distal deflection blocked proximal to His (fifth atrial deflection). In addition, intermittent block also occurred distal to the bundle of His (seventh, ninth and eleventh atrial deflections).

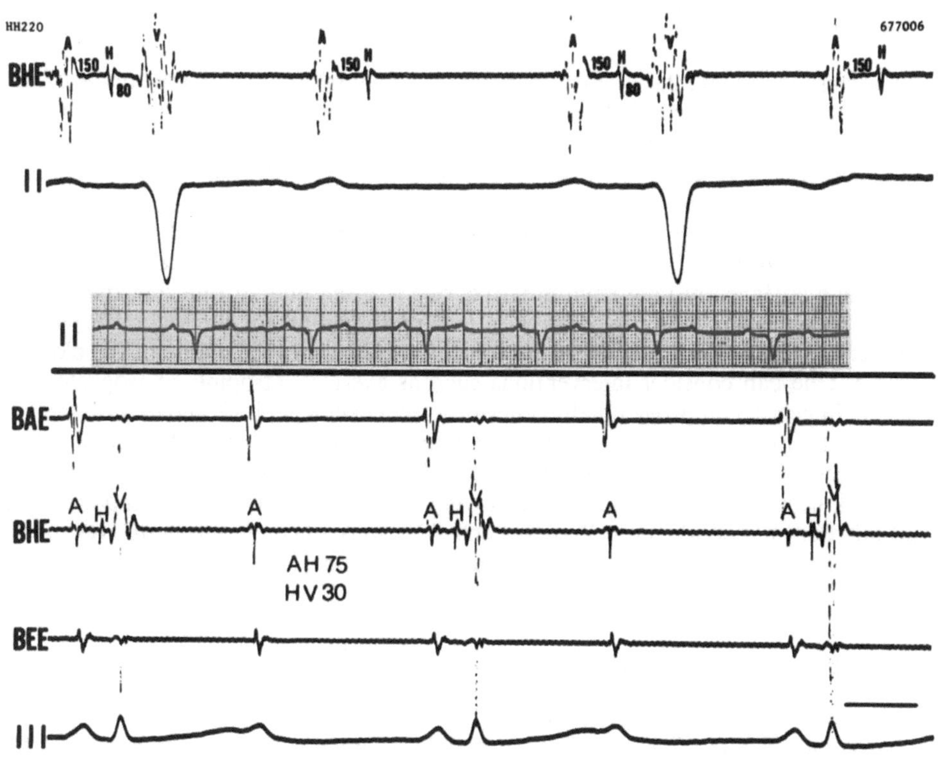

Fig. 17-14. Chronic 2:1 AV block in two different patients. In the top panel, 2:1 AV block occurred distal to the bundle of His. The A-H interval (150 msec) and H-V interval (80 msec) were prolonged. In the lower panel, 2:1 AV block occurred proximal to the bundle of His. The A-H interval (75 msec) and the H-V interval (30 msec) remained constant and normal. In the top panel a bundle branch block was present, while in the bottom panel, the QRS was normal.

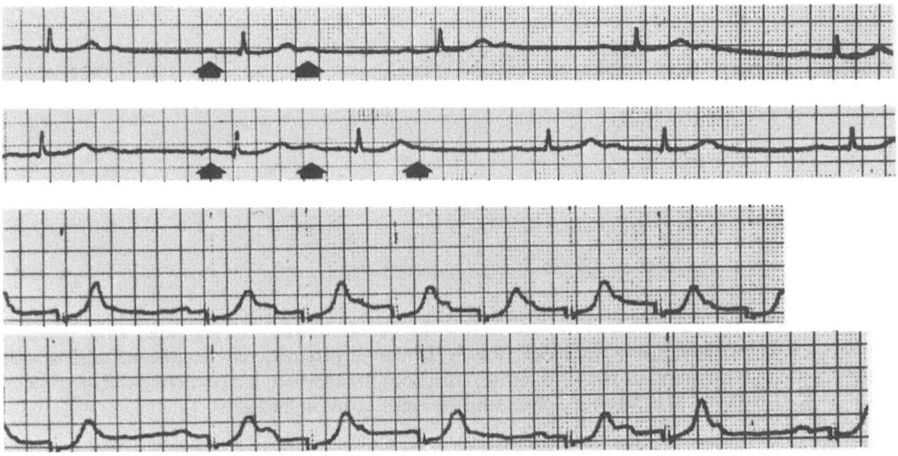

Fig. 17-15. Type 1 (Wenckebach) second-degree AV block. In the top tracing, 2:1 block occurred (P waves indicated by solid arrows). In the second tracing, the 2:1 AV block becomes 3:2 AV block and P-R prolongation for the second P wave in the series can be easily demonstrated (second arrow). The last two recordings illustrate the usual response of Wenckebach AV block to atropine, isoproterenol or exercise, producing an increase in the atrial rate as well as an increase in the ratio of conducted beats.

bundle branch block, 2:1 block may be either proximal or distal to the bundle of His. In such instances, His bundle electrocardiography may be necessary to localize the site of block, which, naturally, would be of considerable prognostic importance in the management of the patient because of the clinical implications mentioned earlier. Before His bundle electrocardiography is attempted, a number of approaches may be tried to establish the type of block, and may eliminate the need for His bundle electrocardiography. For example, if 2:1 AV block is due to Wenckebach block, by recording sufficiently long rhythm strips, one is often able to find that the 2:1 AV block becomes 3:2 at some point, with P-R prolongation for the second P wave in the series (Figure 17-15). The P-R prolongation establishes the nature of the block as type I. One can consider interventions such as exercise, atropine, or isoproterenol, which, in general, improve conduction of the Wenckebach block and do not improve or actually may decrease the ventricular rate associated with type II second-degree AV block. Vagal stimulation may worsen Wenckebach block while improving type II block because of the concomitant slowing of the atrial rate without impairing distal His-Purkinje conduction. Wenckebach AV block uncommonly improves during carotid sinus massage if the decreased atrial rate offsets the vagal-induced delay in AV conduction (Figure 17-16).

Third-Degree (Complete) AV Block

Complete heart block may result from block at the level of the AV node (usually congenital) (Figure 17-17), within the bundle of His, or distal to the bundle of His (usually acquired) in the Purkinje system (Figure 17-18). The first two types of block generally exhibit a normal QRS complex because the escape focus which controls the ventricle arises in the His bundle. Therefore, in such instances His bundle electrocardiography may be useful to differentiate AV nodal block from intra-His block since

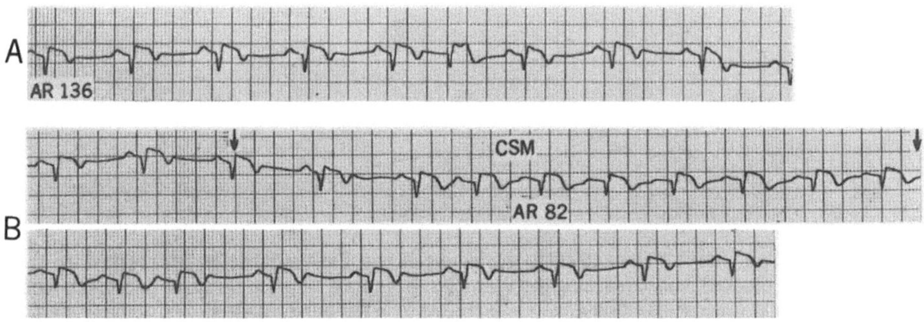

Fig. 17-16. Type I (Wenckebach) second-degree AV block during carotid sinus massage (atypical). In panel A, what appears to be initially sinus rhythm at a rate of 68 beats/min can be documented to be 2:1 AV block on the basis of a 3:2 conduction grouping in the midportion of the tracing. In panel B, carotid sinus massage (CSM) between the inverted arrows slowed the atrial rate to 82 beats/min and achieved 1:1 conduction. Following release of carotid sinus massage, the atrial rate returned to its previous level and 2:1 conduction resumed. AR, atrial rate in beats per minute.

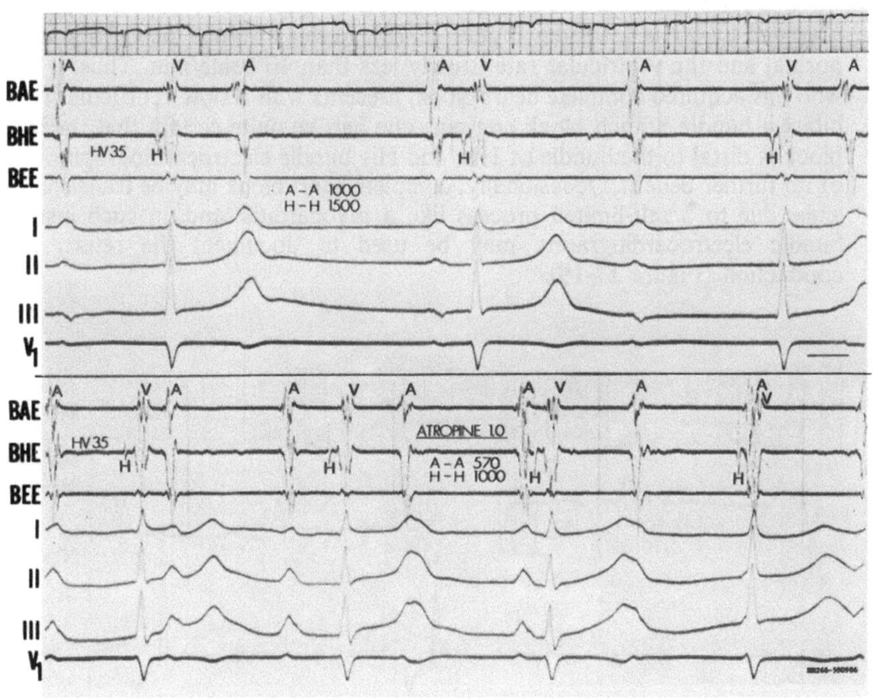

Fig. 17-17. Complete AV block at the level of the AV node. The surface tracing (top) illustrates complete AV block with a normal QRS complex. The top His bundle panel demonstrates the level of this block to be proximal to the His bundle spike, at the level of the AV node. The H-V interval is normal (35 msec). The atrial cycles (1,000 msec) are completely dissociated from the ventricular cycles (1,500 msec). The response to atropine (1 mg IV) is illustrated in the bottom panel. Both the atrial and ventricular rates sped (A-A 570 msec, H-H 1,000 msec), but complete AV block remained.

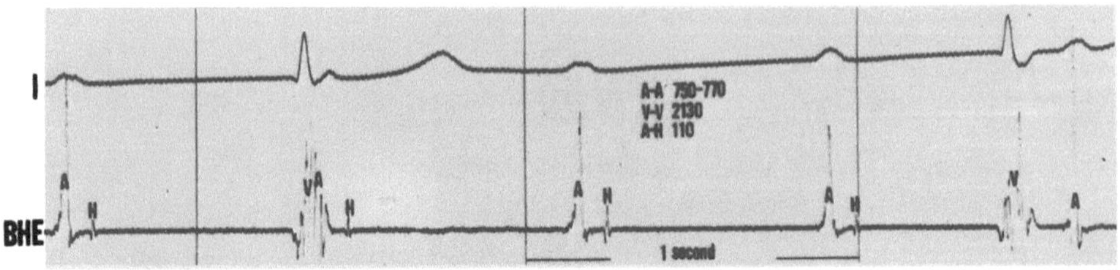

Fig. 17-18. Complete AV block distal to the bundle of His. Each atrial deflection reached the bundle of His and then blocked before reaching the ventricles. Because a ventricular escape pacemaker controlled the ventricles, no ventricular discharge was preceded by a His bundle deflection. Complete AV dissociation due to AV block is present.

the latter may carry more serious prognosis than the former. In patients with AV nodal block, atropine usually speeds the ventricular rate (Figure 17-17), whereas infra-His block may show no acceleration in heart rate after atropine is administered. The most common site of acquired complete heart block is distal to the bundle of His due to trifascicular conduction disturbances caused by degenerative changes in the cardiac skeleton and the His-Purkinje conduction system. Each P wave is followed by a His deflection and the ventricular escape complexes are not preceded by a His defletion (Figure 17-18). In this instance the QRS complex is abnormal and the ventricular rate usually less than 40 beats/min. Thus, if the patient who has acquired complete heart block, presents with a slow ventricular rate and exhibits a bundle branch block contour, one can be quite certain that the level of the block is distal to the bundle of His, and His bundle electrocardiography is probably of no further benefit. Occasionally, complete heart block may be transient and reversible, due to a self-limited process like a myocarditis, and, in such instances, His bundle electrocardiography may be used to document the return to normal conduction (Figure 17-19).

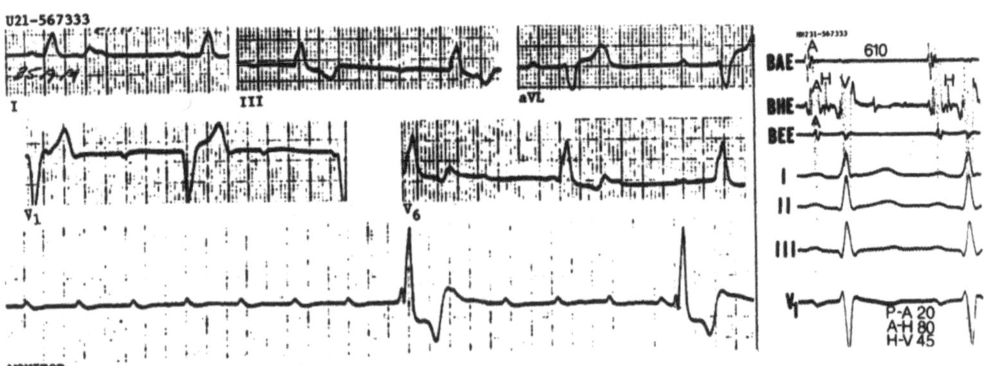

Fig. 17-19. Complete AV block with periods of ventricular asystole due to a myocarditis. The tracings in the left panel were recorded in a young man with flu-like symptoms and signs who presented with pre-syncope. A temporary ventricular pacemaker was inserted. Six weeks later (His bundle recording, panel on the right) conduction had returned entirely to normal and the patient was totally asymptomatic. Permanent pacemaker implantation was not required.

Fascicular Blocks

His bundle electrocardiography may be of benefit in evaluating some patients with fascicular conduction disturbances. For example, consider the elderly patient who has had one or more syncopal spells and now presents with an electrocardiogram demonstrating right bundle branch block and left anterior hemiblock. Are the syncopal spells on the basis of intermittent complete heart block, and is permanent pacemaker insertion indicated for that patient? An evaluation of such a problem includes investigating other causes of syncope plus a period of cardiac monitoring either with portable ECG tape recorder (Figure 17-20) or on a coronary care unit. Although the unequivocal answer to whether asystole caused the syncope would be provided by recording the cardiac rhythm during a syncopal spell, in our experience

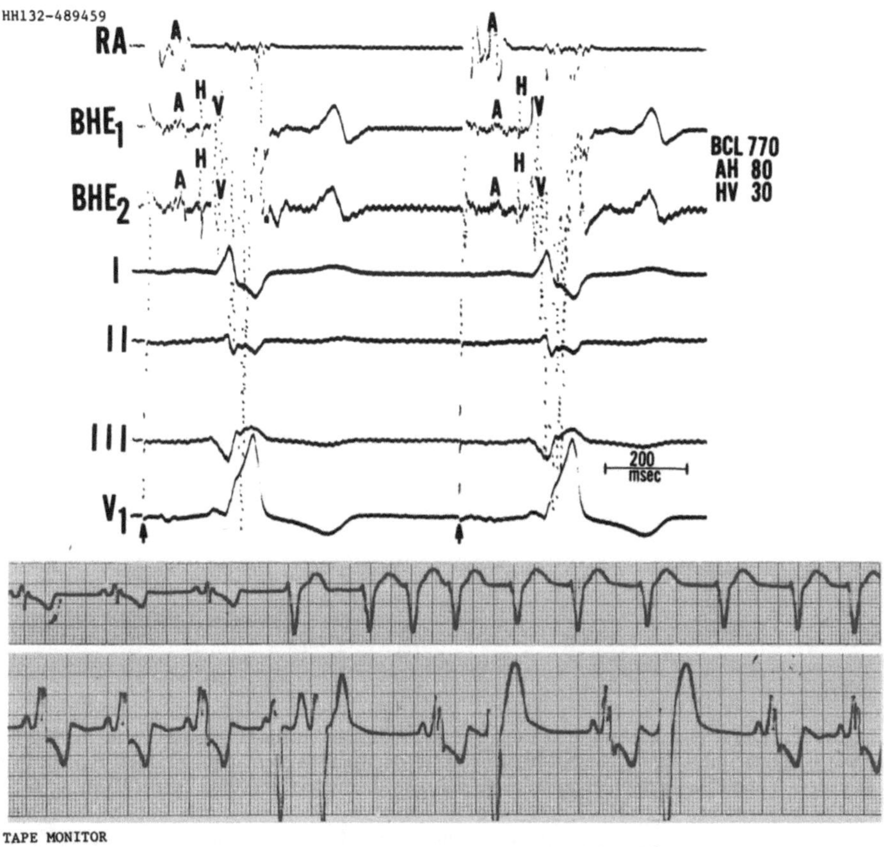

Fig. 17-20. Intermittent ventricular tachycardia in a patient with right bundle branch block, left anterior hemiblock and syncope. This patient with recurrent syncope underwent His bundle electrocardiography because of the electrocardiogram indicating bifascicular block. His bundle study was entirely normal. Prolonged monitoring with a tape recorder (bottom panel) illustrated that the patient experienced intermittent ventricular tachycardia as the possible cause of the syncope. Permanent pacing was not undertaken.

and that of others, prolonged monitoring is generally unrewarding. His bundle electrocardiography may be helpful because preliminary data would suggest that if the H-V interval is greater than 65 or 70 msec, then this patient is at greater risk for developing more advanced AV block and pacemaker insertion should be seriously considered (15). Another recent study (7) is somewhat at variance with the prognostic usefulness of H-V prolongation and suggests that, during the evaluation of syncope in patients with chronic bifascicular block, permanent pacemaker insertion is indicated only if heart block or other serious bradyarrhythmia is documented. If the H-V interval is normal, then other causes for the syncope should be vigorously

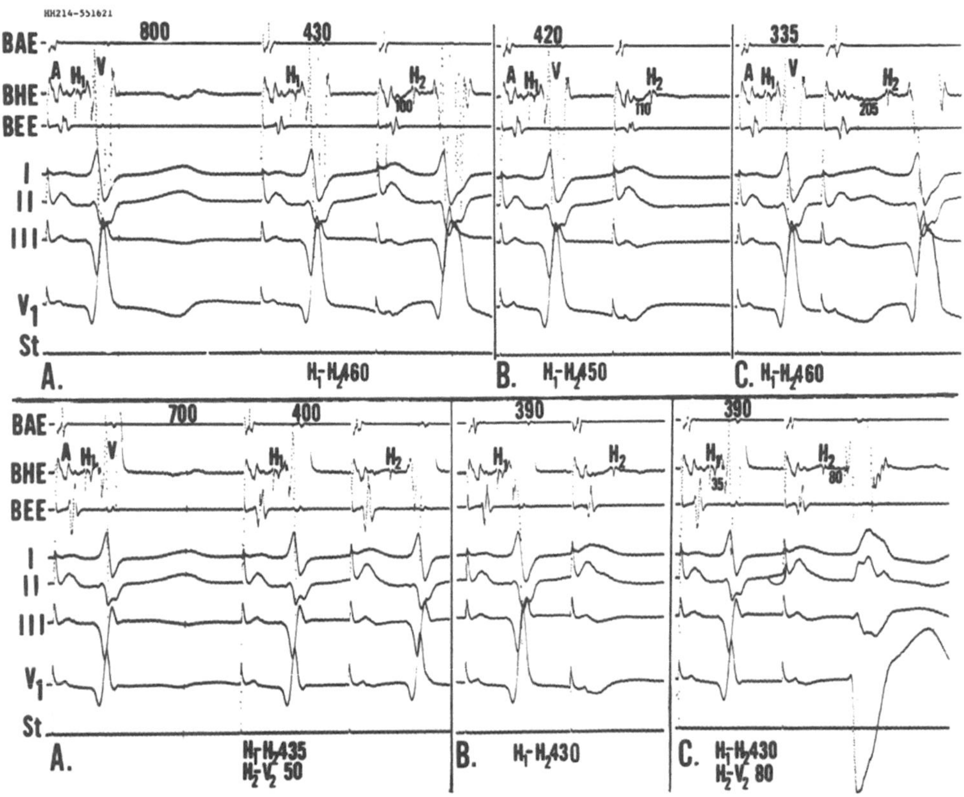

Fig. 17-21. Distal His block elicited using the extrastimulus method. In panel A for both upper and lower portions of this figure, the last basic cycle (H_1-H_1) and the premature cycle (H_1-H_2) are displayed. In panels B and C, only the premature cycle is shown. In the top recording, (panel B) an A_1-A_2 interval of 420 msec resulted in an H_1-H_2 interval of 450 msec and distal His block. In panel C, although the A_1-A_2 interval was shortened to 335 msec, because of A_2-H_2 prolongation to 205 msec, the H_1-H_2 interval actually lengthened to 460 msec and conduction resumed. This is an example of the AV nodal gap phenomenon. In the bottom portion of the figure, conduction occurred at an H_1-H_2 interval of 435 msec because of the shorter basic cycle (700 msec compared to 800 msec for the top half of the figure). At an A_1-A_2 interval of 390 msec in panel B, the resulting H_1-H_2 interval of 430 msec caused block distal to the bundle of His. At the same A_1-A_2 interval of 390 msec, the H_2-V_2 interval lengthened to 80 msec and once again conduction resumed, this time with a left bundle branch block. This observation is an example of distal His gap phenomenon.

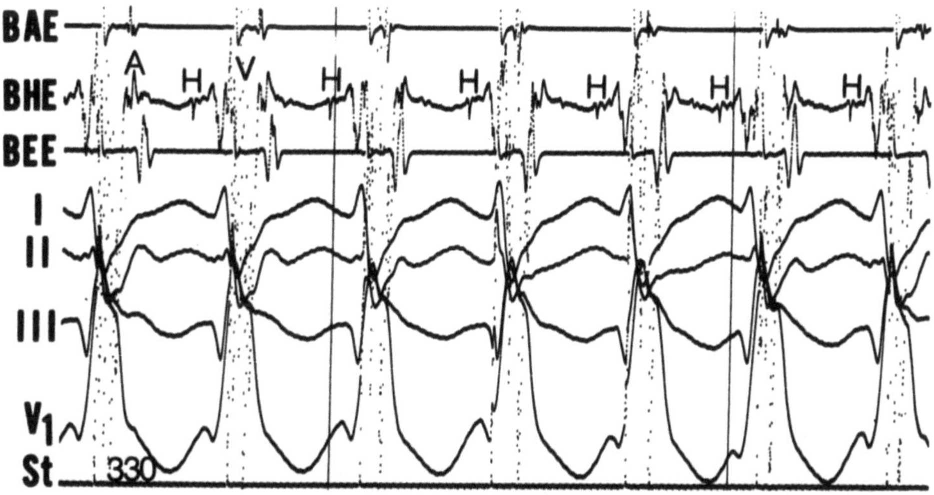

Fig. 17-22. In this patient with distal His block demonstrated in Figure 17-21, 1:1 conduction could occur at very rapid rates (BCL 330 msec, 180 beats/min) in spite of distal His block on other occasions.

searched for, always remembering that a normal H-V interval does not preclude advanced distal His block at other times (5, 12). His bundle electrocardiography may provide information which suggests permanent pacemaker insertion is not indicated in some patients. For example, P-R prolongation which accompanies left anterior hemiblock and right bundle branch block may be shown to represent AV nodal delay rather than increased conduction time in the remaining fascicle, and thus carry a different prognosis. His bundle electrocardiography is the only way to differentiate the site of delay in this instance and does hold some clinical value.

During His bundle electrocardiography, atrial pacing may be useful at times to determine refractory periods of the conducting system by rapid atrial pacing or with the use of the extra stimulus method (Figure 17-21). However, such physiologic stress of the conducting system is more apt to reveal conduction disturbances at the level of the AV node than within the His bundle or distal His-Purkinje system. The latter may conduct 1:1 with a normal H-V interval at very rapid rates and still demonstrate abnormal conduction at other times (Figure 17-22). Rapid atrial pacing may also be used to evaluate sinus node function by determining the duration of overdrive suppression in patients with possible sick sinus syndrome (Figure 17-23).

Tachyarrhythmias

Ventricular Tachycardia Versus Supraventricular Tachycardia With Aberrancy

His bundle electrocardiography may be quite useful in distinguishing tachycardias of ventricular origin from supraventricular origin with aberrant ventricular conduction (10, 32). However, it is important to remember the following when using His bundle electrocardiography to differentiate the origin of tachyarrhythmias.

If an impulse arises in the ventricle and conducts slowly back to the His bundle, the spike representing His bundle activation may be lost within the inscription of the

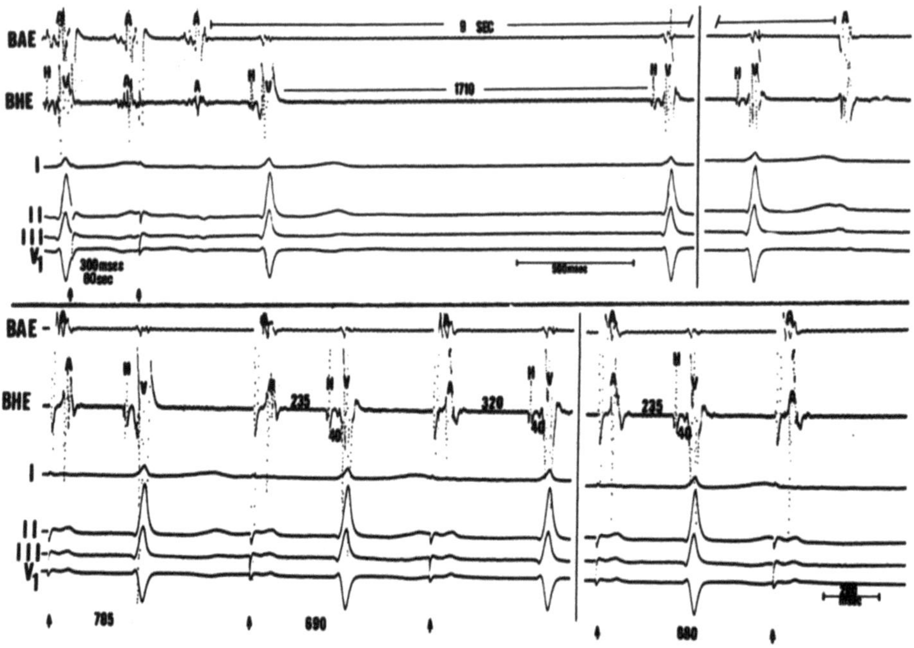

Fig. 17-23. Evaluation of a patient with the sick sinus syndrome. Top panels illustrate the response to rapid right atrial pacing (arrows) for 60 seconds at a cycle length of 300 msec (a marked latency exists between the last stimulus and the succeeding atrial response). Following cessation of rapid atrial pacing, a His bundle escape after 1,710 msec prevents ventricular asystole. However, the normal sinus rhythm did not return for 9 seconds. In the bottom panel is illustrated determination of the effective refractory period of the AV node (ERPAVN) for this patient. The A-H interval during normal pacing is markedly prolonged. In the left portion of the panel, an A_1-A_2 interval of 690 msec conducted to the ventricle. However, shortening this interval to 680 msec (right panel) resulted in block proximal to the bundle of His (ERPAVN). Therefore, this patient had sinus as well as AV nodal disease.

ventricular muscle electrogram. Therefore, when an H deflection fails to precede each V deflection, in spite of optimal catheter position, the tachycardia most likely arose in the ventricles. One must caution against an inaccurately placed His catheter electrode that might fail to register His activation actually present and lead to an erroneous diagnosis of ventricular tachycardia. The His bundle area must be thoroughly explored with the catheter electrode to avoid this mistake. If a clear His deflection, recorded during supraventricular beats that interrupt, precede, or follow the termination of the tachycardia, disappears during the tachycardia (without a change in catheter position), one can feel more secure in the diagnosis of ventricular tachycardia (Figure 17-24).

It is important also to realize that an impulse arising in the ventricle conducts retrogradely toward the His area over Purkinje fibers as well as over ventricular muscle. The upper portion of the right side of the ventricular septum close to the tip of the catheter electrode is not activated by direct contiguity with the His bundle, but depolarizes after initial activation of the epicardial free wall of both ventricles. Although the vector of initial ventricular depolarization and the position of the recording electrode influence recorded ventricular activity, a reduced interelectrode distance (1 to 2 mm) restricts the area from which electrical activity is recorded, so

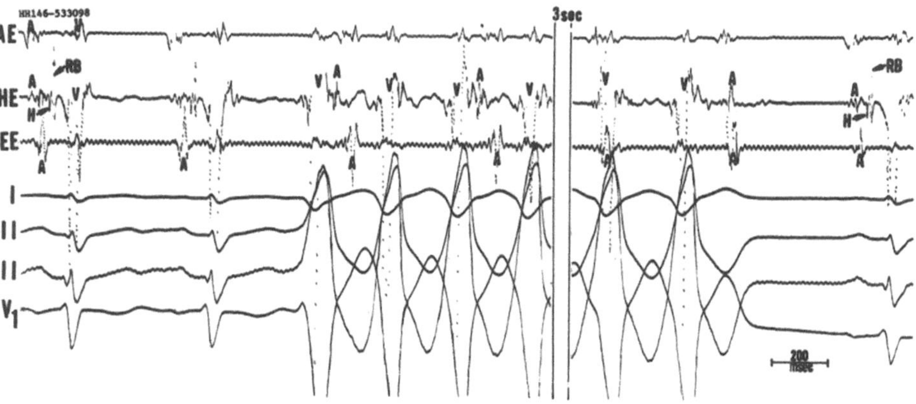

Fig. 17-24. Ventricular tachycardia. His bundle recording during paroxysmal ventricular tachycardia illustrates the loss of the His and right bundle deflections following onset of ventricular tachycardia without moving the electrode catheter. This observation supports the diagnosis of a ventricular tachycardia. A 3-second period of ventricular tachycardia was cut out of the middle portion of the tracing.

that activity may be recorded only, or primarily, from the area close to the electrode. Since the His bundle lies at one end of a rapid transit system composed of bundle branches and Purkinje fibers that conduct an impulse at a velocity of about 3 m/sec compared to ordinary ventricular muscle that conducts at a velocity of 0.5 to 1.0 m/sec, an impulse may originate in the ventricle, enter the Purkinje network, and retrogradely reach and discharge the His bundle before slower intramuscular conduction discharges the underlying ventricular muscle recorded by the same catheter. It can be demonstrated during right ventricular pacing that His bundle activation follows the onset of the QRS complex in one or more leads but may precede local septal muscle activity recorded beneath the His bundle catheter electrode. In Figure 17-25, this event is illustrated in a patient. Panel A records activity during spontaneous sinus rhythm, while panel B displays the results obtained during pacing from the apex of the right ventricle. In spite of the impulse originating from within the ventricle, bundle of His activation preceded local septal muscle activation but *followed* the onset of the QRS complex. The H-V interval is thus determined by the site of origin of the impulse in the ventricle and the *difference* between conduction time from that site to the His bundle and to the ventricular muscle.

If the impulse arose high in one of the bundle branches, at a site close to the bundle of His, it could reach and activate the His bundle very rapidly, ahead of all ventricular muscle activation. The contour of the QRS complex will obviously be altered, but its duration may remain less than 0.12 seconds. The H-V interval will be shorter than normal, though H still precedes ventricular activation. This reasoning may explain one type of aberrantly conducted "junctional" escape beat and the recent report of a ventricular tachycardia with QRS duration of only 100 msec (2).

Therefore, His bundle activation in advance of *locally* recorded ventricular muscle activation does not rule out a ventricular site of origin for the QRS complex in question. One can be reasonably certain that the impulse arose in the ventricle if His discharge occurs after the onset of the QRS complex recorded in multiple leads, or if

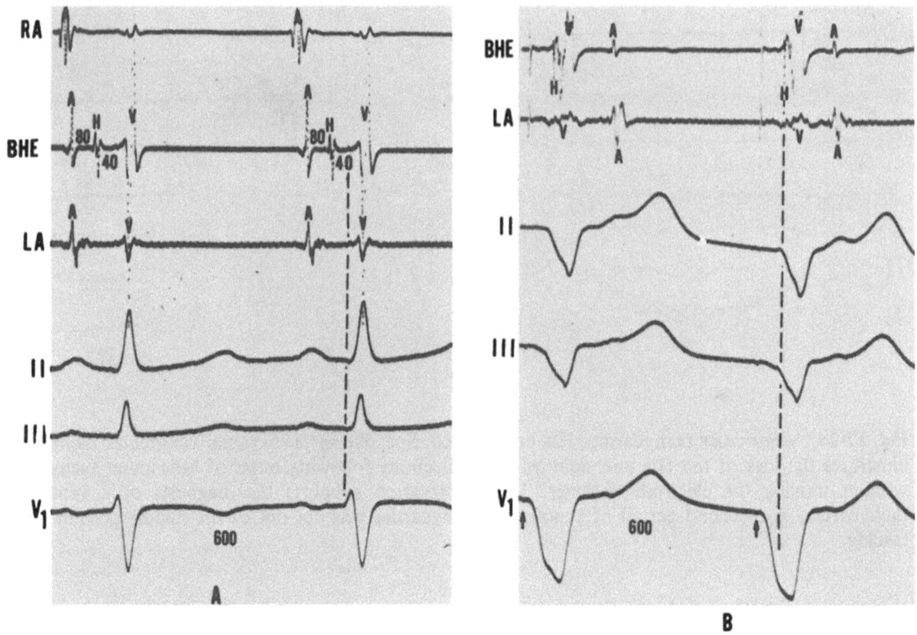

Fig. 17-25. His bundle recording during ventricular pacing. Panel A illustrates that, with a well-positioned His bundle catheter electrode, ventricular septal depolarization is recorded considerably after the onset of the QRS complex (interrupted line). In this example, the H-V interval is measured from the His deflection to the onset of the QRS complex, not to the onset of the ventricular septal depolarization. In panel B, pacing from the apex of the right ventricle resulted in a retrograde His deflection which preceded the onset of ventricular septal depolarization. However, the His deflection (interrupted line) occurred well after the onset of the QRS complex, and confirms the ventricular origin of the QRS complex. LA = left atrium recorded from an esophageal lead. Arrows indicate right ventricular pacing spikes which are better seen in the BHE and LA leads.

the H-V time is shorter than during normal conduction (pre-excitation provides the exception to this statement). As Figure 17-26D demonstrates, during this tachycardia with a wide QRS complex, His bundle activation (interrupted line) followed the earliest ventricular muscle activation recorded in multiple surface tracings (onset of the QRS complex), but preceded activation of local ventricular septal muscle recorded beneath the His electrode catheter. Thus, during this ventricular tachycardia, conduction time from the site of origin of the impulse in the ventricle to the His bundle was less than conduction time from the site of origin of the impulse in the ventricle to the ventricular muscle recorded near the His bundle. The H-V interval represents the difference between these two conduction times, and was thus shortened.

Theoretically, it is possible that an impulse may arise in the His bundle distal to the site at which His activity is being recorded, and conduct retrogradely to the recording site with extreme delay, thus enabling the impulse travelling orthogradely to discharge the ventricles ahead of His activation. This would amount to a supraventricular impulse in which recorded H activity follows the onset of ventricular depolarization.

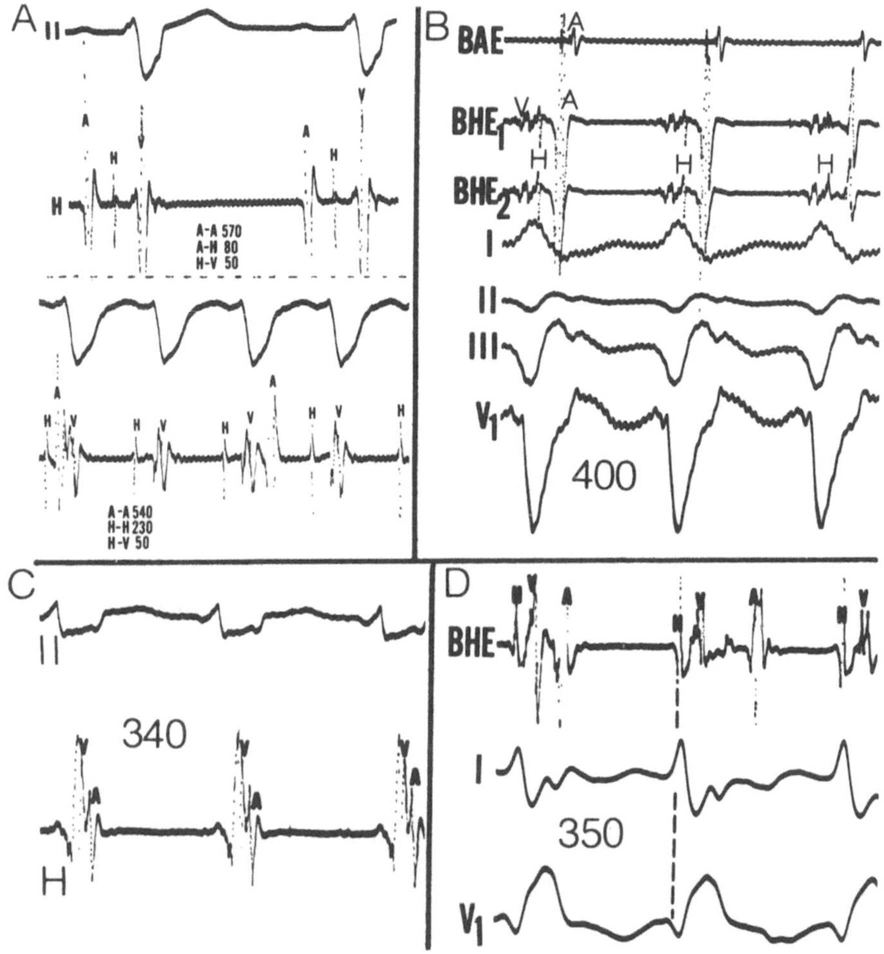

Fig. 17-26. His bundle recording in 4 different patients with tachycardias. Panel A, top portion of the tracing illustrates His bundle recording during sinus rhythm. The H-V interval is 50 msec. Bottom portion of panel A illustrates His bundle recording during tachycardia. The QRS complex and H-V interval are unchanged from those recorded during sinus rhythm. Therefore, this is clearly a supraventricular tachycardia. Of note is the fact that the atria discharged at a different rate (not a multiple) than the ventricular rate; therefore, AV dissociation is present during this *supraventricular* tachycardia. Panel B. His bundle activity occurred after the onset of the QRS complex, during ventricular septal depolarization, which assured the diagnosis of ventricular tachycardia. The R-P interval remained fixed and the atria were captured retrogradely from the ventricles. Therefore, AV dissociation is not present during this *ventricular* tachycardia. Panel C. His bundle activity was not recorded in spite of careful exploration of the His bundle area with the catheter electrode tip. This most likely represents a ventricular tachycardia with 1:1 retrograde atrial capture but one cannot be as certain as for Figure 17-25 or Figure 17-26, panels B and D. Panel D. His bundle activity preceded the onset of ventricular septal depolarization (interrupted line) but followed the onset of the QRS complex. Therefore, this must be a ventricular tachycardia. A retrograde VA Wenckebach (not shown in its entirety) was also present.

The presence of fusion and capture beats provide important evidence in favour of a ventricular origin for the particular tachycardia in question. Other criteria are useful but sometimes His bundle electrocardiography may be the only means for differentiating aberrant supraventricular conduction from ventricular tachycardia with any degree of certainty. The presence or absence of AV dissociation cannot be used to distinguish supraventricular from ventricular tachyarrhythmias because AV dissociation may or may not be present with either tachycardia (Figure 17-26).

Supraventricular Tachycardia

Atrial pacing (14) and His bundle electrocardiography can be quite useful in the analysis of other types of tachycardias, both supraventricular (11) and ventricular (28, 29). One such group of patients involve those with supraventricular tachycardias such as paroxysmal atrial or junctional tachycardia, either with or without the Wolff-Parkinson-White (pre-excitation) syndrome (for references, see review article 33). Stimuli can be delivered at increasing frequencies or, using the extrastimulus method, a test stimulus can be delivered prematurely after a train of eight or ten beats paced at a fixed cycle length. Supraventricular tachycardia can be initiated and terminated in patients with paroxysmal artrial or junctional tachycardia by a precisely timed stimulus delivered to atrium or ventricle. The physiologic parameters of the tachycardia can be determined, and the response to drugs evaluated (Figures 17-27 and 17-28).

In patients with pre-excitation syndrome, excitation of the ventricles can occur predominantly or exclusively over either the normal pathway or the anomalous

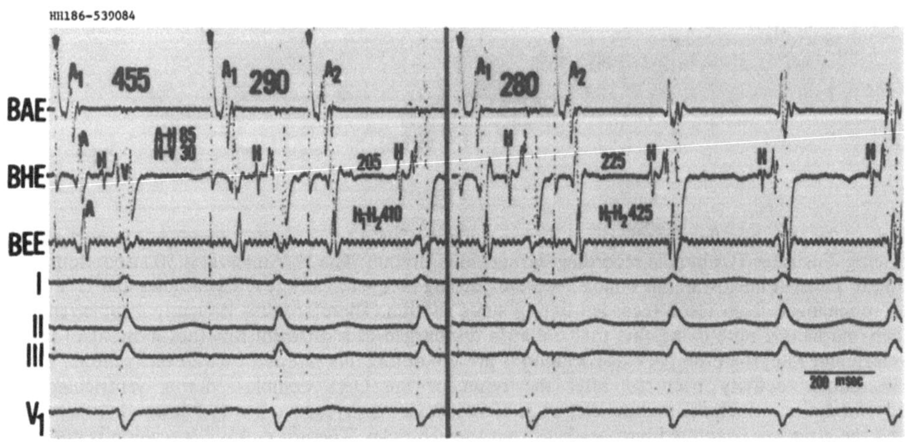

Fig. 17-27. Precipitation of supraventricular tachycardia (paroxysmal junctional tachycardia). In the panel on the left is displayed the last basic cycle (A_1-A_1) and the premature cycle (A_1-A_2). In the panel on the right, only the A_1-A_2 interval is presented. Right atrial pacing spikes indicated by arrows. Following an A_1-A_2 interval of 290 msec, the A-H interval lengthened to 205 msec, the H_1-H_2 interval to 410 msec and supraventricular tachycardia was not precipitated. In the panel on the right, shortening the A_1-A_2 interval by 10 msec to 280 msec resulted in an A_2-H_2 interval of 225 msec, an H_1-H_2 interval of 425 msec and precipitation of a supraventricular tachycardia.

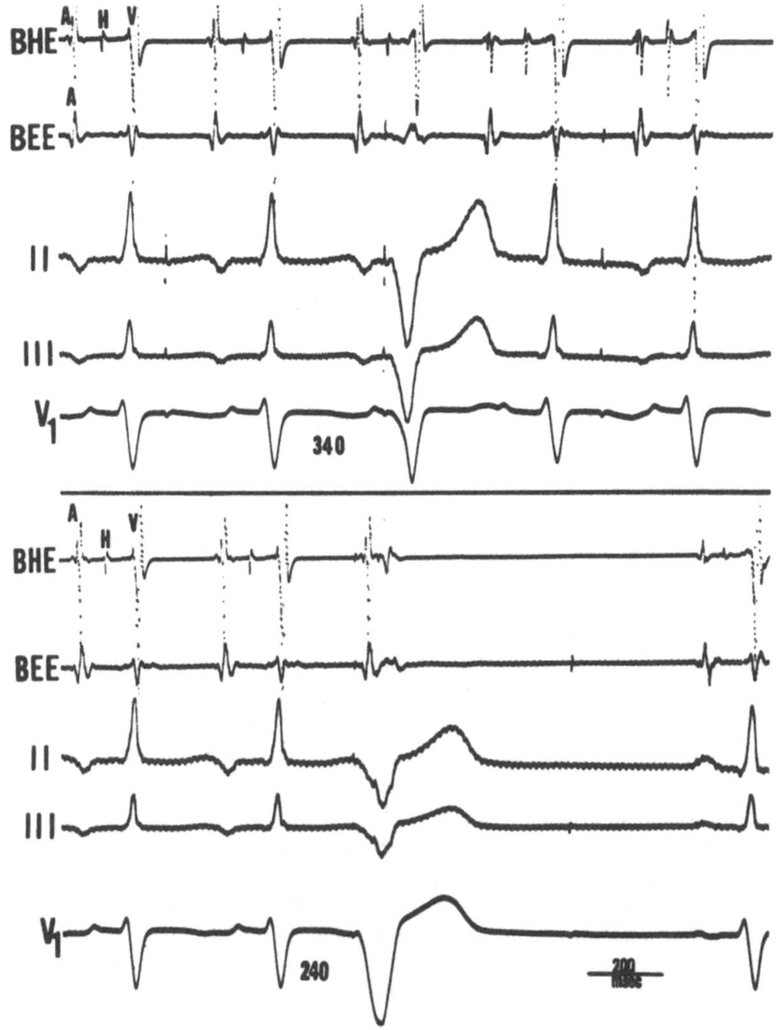

Fig. 17-28. Termination of supraventricular tachycardia with ventricular pacing from the apex of the right ventricle. During the spontaneous supraventricular tachycardia, random right ventricular pacing elicited premature ventricular systoles. In the top panel, when the premature ventricular systole occurred 340 msec after the last QRS complex, the supraventricular tachycardia continued. In the lower panel, when the premature ventricular systole occurred 240 msec after the last QRS complex, the supraventricular tachycardia terminated and sinus rhythm was restored. Presumably, in the lower panel, premature ventricular depolarization retrogradely penetrated the area of reentry, (usually the AV node) made one of the reentrant pathways refractory and terminated the tachycardia.

pathway. Progressively faster atrial rates (Figure 17-29) or earlier premature atrial systoles encounter increasing AV nodal (A-H) delay in conduction but no delay over the bypass. Consequently, the degree of ventricular pre-excitation increases to a maximum due to exclusive bypass conduction. Slightly earlier atrial stimulation finds the bypass refractory and the AV node excitable (Figure 17-30). Exclusive conduction over the normal pathway occurs and elicits a normal QRS. At this moment, a SVT is initiated with orthograde conduction over the normal pathway and retrograde conduction over the anomalous pathway. The P-R interval exceeds the R-P interval during such a tachycardia. Exceptions to this mechanism have been documented. For example, reentry within the AV node, independent of the accessory bundle, may explain some examples of SVT during pre-excitation (31).

Using the extrastimulus method applied to the atrium, the refractory period of the bypass may be established. The interval between the last normal atrial response (A_1) to a train of stimuli delivered regularly for eight or ten beats and the latest premature atrial response (A_2) which conducts solely over the normal pathway as judged by a prolonged P-R interval and normal QRS complex defines the bypass refractory period (Figure 17-30). Patients who have a bypass with a short refractory period may be prone to developing rapid ventricular rates during atrial flutter or fibrillation. Some patients have a bypass with a very long refractory period.

Electrophysiologic pacing studies in patients with the pre-excitation syndrome have demonstrated that: (a) the typical QRS is a fusion beat and exclusive conduction over the bypass or normal AV node-His bundle may occur as a result of premature stimulation; (b) conduction velocity in the bypass exceeds that found in the AV node and bypass conduction is not subject to rate-related delay as is the normal AV node and may conduct in an all-or-none fashion; (c) the refractory period of the bypass often exceeds that of the AV node and in such instances early premature atrial depolarization may find the bypass refractory, conduct slowly over the normal route (producing a completely normal QRS complex preceded by a long P-R interval), and return to the atria over the bypass which has now recovered, thereby initiating a reentrant SVT. Uncommonly during the SVT, orthograde conduction may occur over the bypass and retrograde conduction over the normal pathway. It is theoretically possible that in patients with multiple pathways combinations of James, Mahaim, or Kent fibers may provide reentry circuits that do not require participation of the normal AV node-His bundle. Recent observations suggest that bypass tracts at times may conduct in only one direction (31).

It is important to stress that these pacing procedures must be done cautiously. Precipitation of atrial flutter or fibrillation in a patient with the pre-excitation syndrome may lead to inordinately rapid ventricular rates (250 to 300/min) with hemodynamic decompensation and the need for prompt direct current cardioversion. Rarely, ventricular fibrillation may result.

It is our feeling that such electrophysiologic evaluations may be quite useful, particularly for patients with the pre-excitation syndrome, since the nature of the tachyarrhythmia and the electrophysiologic characteristics of the bypass can be established both in the control setting and in response to drug administration (27). Of particular importance is the duration of the refractory period in the bypass, since this plays a determining role in establishing the ventricular rate during atrial fibrillation and probably atrial flutter as well. A small but definite percentage of patients with the pre-excitation syndrome have sudden death probably due to ventricular fibrillation, in most cases, precipitated by the rapid ventricular response to atrial fibrillation. At the present time, we feel that these studies should be confined to centers clearly invested in doing electrophysiologic research, since the studies require fairly sophisticated pacing and recording equipment as well as a large amount of

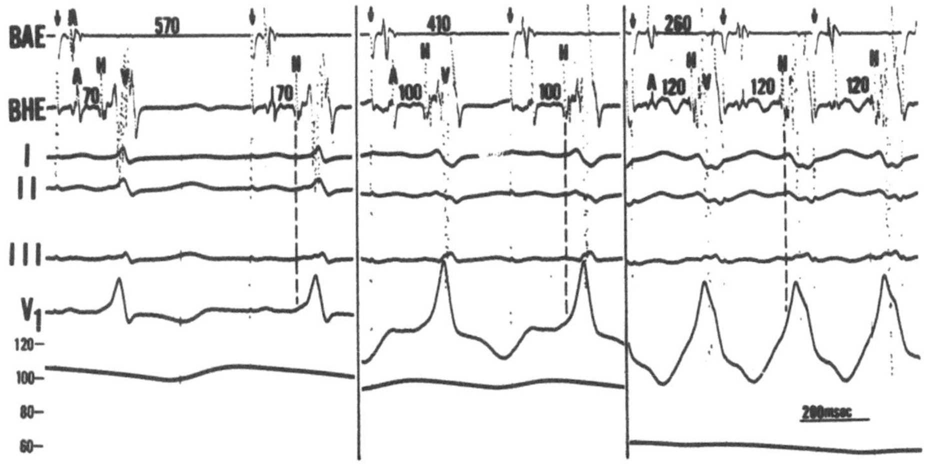

Fig. 17-29. Right atrial pacing in a patient with the pre-excitation (WPW) syndrome, type A. Each panel presents the results of right atrial pacing at gradually increasing rates. Note how the A-H interval lengthened, His bundle activity (interrupted lines) became more and more buried within the QRS complex, and the QRS complexes became more and more anomalous in configuration due to increasing degrees of ventricular excitation over the bypass tract. Note also the decrease in mean systolic blood pressure at the more rapid rates. Compare this tracing with Figure 17-26; note that His bundle excitation can occur after the onset of the QRS complex in the WPW syndrome during *supraventricular* conduction.

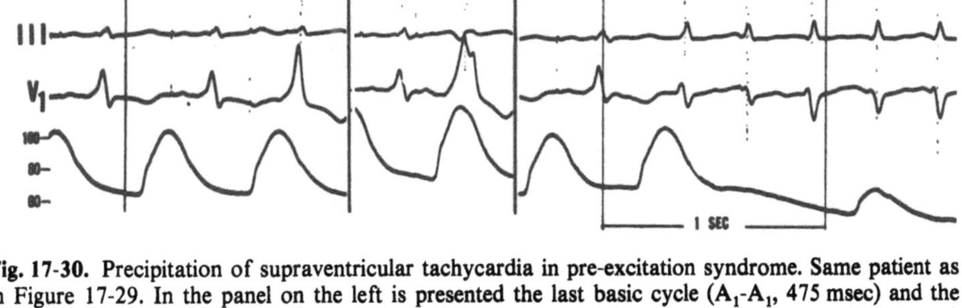

Fig. 17-30. Precipitation of supraventricular tachycardia in pre-excitation syndrome. Same patient as in Figure 17-29. In the panel on the left is presented the last basic cycle (A_1-A_1, 475 msec) and the premature cycle (A_1-A_2, 390 msec). In the middle panel is presented only the A_1-A_2 interval (285 msec) and in the panel on the right is presented the A_1-A_2 interval (265 msec) and the subsequent supraventricular tachycardia. Progressively shorter A_1-A_2 intervals elicited increasing degrees of anomalous ventricular excitation. Finally, at an A_1-A_2 interval of 265 msec (right panel), the refractory period of the bypass tract was reached and conduction occurred normally over the AV node. (The first His deflection was not recorded due to catheter movement.) At the time of block in the bypass tract, a supraventricular tachycardia with a normal QRS resulted because conduction occurred anterogradely over the normal AV node-His bundle pathway and returned over the previously blocked bypass tract to elicit a reentrant supraventricular tachycardia. Right atrial pacing spikes indicated by arrows.

time committed to the study and its subsequent analysis. Such procedures, however, may provide important information regarding the therapeutic use of pacing or surgery to control the arrhythmias but should be relegated to specialized centers devoted to this analysis (26).

Related investigations may be considered in patients with drug-resistant ventricular tachyarrhythmias. Attempts at defining reentrant pathways, for example, may permit a surgical therapeutic approach in selected patients.

Summary

In this paper we have reviewed the technique of His bundle recording, the significance of proximal and distal His bundle delay and block, and the varieties of first-, second-, and third-degree AV block. We have also reviewed the potential usefulness of His bundle electrocardiography to determine the nature and the site of AV block and to distinguish tachycardias of ventricular origin from supraventricular origin with aberrant ventricular conduction. In addition, we have discussed the application of His bundle electrocardiography in the evaluation of patients with supraventricular tachycardia.

In general, we feel the clinical indications for His bundle electrocardiography are as follows:

In the patient with bifascicular block
1. Unexplained syncope.
2. Unexplained bradyarrhythmia.

In the patient with AV block
1. Chronic type I or type II second-degree or third-degree AV block with a normal QRS complex.

Usually, routine electrocardiography provides sufficient information to establish the site and nature of AV block. However, lesions such as intra-His block cannot be diagnosed from the scalar ECG; since intra-His block *may* carry a worse prognosis than proximal His block, His bundle electrocardiography may be considered in instances of chronic second- or third-degree AV block and a normal QRS complex.
2. Chronic type I second degree AV block with a bundle branch block.
3. Chronic 2:1 AV block.
4. Unusual, atypical or exceptional forms of AV block.

It must be remembered that, in the evaluation of patients with conduction disturbances, a patient may have a normal H-V interval and still have trifascicular disease with intermittent distal His block on other occasions. Also, the distal His conduction disturbance may progress from a normal to an abnormal value after the study has been terminated and this may not be predictable.

In the patient with tachycardia
1. Differentiation of ventricular tachycardia from supraventricular tachycardia with aberrant ventricular conduction.
2. Hard-to-control supraventricular tachycardia in order to evaluate mechanisms, response to drug administration or pacing as a therapeutic approach.

3. Evaluation of patients with the pre-excitation syndrome who develop atrial fibrillation with rapid ventricular rates or other hard-to-control supraventricular tachycardias as to mechanisms, response to medical therapy, pacemaker or surgical approach.
4. Symptomatic palpitations without documentation.
5. Hard-to-control ventricular tachyarrhythmias.

It is our feeling that patients with tachycardias should be studied at specialized centers.

Less definite indications for His bundle electrocardiography would be in the evaluation of patients with any type of chronic second or third degree AV block who are candidates for permanent pacemaker implantation, patients with bifascicular or bundle branch block and significant P-R prolongation or patients with acute myocardial infarction and bundle branch block. In general, if the clinical evaluation accurately and adequately supports the decision to implant a permanent pacemaker on the basis of clinical electrocardiography, symptoms, and so on, His bundle electrocardiography usually provides only confirmatory information.

Acknowledgments

This work supported in part by the Herman C. Krannert Fund and by grants HL-06308, HL-05363, and HL-05749 from the National Heart and Lung Institute of the National Institutes of Health, U.S. Public Health Service, the Indiana Heart Association, and the Veterans Administration Hospital, Indianapolis, Indiana.

References

1. Bharati, S., Lev, M., Wu, D., Denes, P., Dhingra, R., and Rosen, K. M. Pathophysiologic correlations in two cases of split His bundle potentials. Circulation, 49:615, 1974.
2. Cohen, H. C., Gozo, E. G., and Pick, A. Ventricular tachycardia with narrow QRS complexes (left posterior fascicular tachycardia). Circulation, 45:1035, 1972.
3. Damato, A. N. Noninvasive methods for recording bundle of His activity. Am. J. Cardiol., 33:444, 1974.
4. Damato, A. N., Varghese, P. J., Caracta, A. R., Akhtar, M., and Lau, S. H. Functional 2:1 A-V block within the His-Purkinje system. Circulation, 47:534, 1973.
5. DeJoseph, R. L. and Zipes, D. P. Normal H-V time in a patient with right bundle branch block, left anterior hemiblock and intermittent complete distal His block. Chest, 63:564, 1973.
6. DePasquale, N. P. and Bruno, N. S. Natural history of combined right bundle branch block and left anterior hemiblock (bilateral bundle branch block). Am. J. Med., 54:297, 1973.
7. Dhingra, R. C., Denes, P., Chuquima, R., Amat-Y-Leon, F., Wyndham, C., and Rosen, K. M. Syncope in patients with chronic bifascicular block significance causative mechanisms, and clinical implications. Ann. Intern. Med., 81:302, 1974.
8. Dhingra, R. C., Denes, P., Wu, D., Chuquimia, R., and Rosen, K. M. The significance of second degree atrial ventricular block and bundle branch block. Circulation, 49:638, 1974.
9. Dreifus, L. S. and Watanabe, Y. Localization and significance of atrioventricular block. Am. Heart J., 82:435, 1971.
10. Fisch, C. and Zipes, D. P. His bundle electrocardiography. Am. Heart J., 86:3, 1973.
11. Goldreyer, B. N. and Bigger, J. T. Site of reentry in paroxysmal supraventricular tachycardia in man. Circulation, 43:15, 1971.
12. Haft, J. I. and Kranz, P. D. Intraventricular conduction intervals during orthograde conduction in patients with complete heart block. Chest, 63:751, 1973.

13. Langendorf, R. and Pick, A. Atrioventricular block type II (Mobitz): Its nature and clinical significance. Circulation, 38:819, 1968.
14. Langendorf, R. and Pick, A. Artificial pacing of the human heart. Its contribution to the understanding of the arrhythmia. Am. J. Cardiol., 5:516, 1971.
15. Narula, D., Gann, D., and Samet, P. Prognostic value of H-V interval in patients with right bundle branch block and left axis deviation following observations from one to six years. Circulation, 49 and 50: Suppl. 3:56, 1974.
16. Narula, D. and Samet, P. Predelection of elderly females for intraHis bundle blocks. Circulation, 49 and 50: Suppl. 3:195, 1974.
17. Narula, O. S. and Samet, P. Wenckebach and Mobitz Type II AV block due to block within the His bundle and bundle branches. Circulation, 41:947, 1970.
18. Narula, O. S., Scherlag, B., Samet, P., and Javier, R. P. Atrioventricular block. Localization and classification by His bundle recordings. Am. J. Med., 50:146, 1971.
19. Ranganathan, N., Dhurandhar, R., Phillips, J. H., and Wigle, E. D. His bundle electrogram in bundle branch block. Circulation, 45:282, 1972.
20. Rosen, K. M., Lobe, H. S., Gunnar, R. M., and Rahimtoola, S. H. Mobitz type II block without bundle branch block. Circulation, 44:1111, 1971.
21. Rosen, K. M., Rahimtoola, S. H., and Gunnar, R. M. Pseudo A-V block secondary to premature nonpropagated His bundle depolarization: documentation by His bundle electrocardiography. Circulation, 42:367, 1970.
22. Rosenbaum, M. B., Elizari, M. V., and Lazzari, J. O. Hemiblocks-Tampa Tracings, 1970.
23. Scherlag, B. J., Lau, S. H., Helfant, R. H., Berkowitz, W. D., Stein, E., and Damato, A. N. Catheter technique for recording His bundle activity in man. Circulation, 39:13, 1969.
24. Schuilenburg, R. M. and Durrer, D. Conduction disturbances located within the His bundle. Circulation, 45:612, 1972.
25. Steiner, C., Lau, S. H., Stein, E., Wit, A. L., Weiss, M. B., Damato, A. N., Haft, J. I., Weinstock, M., and Gupta, P. Electrophysiologic documentation of trifascicular block as the common cause of complete heart block. Am. J. Cardiol., 28:436, 1971.
26. Wallace, A. G., Sealy, W. C., Gallagher, J. J., Svenson, R. H., Strause, H. C., and Kasell, J. Surgical correction of anomalous left ventricular pre-excitation: Wolff-Parkinson-White (Type A). Circulation, 49:206, 1974.
27. Wellens, H. J. J. and Durrer, D. Effect of procainamide, quinidine and ajmaline in the Wolff-Parkinson-White syndrome. Circulation, 50:114, 1974.
28. Wellens, H. J. J., Schuilenburg, R. M., and Durrer, D. Further observations on ventricular tachycardia as studied by electrical stimulation of the heart. Circulation, 49:647, 1974.
29. Wellens, H. J. J., Schuilenburg, R. M., and Durrer, D. Electrical stimulation of the heart in patients with ventricular tachycardia. Circulation, 45:216, 1972.
30. Zipes, D. P. and DeJoseph, R. L. Dissimilar atrial rhythms in man and dog. Am. J. Cardiol., 32:618, 1973.
31. Zipes, D. P., DeJoseph, R. L., and Rothbaum, D. A. Unusual properties of accessory pathways. Circulation, 49:1200, 1974.
32. Zipes, D. P. and Fisch, C. Supraventricular arrhythmia with abnormal QRS complex. Arch. Intern. Med., 129–993, 1972; 130:129, 426, 781, 950, 1972.
33. Zipes, D. P., Rothbaum, D. A., and DeJoseph, R. L. Pre-excitation syndrome. Cardiovasc. Clin., 1:210, 1974.

Chapter 18 Computerized Electrocardiography—Its Practical Value

LEON PORDY, M.D.

General Considerations

Computerized electrocardiography had its inception in the late 1950s with the work of Pipberger (17, 23) and Caceres (5), followed in the early 1960s by Smith (21) and Pordy (19). This initial thrust was extended in other centers, including Arvedson in Sweden. The basic principle involved is the conversion of the analog electrocardiographic (ECG) or vectorcardiograph (VCG), or both signals to digits, using an analog to digital converter. The records in digital format are then processed by the modern digital computers, with proper programming and at incredible speeds to produce analyses of the tracings comparable to that obtained by the human observer.

In the late 1960s, as a spin-off of the above efforts, three channel electrocardiography was introduced into clinical electrocardiographic practice. Thus, the standard 12-lead electrocardiogram, recorded in four-lead sets containing simultaneously leads I, II, and III; AVR, AVL, and AVF; V1, V2, and V3; and V4, V5, and V6, was recorded on analog tape, and this reduced computer processing time by two thirds. Furthermore, by simultaneously recording three leads, the exact onset and offset of the various waves involved could be determined exactly both for the human and for the computer. For example, lead II, which for many years had served as the interval measurement lead, was quickly found to contain many portions of ECG waves perpendicular to it. Only then could the resultant error in measurements of P, QRS, T, and the intervals P-R and QT be appreciated fully. It therefore became obvious that newer and more accurate measurements of various parameters could be obtained easily and errors that had persisted for many years could finally be corrected.

The second major advantage of three-channel electrocardiography was that both the 12-lead electrocardiogram and the component vectorcardiographic leads could be recorded with facility on the same patient, and the diagnostic value of each method could be established readily in huge numbers of cases. The old-fashioned methods for vectorcardiographic recordings by photographing the oscilloscopic Lissajeau loops were now readily replaced by recording component VCG leads simultaneously, followed by rapid computer analysis.

The basic issues then became focused into two main problems: (a) computer ECG analysis both for the standard ECG tracings and for ECG monitoring as compared with human observer interpretation and (b) classic 12 lead electrocardiography as compared with VCG.

Computer Compared with Human Analysis

Most humans are naturally apprehensive about the possibility that computer processing may eventually eliminate them from their specific occupations. In defense of their position, in the case of computer electrocardiography, the human observer is armed with the fantastic ability to recognize patterns. Since routine electrocardiographic interpretation depends on empirical observations of patterns, the diagnositic accuracy of most ECG interpreters ranges in the high 90th percentile. It is interesting to note, however, the famous study of Simonson *et al.* (20) in which the collective accuracy of 10 of the world's foremost ECG and VCG experts was approximately 54 percent for ECG interpretation but less for VCG analysis (47 percent). Furthermore, documented studies have shown an inter- and intraobserver variability of about 20 to 30 percent. Moreover, only a portion of the analyses may be supported by surgical, angiographic, and/or autopsy evidence, since rhythm defects and conduction pathway abnormalities cannot be verified by the aforementioned methods. However, the human, unlike the computer, is subject to fatigue and distractions that may diminish his performance. To compensate for this, he may review the ECG data several times and/or may consult with others before formulating his final analytic judgement in a particular case. On the other hand, the computer is neither subject to fatigue nor to error if it is programmed properly, but the digital data must be presented in a special format to compensate for the computer's inability to recognize patterns. The incredible speed with which mathematical computations are performed covers this latter fault quite adequately for clinical purposes. The final advantage of computer technology in electrocardiography is that vast amounts of accumulated data can be stored on either disk, drum, or digital tape and retained for later statistical or other detailed study. The application of these data will be discussed later in the section on ECG as opposed to VCG.

The use of the computer for ECG monitoring, although involving tremendous programming efforts, has just recently achieved success for clinical application. Here, the fatiguability of the human is well-recognized and combined with the large number of false technical alarms, has even caused unplugging of many monitoring units. In fact, recent studies by Oliver *et al.* (16) and by Nolle *et al.* (15) demonstrated the superiority of computer as compared with human monitoring over the long term. Interestingly, many of the computer ECG monitoring systems include interaction between the human observer and the machine. For example, the human, on computer query, identifies the dominant beat and the program then proceeds.

Current methodology does not place the computer in competition with the human but has evolved in such a manner that the bulk of the tedious work involved is performed by the computer and the physician retains his control by overseeing the results.

Electrocardiography vs. Vectorcardiography

Since the introduction of the Mann monocardiogram, the clinical application of vectorcardiography has attained a status superior to that of the electrocardiogram in our cardiographic diagnostic armamentarium. The change from the original uncorrected, nonorthogonal methods (Burch, Duchosal, Grishman) has occurred so that "corrected, orthogonal" lead systems (Frank, McFee, and others) are in current favor and use. Computerization of both the electrocardiogram and the vectorcardiogram has afforded us large banks of data by which the two methods can be compared and cross-correlated with clinical information. Examination of these data led some observers to question the diagnostic superiority of the vectorcardiogram. Personally, I found that there was not a 1:1 correlation between the classic 12-lead ECG and the Frank VCG. From a theoretic basis, any such correlation would indeed be entirely fortuitous. Examination of thousands of simultaneously recorded ECGs and VCGs showed that the frontal plane, as defined by standard electrocardiography, bore no exact relationship to that of the Frank vector, and therefore the diagnosis of left anterior and/or posterior fascicular block could not be accurately defined using the same angular criteria for both methods. For example, an angle of —45° in the scalar leads may be comparable to —10° in the Frank frontal plane; however, the actual angle with the Frank leads is extremely variable. This is related first, to the location of leads A, C, and I on the chest wall and second, to the fact that the inferior-superior Frank lead set is composed of the foot electrode (F) plus the mid-back (M) minus the head electrode (H). Other inconsistencies included deficiencies of the Frank system in the diagnosis of anteroseptal infarction, left ventricular hypertrophy, and diaphragmatic wall infarction. Such failures of the Frank system are not evident with small numbers of cases, but with the huge numbers recorded and stored with current computer techniques, these inconsistencies became readily apparent.

Computer Programming for ECG Analysis

Program Criteria

The initial efforts concerning programming for computer ECG analysis were obviously based upon empiric criteria used for years for analysis by electrocardiographers, as confirmed by clinical, catheterization, and autopsy data. Although such criteria are not universally agreed upon, this pragmatic approach worked well in the clinical environment. Better correlation could be obtained by using the well-known studies of Sodi-Pallares *et al.* (22), for example, in the more precise definition of the location of myocardial infarctions. This may also be improved by ancillary methods, such as echocardiography (Teichholz *et al.* (4, 24)). Age body build, clinical diagnosis, and drugs, remain extremely important and these factors must be incorporated in computer ECG programs just as they are in the interpretation by humans. Eventually, after enormous amounts of computerized cases are analyzed statistically, the interpretations will be printed by computer together with probabilities for the accuracy of individual diagnostic statements.

Early efforts for programming computer VCG analysis were less effective because of the diverse opinions concerning diagnostic criteria. In fact, many VCG programs were based upon human observer diagnosis for the classic 12-lead ECG in the same case. Unfortunately, however, the degree of overlap between normal and various abnormal diagnostic entities may be greater with VCG than with ECG so as to preclude definitive and accurate differential diagnostic statements. An excellent illustration of this point is an article by Ha, Kraft, and Stein (10), reporting on the inability to distinguish between direct posterior myocardial infarction and normal variation in the Frank VCG.

Measurement Program

It is important at this time to consider computer measurement programs since diagnostic accuracy is totally dependent upon the accuracy of computer measurements. Obviously "clean" records with minimal noise are absolutely essential for proper performance in this field. Baseline drift can be corrected by the program. A concurrence in wave amplitude has been noted in both human and computer measurements. However, most computer programs yield wave parameter measurements that are wider than those made by electrocardiographers. The reason lies in the fact that with the computer program the onset and offset of various waves are detected more accurately. Therefore, in view of this fact, our customary criteria for wave width measurements should be altered. The precision of measurements by computer may be such that printouts contain values to the third decimal place. This "precision" must be distinguished from the "accuracy" of computer measurements. The accuracy of these affects not only the accuracy of the contour diagnostic program but the rhythm analysis as well.

Since clinical requirements for computer electrocardiography include: (a) determination of cardiac rhythm, (b) analysis of the wave-shape or contour, and (c) comparison with previous tracings, the comparative program must be an essential part of the package, if the computer system is to be complete for clinical use.

Second Compared with First Generation Computer Programs

Various studies compared the results of first generation computer programs for both the classic 12-lead ECG and the VCG (8, 9). In this report, the program for classic 12 leads was found to be clinically superior to the Frank VCG. When both ECG and VCG analyses were combined, the diagnostic accuracy improved in 4 percent of the cases. Other observers (17, 21) restricted their programs to VCG analyses.

A different approach to the aforementioned systems was initiated by Pipberger who used second generation computer programming, i.e., multivariate analysis. Basically, the findings most valuable in differentiating tracings of a single or combined pathologic entity from normal are determined by the computer. When the learning set is complete, using records from known abnormal and normal cases, this system is applied to unknown cases with results supposedly achieving a high degree of accuracy when confirmed by objective non-ECG methods. Unfortunately, although this may prove feasible for one to possibly four combined abnormalities, it cannot be used with higher numbers of abnormal findings and therefore, its clinical usefulness is severely limited. In fact, a review presented at the First International Meeting on Electrocardiology in Wiesbaden, Germany in October 1974 reported that in a comparison of many programs both the cardiologist and the results of the multivariate analysis program of the Frank VCG agreed in many abnormal diagnoses (such as posterior wall infarction) where the actual non-ECG data proved the cases were entirely normal. Kornreich (11–14) employed multivariate computer analysis techniques with nine surface leads and compared the results with the Pipberger multivariate analysis program for the Frank VCG. He showed that the orthogonal VCG Frank leads did not contain all of the waveform information detected by the maximal surface leads. Kornreich *et al.* (13) also applied this system in the computer diagnosis of angina pectoris from maximal QRS surface waveform information at rest and achieved startling diagnostic results as compared to the Frank leads. Should the accuracy of this method be confirmed by other workers, the necessity for diagnostic exercise electrocardiographic testing may well be obviated.

Method

The present method for computerized electrocardiography developed at The Mount Sinai Hospital in conjunction with the Cro-Med Bionics Corporation in New York City represents a complete system for application in the clinical environment. The programming is continually updated under the control of an international board of cardiologists so that newer concepts may be incorporated directly after they are appropriately tested and agreed to by members of the board. The concept includes ECG recording on analog tape using three-channel equipment. After extensive study of several hundred thousand cases in which both the classic 12-lead ECG and the Frank VCG were analyzed, the latter method was dropped from the program as a routine, although it is still being continued in the European facilities.

The main thrust is to provide a system in which rhythm analysis, contour analysis, and comparison of previous cases are available. The usual application in the hospital environment is that cases are recorded at the bedside on analog tape. Approximately 35 cases may be taken in a single analog reel. These are then transmitted from the satellite hospitals via ordinary telephone to the computer center where the data are converted by Analog to Digital converters to digits on digital magnetic tape. The cases are processed in batch and the computer printouts are then reviewed by physicians either at the computer site or local hospital. This overview corrects any error in computer diagnostic statements. The results are relayed back to the sending hospital via teletype message with automatic answer so that the technician does not have to be physically present to receive the answers. Emergency cases may be transmitted to the computer center by telephone and the computer report relayed back directly after processing. For preoperative cases, processing is usually done at a specified time at the computer center so that the reports may be placed on the charts of the preoperative patients in the early evening for reference by the anesthesiologist as he makes his rounds. The records, at present, may be stored on digital magnetic tape for later use for the computer comparative program. Fourteen thousand cases may be stored on one digital reel; the retrieval time for all cases is in the order of 9 to 10 minutes and this may be performed in partition on the computer while routine cases are being analyzed simultaneously. The comparative program entails 9 seconds of computer time on the present system. Record storage on disk was used initially but then dropped because space was limited. The present computer disk availability of multi-million bytes makes storage on disk feasible and is a definite improvement because of the disk feature of random access.

Table 18-1. Specific Rhythm Analysis Statements Covering most Clinical Arrhythmia Analyses

Rhythm analysis
Normal sinus rhythm—rate
Sinus tachycardia—rate
Sinus bradycardia—rate
Low atrial or junctional pacemaker—rate
Junctional rhythm—rate
Idioventricular rhythm or junctional rhythm with IV block—rate
Junctional tachycardia—rate
Ventricular tachycardia—rate
Ventricular—complex tachycardia—rate (ventricular or supraventricular with ventricular aberration)
Supraventricular tachycardia—rate
Second-degree atrioventricular conduction defect, Mobitz Type 2, rate
Second-degree atrioventricular conduction defect with Wenckebach phenomenon, Mobitz Type 1, rate
Wandering pacemaker—rate
Atrioventricular dissociation—rate
Third-degree atrioventricular block—rate
Atrial flutter-rate, i.e., ventricular rate
Atrial flutter–fibrillation; ventricular rate
Atrial fibrillation with AV block, ventricular rate
Atrial fibrillation—ventricular rate
Atrial fibrillation with AV block and either junctional rhythm with IV block or idioventricular rhythm—rate
Undetermined rhythm—rate
With sinus arrhythmia
With sinus arrest
With intermittent aberrant ventricular conduction
With atrial premature complex and aberrant ventricular conduction
With a ventricular premature complex
With ventricular premature complexes
Which have variable coupling and variable contour
Which have variable coupling and fixed contour
Which have fixed coupling and variable contour
Which have fixed coupling and fixed contour
With supraventricular premature complex and aberrant ventricular conduction
With supraventricular premature complex
With interpolated ventricular premature complex
With interpolated supraventricular premature complex
With ventricular fusion
With junctional escape
With delayed beat of unknown origin
Electronic pacemaker (amplitudes given for each lead)
First-degree AV block
Type A Wolff-Parkinson-White pattern (QRS initially upward in V_1)
Type B Wolff-Parkinson-White pattern (QRS initially downward in V_1)
Short P-R. Lown-Ganong-Levine syndrome, if history of tachycardia

At present the program is operated on Disk Operating System (DOS) or Operating System (OS), the latter being preferable for multiple program access. The apparatus is either an IBM 360/50 or 370/135 digital computer. The method will be presented by illustrative cases. The rhythm analysis includes all basic cardiac arrhythmias plus any ectopic events that occur (see Table 18-1). The contour criteria

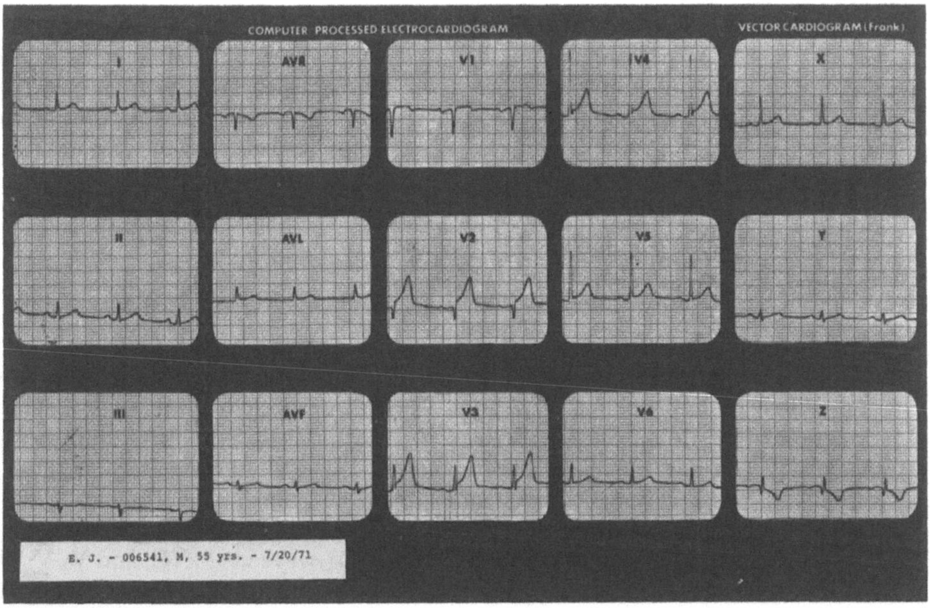

Fig. 18-1A. Male, 55 years; acute anteroseptal myocardial wall infarction; July 20, 1971. Strip chart recording of 12-lead electrocardiogram and component Frank VCG leads.

THE MOUNT SINAI HOSPITAL. NYC - CRO-MED BIONICS CORP. COMPUTER ANALYSIS OF ECG

THIS ANALYSIS IS MADE AVAILABLE FOR USE ONLY UNDER THE DIRECTION OF A PHYSICIAN APPROVED UNDER THIS PROGRAM

PATIENT NUMBER 006541 DATE RECORDED 07/20/71 DATE PROCESSED 07/20/71 RECORD SOURCE 1023 TIME 10 AUX. 0000000000
PATIENT DESCRIPTION - 55 YEAR OLD MALE. 66 INCHES, 160 POUNDS.

***** RHYTHM ANALYSIS *****

NORMAL SINUS RHYTHM, RATE 65

RHYTHM FOR INDIVIDUAL LEADSETS
NORMAL SINUS RHYTHM, RATE 65
NORMAL SINUS RHYTHM, RATE 65
NORMAL SINUS RHYTHM, RATE 62
JUNCTIONAL RHYTHM, RATE 66
JUNCTIONAL RHYTHM, RATE 65

***** ECG MEASUREMENTS *****

LEAD	WIDTHS IN SECONDS						AMPLITUDES IN TENTHS OF MILLIVOLTS								AREA		IRREG SHAPES		
NOS.	Q	R	S	R'	S'	INT	JJ	Q	R	S	R'	S'	P	T	QRSA	QRSTA	RDN	PND	TND
I	0.0	0.072	0.0	0.0	0.0	0.026	0.7	0.0	7.7	0.0	0.0	0.0	0.7	2.2	27.7	47.5	00	00	00
II	0.0	0.052	0.020	0.0	0.0	0.036	0.1	0.0	5.6	-0.8	0.0	0.0	1.1	1.8	13.7	29.9	00	00	00
III	0.0	0.028	0.056	0.0	0.0	0.020	-0.4	0.0	1.0	-3.5	0.0	0.0	0.4	-0.5	-8.4	-11.9	00	00	00
AVR	0.052	0.0	0.0	0.0	0.0	0.0	-0.5	-6.1	0.0	0.0	0.0	0.0	-0.9	-1.8	-15.8	-30.9	00	00	00
AVL	0.0	0.068	0.0	0.0	0.0	0.020	0.4	0.0	4.7	0.0	0.0	0.0	0.1	1.2	15.9	25.9	00	00	00
AVF	0.0	0.040	0.036	0.0	0.0	0.020	0.1	0.0	2.1	-1.7	0.0	0.0	0.6	0.7	1.2	5.8	00	00	00
V1	0.064	0.0	0.0	0.0	0.0	0.0	0.4	-8.5	0.0	0.0	0.0	0.0	0.3	1.0	-27.2	-13.4	00	00	00
V2	0.040	0.0	0.0	0.0	0.0	0.0	2.1	-4.3	0.0	0.0	0.0	0.0	0.4	8.4	-8.6	107.3	00	00	00
V3	0.0	0.048	0.012	0.0	0.0	0.032	3.0	0.0	8.9	-1.5	0.0	0.0	0.4	10.3	20.4	162.5	00	00	00
V4	0.0	0.052	0.0	0.0	0.0	0.032	2.3	0.0	22.2	0.0	0.0	0.0	0.3	7.3	57.7	149.6	00	00	00
V5	0.0	0.052	0.0	0.0	0.0	0.028	0.9	0.0	16.3	0.0	0.0	0.0	0.4	4.2	42.3	95.2	00	00	00
V6	0.0	0.056	0.0	0.0	0.0	0.032	0.1	0.0	6.9	0.0	0.0	0.0	0.3	1.8	19.3	41.9	00	00	00

**OVERALL INTERVALS IN SECONDS **

HRT	QRS	P-R	Q-T	T	P
68	0.074	0.204	0.369	0.176	0.089

** VECTOR ANGLE IN DEGREES **

QRS	T	P	QRST	J
04	17	51	11	NONE

INTERVALS FOR INDIVIDUAL LEADSETS

HRT	QRS	P-R	Q-T	T	P	BEAT
65	0.076	0.208	0.366	0.166	0.114	2
65	0.072	0.191	0.366	0.167	0.088	4
82	0.072	0.214	0.369	0.279	0.090	2
66	0.076	0.0	0.378	0.248	0.0	3
65	0.075	0.0	0.367	0.197	0.0	9

***** CONTOUR ANALYSIS *****

QS OR QS EQUIVALENT IN V2 AND/OR V3
J ELEVATED IN VL, V2 OR V3
COMPATIBLE WITH ANTEROSEPTAL INFARCTION

PLEASE REPEAT ECG TO DETERMINE AGE OF SUSPECTED INFARCTION

Fig. 18-1B. Computer printout of the abnormal 12-lead electrocardiogram illustrated in Figure 18-1A, with matrix measurements and both rhythm and contour analysis.

likewise cover the gamut of possible electrocardiographic diagnoses plus the specific criteria which resulted in that computer statement. The book containing all of these criteria and their order in the program will be published shortly (6). Four of the rhythm statements appear in the contour section of the computer printout because they depend solely on the contour or wave-shape analysis:

1. "Electronic pacemaker"
2. "First degree AV block"
3. "Types A and B Wolff-Parkinson-White Pattern"
4. "Short P-R"

The first illustration represents the computer analysis of the ECG and Frank VCG of a 55-year-old male admitted to the Coronary Care Unit of the Kings County Hospital in Brooklyn, New York. The tracings were transmitted by ordinary telephone to The Mount Sinai Hospital-Cro-Med Bionics Computer Center in New York City. Figure 18-1A represents the mounted strip chart recordings of the conventional 12-lead ECG plus component leads of the Frank VCG. The basic rhythm noted is regular sinus rhythm; the ECG is compatible with anteroseptal infarction, with deep QS wave in V_1 and V_2, absent "septal Q" wave in I, aVL, and V_4-V_6 plus RS-T elevations in I, aVL, and V_1-V_6. The Frank VCG, however, shows merely RS-T deviations and the Z lead discloses prominent early "anterior" forces in the presence of bona-fide anteroseptal infarction, as shown on the ECG and clinical follow-up! Figure 1B presents the complete 12-lead computer analysis printout in this case, including all matrix measurements and final computer diagnoses (Table 18-2). The sixth line gives the final rhythm analysis statement: *normal sinus rhythm, rate 65*. This statement is followed by a listing of the rhythm analysis statements for each of the individual lead sets (the fifth set being the Frank VCG leads in this case). The fourth and fifth individual rhythm statements are printed as *Junctional rhythm* on lines 11 and 12 of the printout and this suppresses P-R and P measurements on the fourth and fifth lines under *Intervals for Individual Leadsets*. However, the voting scheme discounts these two individual leadset rhythm statements, and the final rhythm statement is reported correctly as shown. The next section on the printout lists the detailed matrix ECG measurements for the 12-lead ECG followed by

Table 18-2. Computer Printout Code

Clinical data available	Entered by ECG technician
Rhythm for individual lead sets Intervals for individual lead sets	Go in sequence, 1 to 4
INT	Time of onset of intrinsicoid deflection
JJ	Amplitude of J junction (RS-T segment onset)
QRSA, QRSTA	QRS area, QRST area
RDN	RD = delta wave, RN = notched R
PND	PN = notched P, PD = diphasic P
TND	TN = notched T, TD = diphasic T
HRT	Average heart rate (rate under rhythm analysis is for dominant rhythm only)
Vector angle in degrees	Frontal plane angles, computed from limb leads
Beat	Best number of that lead set selected as typical and used for final measurements

the overall intervals in seconds above the intervals for individual leadsets (the fifth represents the Frank VCG leads). The section labeled *Vector Angle in Degrees* refers to the frontal plane derived from the extremity leads of the 12-lead ECG.

The final contour analysis section of the computer printout lists the contour diagnostic statements for this case, with the applicable criteria directly above each statement: *compatible with anteroseptal infarction; please repeat ECG to determine age of suspected infarction.* In this case clinical data were not available on the record; the appearance of *acute myocardial infarction* or *chest pain* in the clinical data section would cause the final contour statement to read: *Compatible with anteroseptal infarction. Suggests suspected infarction is* acute. *Please repeat.*

Computer diagnosis of the Frank VCG in this case is shown in Figure 18-1C. This printout was produced with the Mayo VCG program of Dr. Ralph Smith—first release. Since the final rhythm was analysed as nodal rhythm, P-R and P durations are reported as zero and all P-wave vector measurements are suppressed. The contour diagnostic statement was *abnormal electrocardiogram*, with no detection of the existence of anteroseptal infarction. The incorrect VCG computer analyses are related in this printout to measurement and programming error for the rhythm analysis and to the basic faulty electrode locations of the so-called *corrected and orthogonal* component leads of the Frank VCG system.

The second case illustrates the use of our automatic comparative ECG program, despite a vast geographic difference in the sites of the ECG recordings. The patient is a 58-year-old male with far advanced coronary artery disease, who has been followed by me since 1955. He sustained an acute diaphragmatic myocardial infarction (with right bundle branch block and left axis deviation) in 1971. On September 21, 1972, he reentered The Mount Sinai Hospital Ames Coronary Care Unit with a

PATIENT NUMBER 006541 DATE RECORDED 07/20/71 DATE PROCESSED 07/22/71
PR DUR= 0, R DUR= 76, RT DUR= 367, P DUR= 0 SEC
ABNORMAL ELECTROCARDIOGRAM
NODAL RHYTHM,RATE 65

SEGMENT	RHO	FRONTAL		SAGITTAL		HORIZONTAL	
ROR3	335	334	302	317	199	61	306
RR	379	346	378	284	92	86	368
RER4	366	357	349	191	111	107	365
RMAX	1115	344	1085	311	402	75	1073
R(1)	60	296	50	306	56	33	39
R(2)	227	323	184	320	174	47	197
R(3)	741	339	690	317	370	67	697
R(4)	1074	344	1046	310	383	76	1033
R(5)	679	353	662	209	174	103	674
R(6)	418	17	236	169	352	147	412
R(7)	105	30	77	152	81	137	97
R(E)	102	352	61	354	82	36	102
T(1)	146	324	64	344	137	21	141
T(2)	194	315	82	342	185	18	185
T(3)	252	320	127	340	233	24	238
T(4)	351	324	181	341	319	26	334
T(5)	487	328	264	341	432	28	465
T(6)	601	331	353	341	516	32	574
T(7)	533	329	370	334	430	39	497
T(8)	265	324	215	321	201	48	233

Fig. 18-1C. Computer printout of the Frank vectorcardiogram illustrated in Figure 18-1A, with planar and spatial measurements and computer VCG analysis.

second severe acute anteroseptal and anterior wall myocardial infarction and required temporary transvenous cardiac pacing. On September 25, 1972, his 12-lead ECG disclosed normal sinus rhythm, abnormal left axis deviation, right bundle branch block, acute anteroseptal and anterior wall infarction with RS-T and T abnormalities (Figure 18-2A). It is interesting to note that the Q waves in leads II, III, and AVF from his previous diaphragmatic myocardial wall infarction disappeared with the onset of this new infarction. After recovery, he traveled to Hollywood, Florida for recuperation and entered the Golden Isle Hospital there on December 28, 1972 because of a recurrence of prolonged, severe anterior chest pain. His record on that day was processed at our computer center in New York, since we service the Golden Isle Hospital for computer ECG analysis. This ECG tracing (Figure 18-2C) revealed normal sinus rhythm, unusual superior axis deviation, right bundle branch block, anteroseptal and anterior wall infarction. There was probably an extension of the infarction and the progressive changes of the RS-T segments and T waves as seen customarily following acute myocardial infarction.

The computer printout for the ECG record on September 25, 1972 in New York is shown in Figure 18-2B. The clinical data available listed *Acute myocardial infarction and pronestyl*; the patient was receiving this drug at that time for control of ventricular premature beats. On line 9 of the printout, in the rhythm analysis section, the rhythm is stated correctly as *Normal sinus rhythm, rate 92.* Following the detailed matrix listing of ECG measurements, the contour analysis section prints the correct diagnostic statements: *Abnormal left axis deviation* (–57°), *suggests right*

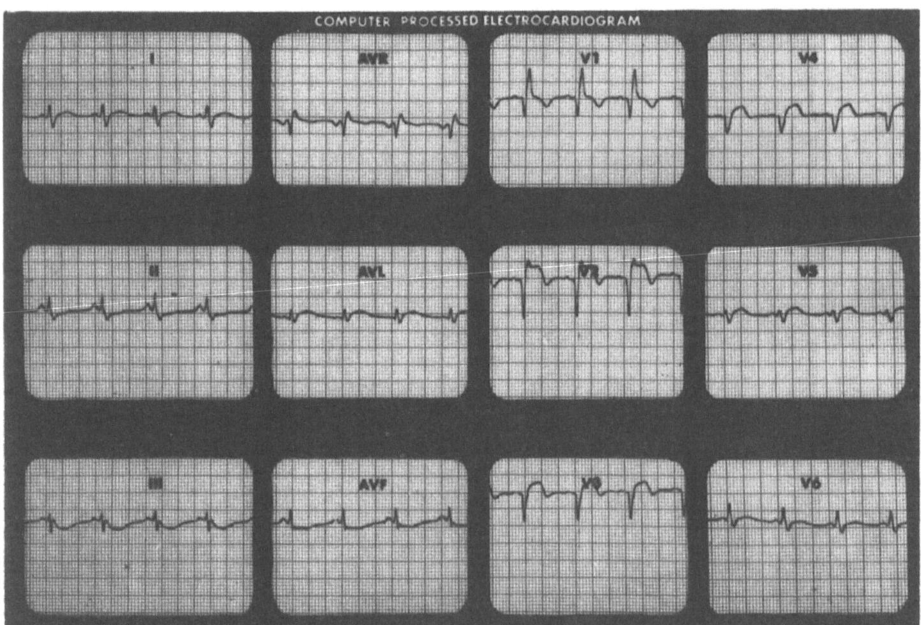

Fig. 18-2A. Male, 58 years; September 25, 1972; acute anteroseptal and anterior infarction, right bundle branch block, left axis deviation, bilateral bundle branch block, and RS-T and T abnormalities. Strip chart recording of 12-lead electrocardiogram.

```
                    THE MOUNT SINAI HOSPITAL, NYC - CRO-MED BIONICS CORP. COMPUTER ANALYSIS OF ECG

          THIS ANALYSIS IS MADE AVAILABLE FOR USE ONLY UNDER THE DIRECTION OF A PHYSICIAN APPROVED UNDER THIS PROGRAM

PATIENT NUMBER 000029   DATE RECORDED 09/25/72  DATE PROCESSED 01/05/73   RECORD SOURCE 1171  TIME  0   AUX. 0000000009
PATIENT DESCRIPTION  -  58 YEAR OLD MALE.  70 INCHES. 200 POUNDS.
        CLINICAL DATA AVAILABLE -
                 ACUTE MYOCARDIAL INFARCTION
                 PRONESTYL

***** RHYTHM ANALYSIS *****

NORMAL SINUS RHYTHM, RATE  92

   RHYTHM FOR INDIVIDUAL LEADSETS
NORMAL SINUS RHYTHM, RATE  92
NORMAL SINUS RHYTHM, RATE  92
NORMAL SINUS RHYTHM. RATE  92
NORMAL SINUS RHYTHM, RATE  93


***** ECG MEASUREMENTS *****

LEAD            WIDTHS IN SECONDS                         AMPLITUDES IN TENTHS OF MILLIVOLTS            AREA          IRREG SHAPES
NOS.     Q      R     S     R'     S'    INT         JJ   Q    R    S    R'   S'   P    T          QRSA QRSTA        RON PND TND
  I     0.0   0.052 0.052 0.0    0.0   0.028        0.7  0.0  3.9 -2.8  0.0  0.0  0.7  0.5          2.9   7.1        00  00  00
 II     0.0   0.040 0.084 0.0    0.0   0.024       -1.4  0.0  5.4 -3.4  0.0  0.0  1.5 -0.8         -3.4 -11.5        00  00  00
III     0.0   0.032 0.092 0.0    0.0   0.020       -2.3  0.0  2.3 -3.5  0.0  0.0  0.9 -1.2        -12.5 -24.7        00  00  00
AVR     0.060 0.064 0.0   0.0    0.0   0.084       -0.3 -4.6  2.7  0.0  0.0  0.0 -1.2  0.5         -5.2  -1.2        00  00  00
AVL     0.0   0.036 0.044 0.0    0.0   0.016        1.2  0.0  3.1 -1.6  0.0  0.0 -0.1  0.7          2.0   9.0        00  00  00
AVF     0.0   0.044 0.084 0.0    0.0   0.028       -1.1  0.0  3.8 -2.6  0.0  0.0  1.2 -0.8         -2.6 -10.6        00  00  00
 V1     0.060 0.075 0.0   0.0    0.0   0.092        0.4 -6.6  8.8  0.0  0.0  0.0  0.4 -2.1         13.6 -11.1        00  00  00
 V2     0.060 0.080 0.0   0.0    0.0   0.104        3.2-12.0  4.9  0.0  0.0  0.0  0.3  3.5        -16.4  24.9        00  00  01
 V3     0.084 0.0   0.0   0.0    0.0   0.0          2.8 -7.5  0.0  0.0  0.0  0.0  0.3  3.5        -31.5   9.8        00  00  01
 V4     0.0   0.016 0.068 0.0    0.0   0.008        2.5  0.0  0.7 -4.7  0.0  0.0  0.4  3.0        -15.4  10.4        00  00  00
 V5     0.0   0.044 0.060 0.0    0.0   0.032        1.6  0.0  1.7 -2.3  0.0  0.0  0.6  1.4         -3.2   8.8        00  00  00
 V6     0.0   0.055 0.060 0.0    0.0   0.032        0.4  0.0  4.6 -1.8  0.0  0.0  0.6  0.3          7.4   9.2        00  00  00

** OVERALL INTERVALS IN SECONDS **                      ** VECTOR ANGLE IN DEGREES **
HRT   QRS   P-R   Q-T    T     P                              QRS   T    P  QRST   J
 92 0.120 0.122 0.329 0.200 0.077                             -57  -70   62  -65  -63

   INTERVALS FOR INDIVIDUAL LEADSETS
HRT   QRS   P-R   Q-T    T     P     BEAT
 92 0.115 0.127 0.327 0.200 0.080    2
 92 0.115 0.121 0.327 0.203 0.071    2
 92 0.128 0.115 0.371 0.236 0.079    2
 93 0.120 0.126 0.292 0.164 0.078    2


***** CONTOUR ANALYSIS *****

        ABNORMAL LEFT AXIS DEVIATION

        QRS INTERVAL GREATER THAN OR EQUAL TO 0.120 SEC.
        S IN I OR THE WIDER OF R AND R-PRIME IN AVR GREATER THAN OR EQUAL TO 0.030 SEC.
        ONSET OF INTRINSICOID DEFLECTION IS GREATER THAN OR EQUAL TO 0.040 SEC. IN V1 OR V2
SUGGESTS RIGHT BUNDLE BRANCH BLOCK

        QRS ANGLE BETWEEN -30 AND -120 DEGREES INCLUSIVE
SUGGESTS BILATERAL BUNDLE BRANCH BLOCK

        ABNORMAL Q OR Q EQUIVALENT IN V2 OR V3
        QS OR QS EQUIVALENT IN V2 AND/OR V3
        J ELEVATED IN V1, V2 OR V3
        T WAVE INVERTED OR DIPHASIC IN V1. V2, OR V3
COMPATIBLE WITH ANTEROSEPTAL INFARCTION

        ABNORMAL Q OR Q EQUIVALENT IN V4
        J ELEVATED
COMPATIBLE WITH ANTERIOR INFARCTION

SUGGESTS SUSPECTED INFARCTION IS ACUTE. PLEASE REPEAT ECG

        T WAVE INVERTED IN LEADS  II. III. AVF,  V1.
        T WAVE LOW OR DIPHASIC IN LEADS  V2,  V3,  V6.
        J DEPRESSION AT LEAST 1 TENTH OF MVOLT IN LEADS  II, III, AVF.
S-T AND T ABNORMALITIES
```

Fig. 18-2B. Computer printout of the abnormal 12-lead electrocardiogram illustrated in Figure 18-2A, with matrix measurements and both rhythm and contour analyses.

bundle branch block; suggests bilateral bundle branch block, compatible with anteroseptal infarction, compatible with anterior infarction, suggests suspected infarction is acute. Please repeat ECG, and ST and T abnormalities.

Likewise, Figure 18-2D lists the computer analysis for the second ECG record of this patient on December 28, 1972 in Florida. The patient number at the Golden Isle Hospital is shown as 464400; whereas his New York patient number is 000029. The clinical data available are listed as *Acute myocardial infarction* since that was his admission diagnosis in Florida. Although the third lead set shows atrial fibrillation for the rhythm analysis, the voting scheme allows for the final rhythm analysis statement to list correctly: *Normal sinus rhythm, rate 66.* Following the ECG measure-

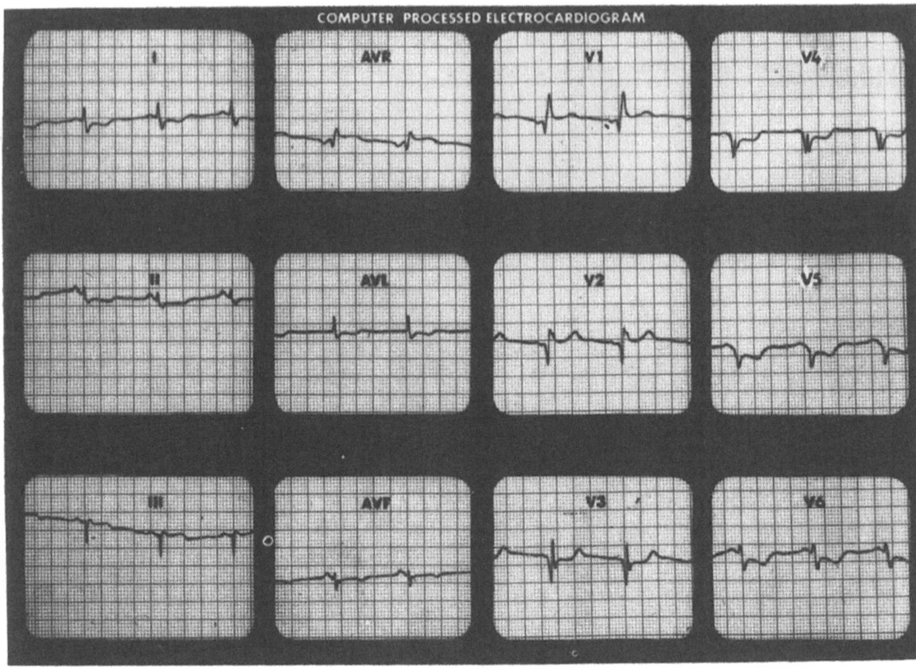

Fig. 18-2C. Male, 58 years; December 28, 1972 (same patient as in Figure 18-2A); subacute anteroseptal and anterior infarction, right bundle branch block, unusual axis deviation, bilateral bundle branch block, and RS-T and T abnormalities. Strip chart recording of 12-lead electrocardiogram.

ments matrix, the contour analysis section lists the appropriate diagnostic statements: *Unusual electrical axis (—101°), suggests right bundle branch block, suggests bilateral bundle branch block, compatible with anteroseptal infarction, compatible with anterior infarction, please repeat ECG to determine age of suspected infarction, and ST and T abnormalities.* In both Figures 18-2B and 18-2D, the criteria for each contour diagnostic statement is printed directly above that statement.

So that the direct computer comparison of the two ECG records can be performed correctly in this particular case, both patient numbers were entered in the request for comparison. Customarily, the patient number is identical for individual cases, and the computer request requires merely the dates of the tracings to be compared.

Figure 18-2E lists the input data plus the detailed computer differences of all stored measurements of both the new tracing versus the previous record. Although this format displays the method for the computer comparison, it is not useful as such for practical clinical purposes. Therefore, this information is listed in the final computer printout in English format (Figure 18-2F). Here we find the patient identification numbers, clinical data and comparison of overall intervals, vector angle values, and heart rate. Note that the frontal plane ECG angle has changed from —57° in the previous record to —101° in the later tracing. The rhythm analysis comparison shows no change; normal sinus rhythm is still present, and both rates are stated. The contour analysis section shows unusual electrical axis *now present*; lists all diagnoses *still present* in the new record, and also gives those statements *no longer present.* For

```
                 THE MOUNT SINAI HOSPITAL, NYC - CRO-MED BIONICS CORP. COMPUTER ANALYSIS OF ECG

       THIS ANALYSIS IS MADE AVAILABLE FOR USE ONLY UNDER THE DIRECTION OF A PHYSICIAN APPROVED UNDER THIS PROGRAM

PATIENT NUMBER 464400   DATE RECORDED 12/28/72  DATE PROCESSED 01/05/73   RECORD SOURCE 3051  TIME  0   AUX. 0000000000
PATIENT DESCRIPTION  -  58 YEAR OLD MALE,  72 INCHES, 180 POUNDS.
        CLINICAL DATA AVAILABLE -
                ACUTE MYOCARDIAL INFARCTION

***** RHYTHM ANALYSIS *****

NORMAL SINUS RHYTHM, RATE  66

   RHYTHM FOR INDIVIDUAL LEADSETS
NORMAL SINUS RHYTHM, RATE  68
NORMAL SINUS RHYTHM, RATE  65
ATRIAL FIBRILLATION, VENTRICULAR RATE  65
NORMAL SINUS RHYTHM, RATE  67


***** ECG MEASUREMENTS *****

LEAD            WIDTHS IN SECONDS                           AMPLITUDES IN TENTHS OF MILLIVOLTS             AREA        IRREG SHAPES
NOS.     Q     R     S     R'    S'    INT          JJ    Q    R    S    R'   S'   P    T          QRSA  QRSTA      RON PNO TNO
  I    0.0   0.044 0.064 0.0   0.0   0.028        -0.8  0.0  4.2 -3.5  0.0  0.0  0.7 -1.2        -2.0 -17.8      00  00  00
 II    0.0   0.028 0.080 0.0   0.0   0.016        -0.6  0.0  2.3 -2.6  0.0  0.0  1.5 -0.4        -7.2 -10.8      00  00  00
III    0.0   0.020 0.028 0.060 0.0   0.056         0.3  0.0  0.8 -5.3  1.1  0.0  0.9  0.9        -3.3   7.1      00  00  00
AVR    0.044 0.060 0.0   0.0   0.0   0.072         1.0 -2.4  2.9  0.0  0.0  0.0 -0.8  0.6         3.5  11.4      00  00  00
AVL    0.0   0.040 0.056 0.0   0.0   0.020        -0.8  0.0  4.9 -2.4  0.0  0.0  0.1 -1.1         3.1 -11.4      00  00  00
AVF    0.0   0.024 0.080 0.0   0.0   0.012        -0.1  0.0  1.3 -3.6  0.0  0.0  0.8  0.5       -12.9  -6.7      00  00  00
 V1    0.048 0.084 0.0   0.0   0.0   0.088         0.9 -3.5  8.8  0.0  0.0  0.0  0.1  0.7        28.5  34.2      00  00  00
 V2    0.052 0.083 0.0   0.0   0.0   0.064         0.8 -5.8  5.3  0.0  0.0  0.0  0.3  1.8         8.3  21.9      00  00  00
 V3    0.060 0.020 0.064 0.0   0.0   0.064        -0.4 -7.0  4.2 -1.1  0.0  0.0  0.3  1.2       -20.3 -10.5      00  00  00
 V4    0.124 0.0   0.0   0.0   0.0   0.0          -1.1 -5.5  0.0  0.0  0.0  0.0  0.2 -2.3       -34.1 -64.4      00  00  00
 V5    0.124 0.0   0.0   0.0   0.0   0.0          -1.8 -5.8  0.0  0.0  0.0  0.0  0.4 -2.5       -35.9 -71.9      00  00  00
 V6    0.0   0.036 0.068 0.0   0.0   0.012        -1.8  0.0  1.9 -4.6  0.0  0.0  0.5 -2.2       -12.2 -43.8      00  00  00

** OVERALL INTERVALS IN SECONDS **                       ** VECTOR ANGLE IN DEGREES **
 HRT   QRS   P-R   Q-T    T     P                              QRS   T    P  QRST   J
  66 0.123 0.151 0.396 0.257 0.085                            -101  162   62 -171 -173

   INTERVALS FOR INDIVIDUAL LEADSETS
 HRT   QRS   P-R   Q-T    T     P      BEAT
  67 0.099 0.147 0.371 0.228 0.091      3
  65 0.094 0.155 0.365 0.260 0.092      2
  66 0.124 0.0   0.436 0.166 0.0        2
  67 0.122 0.112 0.414 0.283 0.072      4


***** CONTOUR ANALYSIS *****

        UNUSUAL ELECTRICAL AXIS

        QRS INTERVAL GREATER THAN OR EQUAL TO 0.120 SEC.
        S IN I OR THE WIDER OF R AND R-PRIME IN AVR GREATER THAN OR EQUAL TO 0.030 SEC.
        ONSET OF INTRINSICOID DEFLECTION IS GREATER THAN OR EQUAL TO 0.040 SEC. IN V1 OR V2
SUGGESTS RIGHT BUNDLE BRANCH BLOCK

        QRS ANGLE BETWEEN -30 AND -120 DEGREES INCLUSIVE
SUGGESTS BILATERAL BUNDLE BRANCH BLOCK

        ABNORMAL Q OR Q EQUIVALENT IN V2 OR V3
COMPATIBLE WITH ANTEROSEPTAL INFARCTION

        ABNORMAL Q OR Q EQUIVALENT IN V4
        T WAVE INVERTED OR DIPHASIC
        ABNORMAL Q OR Q EQUIVALENT IN V5
        T WAVE INVERTED OR DIPHASIC
COMPATIBLE WITH ANTERIOR INFARCTION

PLEASE REPEAT ECG TO DETERMINE AGE OF SUSPECTED INFARCTION

        T WAVE INVERTED IN LEADS   I,  II, AVL,  V4,  V5,  V6.
        J DEPRESSION AT LEAST 1 TENTH OF MVOLT IN LEADS  V4,  V5,  V6.
        J DEPRESSION AT LEAST 0.5 TENTHS OF MVOLT IN LEADS   I,  II, AVL.
S-T AND T ABNORMALITIES
```

Fig. 18-2D. Comptuer printout of the abnormal 12-lead electrocardiogram illustrated in Figure 18-2C, with matrix measurements and both rhythm and contour analyses.

example, the axis is now *unusual* and no longer *left* and the acute infarction noted in the first record is no longer considered acute because of the long time interval between the two records. Finally, the *comparative measurements analysis* section prints those changes in the T waves and RS-T segments considered clinically significant, each followed by the comparison conclusion: *These are progressive changes seen following acute myocardial infarction.* Thus, the automatic computer comparison printouts are not merely percentage measurement changes, but have been programmed to perform in clinical situations in a manner similar to that used today in the modern heart station.

EXPERIMENTAL COMPUTER CCMPARISON OF ELECTROCARDIOGRAMS 01/05/73

	PATIENT NO.	RECCRDEC	PRCCESSEC	CLINICAL	AGE	SEX	HEIGHT	WEIGHT	SOURCE	TIME	AUX.
NEW	4644C0	12/28/72	C1/C5/73	200	58	1	72	18C	3051	C	0C0000000C0
CCMPARED WITH	000029	09/25/72	01/05/73	208	58	1	70	200	1171	0	0000000009

ECG MEASUREMENTS

LEAC NOS.	WICTHS IN SECCNDS Q	R	S	RP	SP	INT	AMPLITUDES IN TENTHS CF MILLIVCLTS ST	C	R	S	RP	SP	P	T	QRSA	QRSTA	IRREG SHAPES RDN	PND	TND
I	0.0	C.044	C.C64	0.C	C.C	0.028	-0.8	0.0	4.2	-3.5	0.0	0.0	0.7	-1.2	-2.0	-17.8	00	00	C0
NEW-CLC	0.0	-0.C08	C.C12	0.C	C.0	0.C	-1.5	0.0	0.3	-0.7	0.0	0.0	0.0	-1.7	-4.9	-24.9	00	00	00
II	0.0	0.C28	C.C8C	0.0	C.0	C.C16	-C.6	0.0	2.3	-2.6	0.0	0.0	1.5	-0.4	-7.2	-10.8	C0	0C	00
NEW-OLD	0.0	-0.012	-C.C04	0.0	C.0	-0.008	C.8	0.0	-3.1	0.8	0.0	0.0	0.0	0.4	-3.8	C.7	C0	0C	00
III	0.0	C.02C	C.C28	C.C60	C.C	C.C56	0.3	0.0	0.8	-5.3	1.1	0.0	0.9	0.9	-3.3	7.1	00	CC	00
NEW-OLD	0.0	-0.012	-0.C64	0.C60	0.0	C.036	2.6	0.0	-1.5	-1.8	1.1	0.0	0.0	2.1	9.2	31.8	0C	0C	00
AVR	0.C44	0.C6C	C.C	0.0	C.C	0.072	1.0	-2.4	2.9	0.0	0.0	0.0	-0.8	0.6	3.5	11.4	C0	0C	00
NEW-OLC	-0.C16	-0.004	C.C	0.C	C.0	-0.012	1.3	2.2	0.2	0.0	0.0	0.0	0.4	0.1	8.7	12.6	C0	00	00
AVL	0.C	0.C4C	0.C56	0.C	C.0	0.C20	-0.8	0.0	4.9	-2.4	0.0	0.0	0.1	-1.1	3.1	-11.4	CC	00	00
NEW-CLD	0.0	0.C04	0.C12	0.0	0.C	C.C04	-2.0	0.0	1.8	-0.8	0.0	0.0	0.2	-1.8	1.1	-20.4	C0	00	00
AVF	C.0	0.024	C.C8C	C.C	0.0	0.C12	-0.1	0.0	1.3	-3.6	0.0	0.0	0.8	0.5	-12.9	-6.7	C0	00	00
NEW-OLD	0.0	-0.02C	-C.C04	C.C	C.0	-0.016	1.0	0.0	-2.5	-1.0	0.0	0.0	-0.4	1.3	-10.3	3.9	0C	00	00
V1	0.048	0.C84	0.C	0.C	0.C	C.C88	C.9	-3.5	8.8	0.0	0.0	0.0	0.1	0.7	28.5	34.2	CC	C0	00
NEW-OLD	-0.012	0.C08	C.C	0.C	0.C	-C.C04	C.5	3.1	0.0	0.0	0.0	0.0	-0.3	2.8	14.9	45.3	00	00	00
V2	0.052	0.C8E	C.C	C.C	C.C	0.064	C.8	-5.8	5.3	0.0	0.0	0.0	0.3	1.8	8.3	21.9	00	00	00
NEW-OLD	-0.C08	0.C08	C.0	C.C	C.C	-0.C40	-2.4	6.2	0.4	0.0	0.0	0.0	0.0	-1.7	24.7	-3.0	00	00	01
V3	0.C60	0.020	-0.C64	0.C	C.0	0.064	-0.4	-7.0	4.2	-1.1	0.0	0.0	0.3	1.2	-20.3	-10.5	00	00	00
NEW-OLD	-0.024	0.02C	0.C64	0.C	C.C	C.064	-3.2	0.5	4.2	-1.1	0.0	0.0	0.0	-2.3	11.2	-20.3	C0	00	01
V4	0.124	0.0	C.C	0.C	C.C	0.C	-1.1	-5.5	0.0	0.0	0.0	0.0	0.2	-2.3	-34.1	-64.4	C0	00	00
NEW-CLD	C.124	-0.016	-C.C68	C.C	C.0	-0.008	-3.6	-5.5	-0.7	4.7	0.0	0.0	-0.2	-5.3	-18.7	-74.8	00	00	00
V5	0.124	0.0	C.C	0.C	0.C	C.C	-1.8	-5.8	0.0	0.0	0.0	0.0	0.4	-2.5	-35.9	-71.9	C0	0C	00
NEW-CLD	0.124	-0.044	-C.C6C	0.C	0.0	-0.C32	-3.4	-5.8	-1.7	2.3	0.0	0.0	-0.2	-3.9	-32.7	-80.7	00	00	00
V6	0.0	0.C36	C.C68	C.C	C.0	C.012	-1.8	0.0	1.9	-4.6	0.0	0.0	0.5	-2.2	-12.2	-43.8	C0	00	00
NEW-OLD	0.0	-C.020	C.CC8	C.C	0.0	-C.020	-2.2	0.0	-2.7	-2.8	0.0	0.0	-0.1	-2.5	-19.6	-53.0	00	00	00

Fig. 18-2E. Computer comparison of electrocardiograms in Figure 18-2C with Figure 18-2A on same patient. List of comparisons of ECG matrix measurements.

Summary and Conclusion

The value of computer electrocardiography compared with human electrocardiographers has been presented and discussed both for routine electrocardiography in the hospital heart station and for ECG monitoring in the coronary care and other intensive care units. From the standpoint of routine electrocardiography, the combination of automatic computer printouts plus physician review appears to be the current method of choice. The advantage of such computer automated hospital heart stations is that physician review of large ECG loads may be performed in a fraction of the time required with the human observer method, thereby freeing the cardiologist or internist for his most important duties relative to direct patient care. The computer system also serves as a great teaching tool, since the criteria for a diagnosis are listed in the computer printout directly above that diagnostic statement. Furthermore, the ease with which huge numbers of cases can be stored and retrieved facilitate statistical studies heretofore not humanely possible.

The advantages and disadvantages of the ECG, VCG, or both computer programs in routine cardiography were considered. Reference was made to the possible application of new "total" surface waveform computer systems using nine surface leads for the future. First- and second-generation computer methods were compared, wtih a personal opinion that if indeed a generation gap exists in this field, for practical purposes the oldfashioned programming of the classic 12-lead ECG yields the most practical results at present.

```
                         EXPERIMENTAL COMPUTER COMPARISON OF ELECTROCARDIOGRAMS                                01/05/73
                         ------------------------------------------------------

         PATIENT NO.   RECORDED   PROCESSED   CLINICAL   AGE   SEX   HEIGHT   WEIGHT   SOURCE   TIME    AUX.

          NEW  4644CO  12/28/72   01/05/73      200      58     1      72      180      3051      0    0000000000
COMPARED WITH  000029  09/25/72   01/05/73      208      58     1      70      200      1171      0    0000000009


                 OVERALL INTERVALS                                  VECTOR ANGLE VALUES        HRT
           QRS   P-R   Q-T    T     P                            QRS   T     P QRST    J      RATE

          0.123 0.151 0.396 0.257 0.085                    NEW  -101  162   62 -171 -173      66
NEW-OLD   0.003 0.029 0.067 0.057 0.008                    OLD   -57  -70   62  -65  -63      92


RHYTHM ANALYSIS

   STILL PRESENT -
                   NORMAL SINUS RHYTHM


CONTOUR ANALYSIS

   NOW PRESENT -
                   UNUSUAL ELECTRICAL AXIS

   STILL PRESENT -
                   SUGGESTS RIGHT BUNDLE BRANCH BLOCK

                   SUGGESTS BILATERAL BUNDLE BRANCH BLOCK

                   COMPATIBLE WITH ANTEROSEPTAL INFARCTION

                   COMPATIBLE WITH ANTERIOR INFARCTION

                   S-T AND T ABNORMALITIES

   NO LONGER PRESENT -
                   LEFT AXIS DEVIATION

                   SUGGESTS SUSPECTED INFARCTION IS ACUTE. PLEASE REPEAT ECG


COMPARATIVE MEASUREMENTS ANALYSIS

   T WAVE NOW INVERTED IN LEAD  V4,  V5.
                        THESE ARE PROGRESSIVE CHANGES SEEN FOLLOWING ACUTE MYOCARDIAL INFARCTION

   T WAVE NOW UPRIGHT IN LEAD III, AVF,  V1

   S-T SEGMENT DEPRESSION NOW LESS MARKED IN LEADS  II, AVF

   S-T SEGMENT DEPRESSION NOW MORE MARKED IN LEADS   I, AVL,  V2,  V3,  V4,  V5,  V6

   S-T NOW DEPRESSED IN LEAD  V4,  V5.
                       THESE ARE PROGRESSIVE CHANGES SEEN FOLLOWING ACUTE MYOCARDIAL INFARCTION
```

Fig. 18-2F. Computer comparison of electrocardiograms in Figure 18-2C with Figure 18-2A on same patient. English text comparison with different patient numbers and clinical data; comparison of both rhythm and both contour analyses plus English comparative measurement analysis and comparative conclusion.

The recent editorial in the journal Circulation entitled *What ECG computer program to choose for clinical application; the need for consumer protection* (18), should be considered. The point taken relative to the certification of programs, such as the MSDL cannot be overemphasized, since the certified program merely refers to reduplication by a user of the same results as the test cases supplied. This is in sharp contrast to findings of Bailey *et al.* (1–3) as to the unreliability of these computer programs. Performance evaluation however, by non-ECG methods, such as cardiac catheterization, cardiac surgery and/or autopsy information are inadequate in that only portions of contour analyses may be verified in this manner and not disturbances of cardiac rhythm, conduction abnormalities, or both. The inter- and intraobserver variability of human interpreters further complicates the attempt at diagnostic verification. Despite these facts, there is little disagreement as to where the needs are greatest. For the acute coronary episodes, sequential changes customarily observed are sufficient verification of the accuracy of diagnostic statements for practical purposes. On the other hand, most computer ECG programs have an accuracy rate of over 99 percent generally for the identification of normal subjects, such as in population studies. Correlation of patient's age, clinical diagnosis, and drugs employed should be a vital part of any clinically acceptable computer ECG program, just as it has been in nonautomated hospital heart stations. The question should not only be *what represents a correct ECG interpretation or diagnosis?* but what system provides a logical and practical solution to the processing of immense numbers of ECG recordings both in the hospital heart station with adequate electrocardiographic expertise and more important the large number of institutions throughout the world where facilities for adequate analyses of ECGs are completely lacking. An interesting discourse on the status of ECG versus VCG interpretation by computer has been presented (7) and the reduction in cost of computer systems to acceptable prices is emphasized.

Despite controversies and disagreements in the field of electrocardiography and vectorcardiography, computerized electrocardiography both for routine electrocardiographic diagnosis as well as rhythm monitoring in the acute and/or ambulatory patient presents a practical, cost-effective methodology for direct clinical application today.

References

1. Bailey, J. J., Horton, M., and Itscoitz, S. B. A method for evaluating computer programs for electrocardiographic interpretation. III. Reproducibility testing and the sources of program errors. Circulation, 50:88, 1974.
2. —— Itscoitz, S. B., Grauer, L. E., Hirshfeld, J. W. Jr., and Horton, M. R. A method for evaluating computer programs for electrocardiographic interpretation. II. Application to version D of the PHS program and the Mayo clinic program of 1968. Circulation 50:80, 1974.
3. —— —— Hirshfeld, J. W. Jr., Grauer, L. E., and Horton, M. R. A method for evaluating computer programs for electrocardiographic interpretation. I. Application to the experimental IBM program of 1971. Circulation, 50:73, 1974.
4. Brik, H., Joffe, C. D., Teichholz, L. E., and Herman, M. V. The electrocardiogram—A poor method of detecting septal involvement in anterior myocardial involvement. Unpublished data.
5. Caceres, C. A., Steinberg, C. A., Abraham, S., Carberry, W. J., McBride, J. M., Tolles, W. E., and Rikli, A. E. Computer extraction of electrocardiographic parameters. Circulation, 25:356, 1962.
6. Computer electrocardiography: Present status and computer criteria for electrocardiography. Pordy, L. (ed.). Futura Publishing Co., Mt. Kisco, New York, 1975.
7. E.C.G. Interpretation by computer. Editorial. Br. Med. J., 3:702, September 21, 1974.
8. Enderle, J., Pordy, L., Chesky, K., Jaffe, H. L., and Friedberg, C. K. Clinical applications of computer analysis of vectorcardiograms. Proceedings of the Satellite Symposium of the XXVth International Congress of Physiological Sciences and the XIIth International Colloquium Vectorcardiographicum. Presses Academiques Européennes, Brussels, 1972, p. 136.
9. —— and Telerman, M. Progression de l'analyse automatique de l'electro- et du vectocardiogramme par ordinateur (20,019 traces). Acta Cardiol., 28:576, 1973.
10. Ha, D., Kraft, D. I., and Stein, P. D. The anteriorly oriented horizontal vector loop: The problem of distinction between direct posterior myocardial infarction and normal variation. Am. Heart J., 88:408, 1974.
11. Kornreich, F. The missing waveform information in the orthogonal electrocardiogram (Frank leads): I. Where and how can this missing waveform information be retrieved? Circulation, 48:984, 1973.

12. —— The missing waveform information in the orthogonal electrocardiogram (Frank leads): II. Diagnosis of left ventricular hypertrophy and myocardial infarction from "total" surface waveform information. Circulation, 48:996, 1973.
13. —— Block, P., and Brismee, D. The missing waveform information in the orthogonal electrocardiogram (Frank leads): III. Computer diagnosis of angina pectoris from "maximal" QRS surface waveform information at rest. Circulation, 49:1212, 1974.
14. —— —— —— The missing waveform information in the orthogonal electrocardiogram (Frank leads): IV. Computer diagnosis of biventricular hypertrophy from "maximal" surface waveform information. Circulation 49:1223, 1974.
15. Nolle, F. M., Oliver, G. C., Kleiger, R. E., Cox, J. R., Clark, K. W., and Ambos, H. D. The Argus/H system for rapid analysis of ventricular arrhythmias. Proceedings, Conf. on Computers in Cardiology, National Institutes of Health, Bethesda, Md. October 2–4, 1974, p. 37.
16. Oliver, G. C., Kleiger, R. E., Krone, R. J., Martin, T. F., Miller, J. P., Nolle, F. M., and Cox, J. R. Application of high speed analysis of ambulatory electrocardiograms. Proceedings, Conf. on Computers on Cardiology, National Institutes of Health, Bethesda, Md. October 2–4, 1974, p. 43.
17. Pipberger, H. V., Stallman, F. W., and Berson, A. S. Automatic analysis of the P-QRS-T complex of the electrocardiogram by digital computer. Ann. Intern. Med. 57:776, 1962.
18. Pipberger, H. V. and Cornfield, J. What ECG computer program to choose for clinical application; the need for consumer protection. Editorial, Circulation, 47:918, 1973.
19. Pordy, L., Jaffe, H., Chesky, K., Friedberg, C. K., Bonner, R. E., Schwetman, H. D., and Alexander, D. Computer analysis of the electrocardiogram: A joint project. J. Mt. Sinai Hosp. (N.Y.), 24:69, 1967.
20. Simonson, E., Tuna, N., Okamoto, N., and Toshima, H. Diagnostic accuracy of the vectorcardiogram and electrocardiogram. A cooperative study. Am. J. Cardiol., 17:829, 1966.
21. Smith, R. E. and Hyde, C. M. A computer system for electrocardiographic analysis. Proc. 3rd Annual Rocky Mountain Bio-Engineering Symposium. Univ. of Colorado, Boulder, May 2–3, 1966.
22. Sodi-Pallares, D., Medrano, G. A., Bisteni, A., and Ponce de Leon, J. Deductive and polyparametric electrocardiography. National Institute of Cardiology, Mexico City, Mexico, D.F., 1970.
23. Taback, L., Marden, E., Mason, H. L., and Pipberger, H. V. Digital recording of electrocardiographic data for analysis by a digital computer. IRE. Trans. Med. Elect., ME-6:167, 1959.
24. Teichholz, L. E., *et al.* Unpublished data.

Chapter 19 Echocardiography—Its Practical Value

ARTHUR D. HAGAN, M.D., F.A.C.C.

General Considerations

Echocardiography is a valuable noninvasive technique for the evaluation of congenital and acquired heart disease. Its practical value as a diagnostic procedure depends entirely on the technical skill of the examiner and the expertise of the physician who interprets the echocardiogram. Significant improvements have been achieved in ultrasound recording equipment since Elder and Hertz (16) first employed reflected ultrasound to examine the heart. Only the conventional, single-crystal transducer echocardiography will be covered in this chapter, other echocardiographic systems, including two-dimensional sector scanning and the multiple-crystal system, will not be discussed.

Echocardiographic records have been markedly enhanced by employing a continuous recording technique instead of Polaroid exposures. The 2.25 mHz transducer, focused at 5.0 or 7.5 cm, is most often used to examine adults. However, better quality studies can usually be obtained in obese individuals and in patients with increased anterior-posterior diameter of the chest by using a 1.6 mHz transducer focused at 10 cm. A 3.5-mHz transducer is often preferable for small children and a 5.0 or 7.5 mHz nonfocused transducer is necessary for newborn infants. Despite technologic improvements in available hardware, significant difficulty may still be encountered in performing an examination. Considerable skill is essential to conduct a complete echocardiographic study, much more than is normally required for any other type of medical machine technician. The technician or physician performing the examination should not only be familiar with cardiac anatomy, physiology, pathology, and congenital malformations, but he must possess knowledge of the working diagnosis in each patient studied. The position of the patient and location of the transducer will vary in each patient, depending on the difficulties encountered. Although the conventional position of the transducer is the second to fifth intercostal space along the left sternal border other more unusual locations may be necessary, such as further lateral over the left precordium, over the left ventricular apex, in the suprasternal notch, along the right sternal border, or in the epigastrum pointing superior and leftward through the diaphragm. In contrast to adults, the transducer beam can be directed through the ribs or sternum in newborn infants since these structures have not yet calcified. The usual position of the patient is supine or turned to the left side. Sometimes the study is easier to perform by elevating the head of the bed 20° to 30°. On rare occasions, some patients with thick chests or hyperinflated lungs can be studied better if they are sitting up, leaning forward, and breathing out, in held expiration, which brings the heart closer to the anterior chest wall. However, care should be taken to avoid initiating a Valsalva maneuver, which usually creates more artifacts and interferences in the echocar-

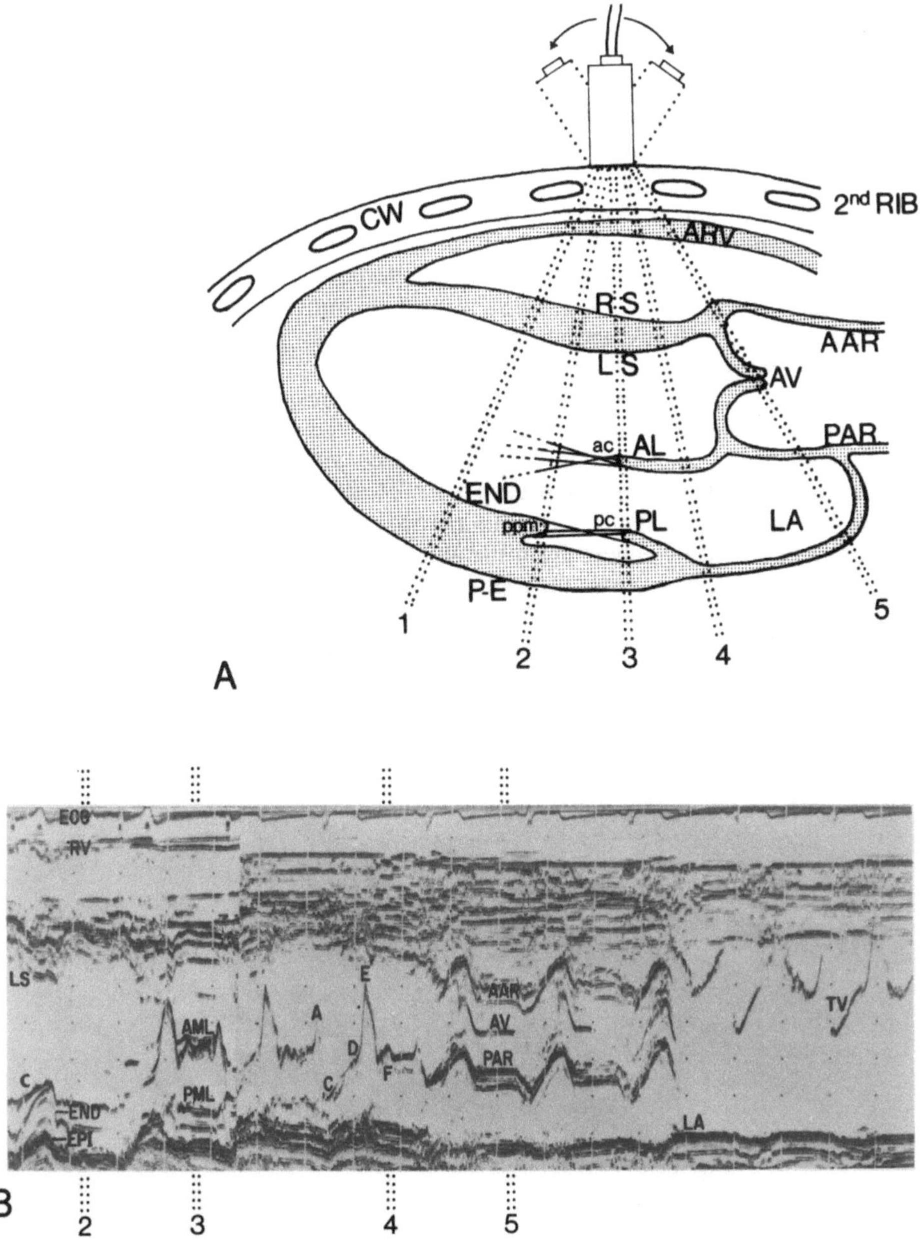

Fig. 19-1. A. Diagram of the heart in sagittal cross-section. B. Continuous echocardiographic recording of a normal adult heart scanning from the left ventricle at the level of the chordae tendineae (position 2) through the mitral valve to the base (position 5) where the aortic valve and left atrium are seen. As the transducer beam is directed medial and inferior from the aortic valve, the tricuspid valve can be identified. ARV = anterior right ventricular wall, RS = right side of septum, LS = left side of septum, AAR = anterior aortic root, AV = aortic valve, PAR = posterior aortic root, AL or AML = anterior mitral leaflet, PL or PML = posterior mitral leaflet, ac = anterior chordae tendineae, pc = posterior chordae tendineae, ppm = posterior papillary muscle, END = endocardium, P-E = pericardium-epicardium, EPI = epicardium, C = chordae, LA = left atrium, TV = tricuspid valve.

diogram. The examiner must constantly be aware of and able to identify cardiac echoes from different transducer locations in conjunction wtih the altered positions of the patient.

When the examiner places the transducer in the third or fourth intercostal space along the left sternal border, the ultrasonic beam can be swept in an arc from the left ventricular cavity (position 1, Figure 19-1A) through the mitral valve apparatus (positions 2, 3, and 4, Figure 19-1A) to the base of the heart (position 5, Figure 19-1A) where the aortic valve and left atrium are recorded. An electrocardiogram is always recorded simultaneously for timing purposes. The corresponding positions diagramed in Figure 19-1A are displayed in Figure 19-1B.

The pulmonary artery and valve, which are usually very difficult to record in an adult, are recognized easily in an infant by directing the transducer superior and slightly lateral to the aortic root (Figure 2). The tricuspid valve can be seen in most patients by directing the ultrasonic beam slightly medial from the plane of the mitral valve or medial and inferior from the aortic valve. The contour and motion characteristics of the anterior tricuspid leaflet are the same as the anterior mitral valve leaflet, however the echoes from the tricuspid valve in diastole are frequently partially obscured by echoes from the anterior right ventricular wall. The tricuspid valve, including echoes from the septal leaflet, is easily recorded in the presence of right ventricular dilatation. The tricuspid and mitral valves are frequently recorded simultaneously in newborn infants (Figure 19-3); this is not true for adults except those in whom the tricuspid valve is displaced toward the left, as in Ebstein's anomaly.

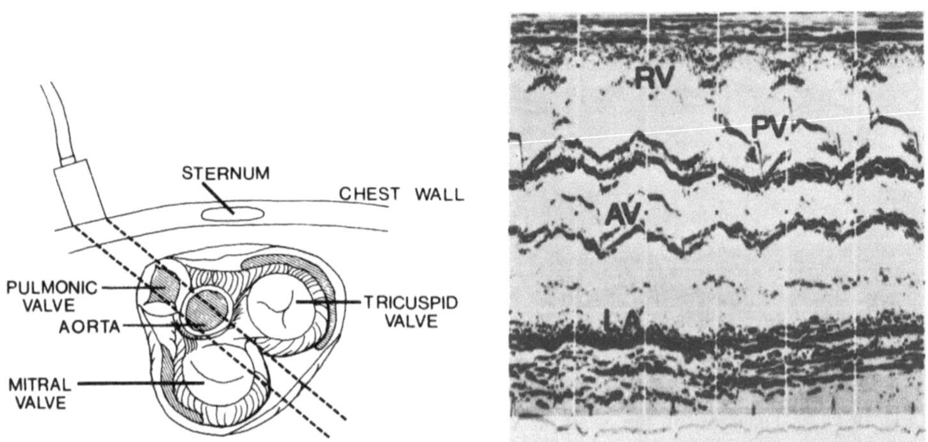

Fig. 19-2. The diagram to the left depicts the heart in coronal view. The pulmonary artery is anterior and lateral to the aorta. The mitral and tricuspid valves are inferior to both pulmonic and aortic valves, therefore they cannot be visualized simultaneously. The diagram shows their respective positions from a right-left and anterior-posterior relationship. The echocardiogram in a normal infant shows the right ventricular wall (RV) and aortic valve (AV); by directing the beam slightly lateral, the pulmonary artery with pulmonic valve (PV) are recorded anterior to the aortic root. LA = left atrium.

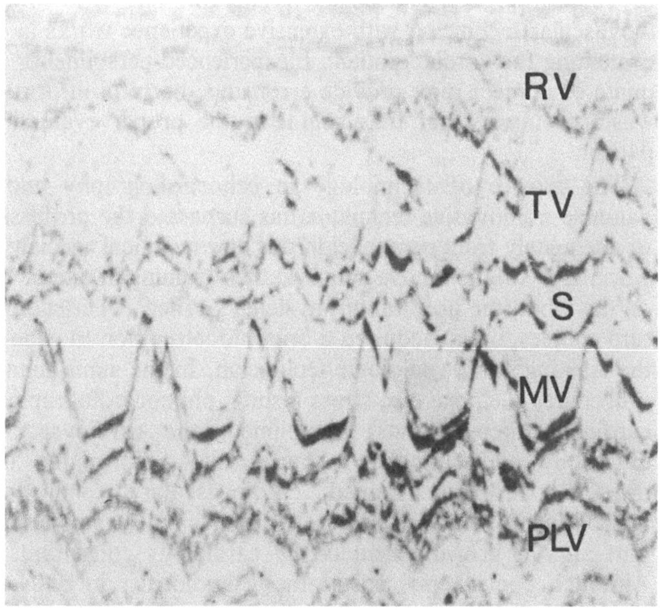

Fig. 19-3. Simultaneous recording of both tricuspid and mitral valves in a normal newborn infant. RV = right ventricular wall, TV = tricuspid valve, S = interventricular septum, MV = mitral valve, PLV = posterior left ventricular wall.

Problems in Training

Most technical problems encountered in obtaining good quality echocardiograms are due to the examiner's lack of experience or inadequate understanding of the clincial considerations in the individual patient. Like many other diagnostic procedures, the physician or cardiovascular technician must have as much information as possible about the patient's cardiac status in order to take the appropriate additional steps necessary to obtain the most useful information. The examiner should know the size of the heart and its position on x-ray films, be aware of the results of cardiac ascultation, and appreciate tentative cardiac diagnoses being considered. Professional interpretation of the echocardiograms cannot be separated from the individuals conducting the study, since interpretation is based upon knowing the location of the transducer and the position of the patient for various recordings, awareness of the images and structures visualized on the oscilloscope, which may not have been recorded on paper, and finally an understanding of other technical difficulties encountered during the procedure. Not all structures can be recorded in all patients at all times; therefore certain key information is required in each case to provide clinically useful recordings. Similar to the cardiac catheterization laboratory, certain essential information is necessary to establish any given diagnosis and to properly evaluate the abnormality. Since the physician caring for the patient, or the cardiologist to whom the patient is referred, normally does not have time to conduct all echocardiographic examinations, the technician performing the study must have extensive knowledge of cardiovascular disorders and preferably conduct the procedure in close proximity to the physician seeing the patient. The practical value of echocardiography depends heavily on this type of arrangement, i.e., a cardiovascular technician with extensive experience works in support of the consultant evaluating the cardiac patient. Inexperienced personnel or personnel who use inadequate equipment may provide erroneous, harmful information, which is not only a waste of money but detrimental to the proper evaluation and treatment of the patient.

The growth of technology in echocardiography and the application of this valuable noninvasive technique has surpassed the professional community's ability to adequately train personnel in this new technical specialty. Most of the technicians working in the field have acquired their training in one of the following manners: (a) on-the-job in the hospital or physician's office, (b) attending short workshops or lecture courses, or (c) acquired a brief indoctrination to echocardiography as a part of the training for a radiologic technician. In the same manner that other diagnostic procedures (i.e., exercise stress testing, phonocardiography with pulse tracings, and cardiac catheterizations) compliment the cardiovascular evaluation, echocardiography adds important supplemental information to the consultant's final decision. Properly trained cardiovascular technicians, or probably more appropriately identified as cardiovascular physician's assistants, are needed to support an ever-growing demand by cardiology consultants throughout the country. Although controversy exists among authorities in both cardiology and radiology specialties as to where this diagnostic procedure should be conducted, the answer for the present time is simple, by those in any institution or hospital who are most qualified. However, to meet present and future demands, medical schools and training institutions need to implement programs to graduate noninvasive cardiovascular technicians with expertise in echocardiography.

It is important to note, when discussing training responsibilities in the field of echocardiography, that pulsed wave ultrasound, used for this purpose, has proved entirely safe for human tissue (55).

Technical Difficulties

Echoes are not always obtained from the same position of the transducer or in the same manner from all patients. It is usually very difficult, and at times impossible, to achieve satisfactory recordings in obese patients or in individuals with large, barrel chests. In these patients a 1.6 mHz transducer, focused at 10 cm is better than the more commonly used 2.25-mHz transducer. In addition, there is an occasional advantage in placing the transducer on the epigastrium and directing the beam through the diaphragm to the heart in a superior, lateral direction. In tall, slender patients with vertical hearts, the transducer is placed lower than usual along the left sternal border. In contrast however, the transducer must be positioned more superior or farther lateral over the precordium when the heart is enlarged or shifted more than normal into the left chest. It is often difficult to obtain complete echoes from each of the structures, and interpretation should be based only on what can be definitely identified. Making judgments from incomplete echoes are to be avoided. Meticulous attention must be given to the simultaneous adjustment of machine controls, location of the transducer and the direction and position of the patient. Rapid respirations and, at times, even normal breathing will interfere with cardiac echoes; intermittent recordings during held respiration and avoiding the Valsalva maneuver usually eliminate that problem. Because of numerous potential difficulties encountered in obtaining good quality echocardiograms, no one can actually appreciate the value or the limitations of this procedure, unless he possesses a good understanding of the technique of echocardiography.

Mitral Valve

When introducing a discussion of the practical value of echocardiography, in addition to pointing out the limitations and controversies in certain areas, it is appropriate to begin with the mitral valve.

Mitral Stenosis

Edler (15) was the first to report on the clinical application of echocardiography when he described the abnormal echoes from the anterior leaflet of the mitral valve in the presence of mitral stenosis. However, it was not until 17 years later when Duchak *et al.* (13) described the normal and abnormal motion of the posterior mitral leaflet that a more accurate assessment of mitral stenosis could be made. No effort will be made to discuss echoes from the normal mitral valve, as seen in the M-mode scanning technique, since this has already been thoroughly described (17). It is now possible to evaluate the severity of mitral stenosis in a far more sophisticated manner by echo than was possible only 3 to 4 years ago. The posterior mitral valve leaflet must be recorded together with the anterior leaflet in order to establish the diagnosis of mitral stenosis from the echocardiogram.

Three main parameters are employed to quantitate the degree of mitral stenosis: (a) the velocity of the anterior leaflet is measured by determining the E to F slope, (b) the pliability of the anterior leaflet is measured by determining the amplitude between closed and open position (D to E points), and (c) the extent to which both the anterior and posterior leaflets are thickened are noted. A velocity of the anterior mitral leaflet less than 15 mm/sec indicates severe mitral stenosis; moderate mitral stenosis is indicated by a velocity of 15 to 25 mm/sec, and mild mitral stenosis is suggested by a velocity of 25 to 40 mm/sec. The velocity appers to change from beat to beat in the presence of atrial fibrillation. Other factors that influence leaflet velocity include the overall quality of the recording and the given location through which the echo beam passes through the leaflet. In other words, if the beam intersects the leaflet near the annulus, the velocity will be slower than that measured when the beam crosses the leaflet near its free margin. The amplitude or excursion of the anterior leaflet is also greater when measured at the tip, in contrast to the distance recorded near the annulus. The maximum obtainable excursion and velocity of the leaflet are the most reliable measurements. A normal excursion (greater than 20 mm) in the presence of severe mitral stenosis suggests that the patient is a candidate for mitral commissurotomy. Evidence of a calcified valve in the presence of poor excursion or leaflet pliability is very suggestive that valve replacement will be necessary. The examiner must be constantly aware that false slowing and decreased excursion may be noted due to faulty recording technique. It is essential that the posterior mitral leaflet be recorded to confirm the presence of mitral stenosis, since several other conditions can cause a decreased velocity of the anterior mitral leaflet, such as idiopathic hypertrophic subaortic stenosis, valvular aortic stenosis, pulmonary hypertension, cardiomyopathy, or any condition causing significant elevation of the left ventricular diastolic pressure or decreased compliance of the left ventricle. Although the posterior mitral leaflet characteristically moves anteriorly during diastole in mitral stenosis, occasionally the posterior leaflet may not move significantly in either direction (Figure 19-4A and B). This may be found in patients following mitral commissurotomy as well as in individuals with mild mitral stenosis in association with aortic valve disease or significant left ventricular dysfunction. Lack of any specific diastolic motion of the posterior leaflet requires that other clinical information be considered in the final interpretation of the echocardiogram to avoid making a false-positive or false-negative diagnosis of mitral stenosis.

Any patient who develops unexplained atrial fibrillation should have an echocardiogram to exclude the possibility of clinically unsuspected mitral stenosis. On rare occasions older patients with mitral stenosis may present with findings of pulmonary edema and severe pulmonary hypertension but have no audible opening snap or diastolic murmur. The diagnosis can be established quickly at the bedside with an echocardiogram (Figure 19-5).

The improved resolution of echoes afforded by the continuous recording technique, compared to the obsolete method of Polaroid exposures, has greatly enhanced the examiner's ability to detect leaflet thickening and the presence of calcification. The examiner must be particularly careful when evaluating leaflet thickness, since faulty technique due to excessively high gain control or improper angle of the echo beam intersecting the leaflet may cause multiple echoes or "parallel layering" of echoes, which can falsely simulate leaflet thickening. Although it remains to be confirmed by other investigators, Nanda (42) has reported that echocardiography is more sensitive than fluoroscopy for the detection of calcium in the mitral valve.

Mitral Regurgitation

Burgess and his coinvestigators (4) described the echocardiographic findings in different types of mitral regurgitation. Although it has long been recognized that the velocity of the anterior mitral leaflet may be increased in the presence of mitral regurgitation, no echo finding is specific enough to confirm or exclude this diagnosis when its etiology is rheumatic or papillary muscle dysfunction. Obtaining serial echocardiograms to determine the changing velocity of the anterior mitral leaflet has little, if any, practical value for evaluating the degree of mitral regurgitation. Vast differences in actual or apparent velocities in normal mitral valves can be caused by improper recording technique, change in heart rate, and failure to record echoes from the same point on the leaflet each time. Another nonspecific finding may be encountered—increased amplitude (>30 mm) of the leaflet excursion (D to E).

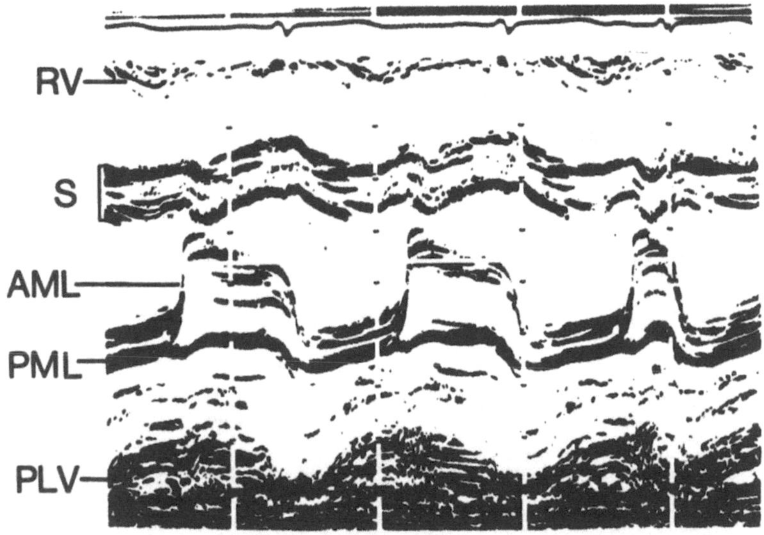

A

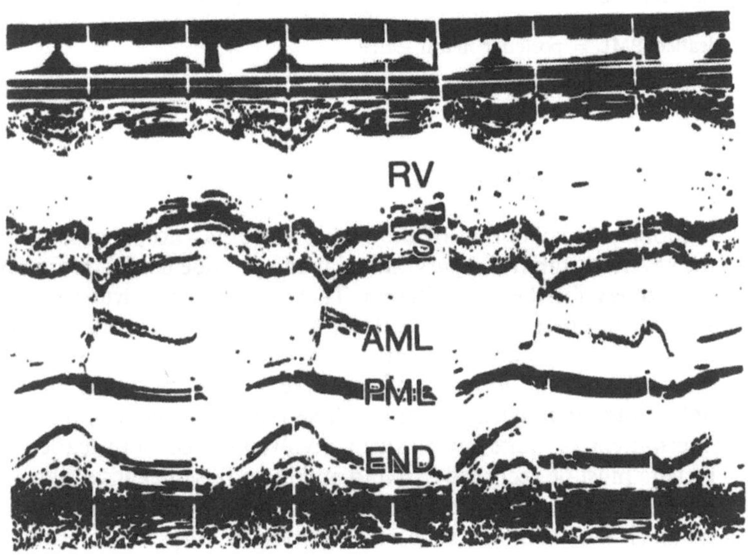

B

Fig. 19-4. A. Typical echocardiogram in a patient with mitral stenosis showing slow velocity of the anterior leaflet and anterior motion of the posterior leaflet during diastole. B. Mitral valve in a patient with neither anterior nor posterior movement of the posterior leaflet during diastole. This patient is 10 years postmitral commissurotomy and has mild residual mitral stenosis. RV = right ventricle, S = septum, AML = anterior mitral leaflet, PML = posterior mitral leaflet, PLV = posterior left ventricle, END = endocardium.

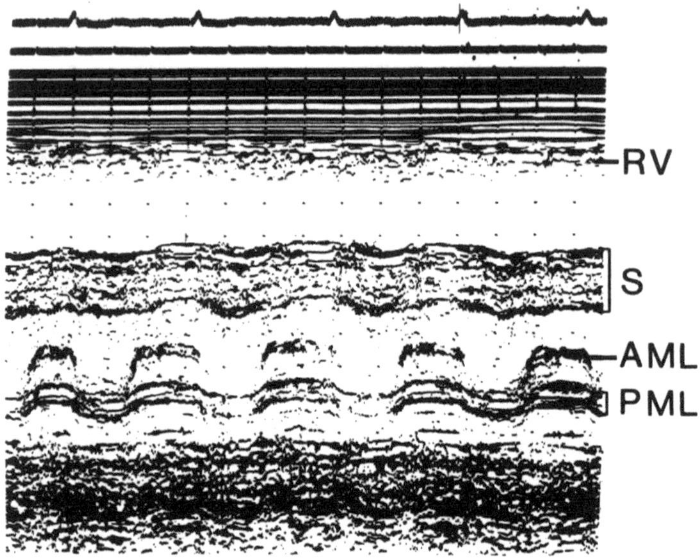

Fig. 19-5. Echocardiogram of the mitral valve showing severe mitral stenosis in an elderly patient with no ascultatory evidence of mitral stenosis (compliments of Dr. Howard Wayne, Sharp Memorial Hospital, San Diego, California). RV = right ventricular wall, S = septum, AML = anterior mitral leaflet, PML = posterior mitral leaflet.

Mitral Valve Prolapse

Although an echogram of the mitral valve has no particular value for quantitating the severity of mitral regurgitation, it can provide useful information to help establish an etiology for the regurgitation. This is particularly true with prolapse of either the anterior or posterior mitral leaflets, a condition commonly found in young to middle age adults and, more frequently, in women. The echogram is a very sensitive technique to detect mild forms of mitral valve prolapse and may be seen in patients having only midsystolic clicks but no audible regurgitation. The prolapse may be mild and intermittent or quite severe, with involvement of both leaflets (Figure 19-6). Both leaflets must be recorded to avoid making a false-negative diagnosis, since frequently only the posterior leaflet will exhibit prolapse. Special maneuvers may be required to establish the diagnosis, such as inhalation of amyl nitrite or recording the echogram with the patient sitting or standing.

We have observed the same findings reported by DeMaria *et al.* (10), i.e., neither the presence nor the degree of mitral regurgitation correlates with the echo pattern of mitral valve prolapse. We have also diagnosed the prolapsed mitral valve syndrome from echocardiograms in patients with Marfan's syndrome as well as in individuals with no abnormal cardiac findings. In addition, we have observed an incidental occurrence of mitral valve prolapse in both adults and children with secundum atrial septal defects. Although the frequency of this association has not yet been established, it should be checked for in each patient with an atrial septal defect since

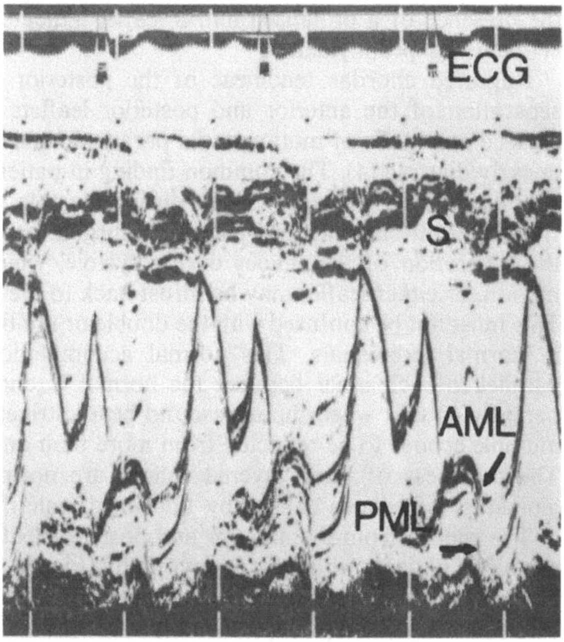

Fig. 19-6. Prolapse of both anterior and posterior mitral leaflets. The bottom arrow shows the posterior leaflet prolapsing all the way to the left atrial wall, which may be noted in some of the more severe forms. S = septum, AML = anterior mitral leaflet, PML = posterior mitral leaflet.

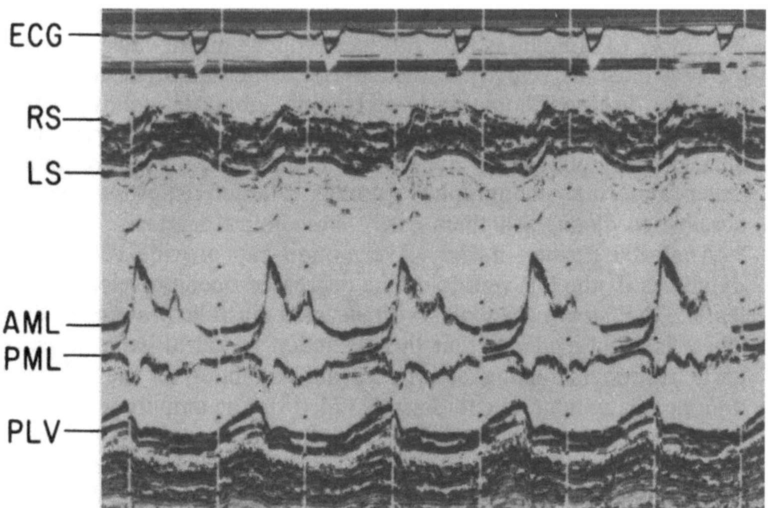

Fig. 19-7. Typical appearance of the mitral valve in a young man with a cardiomyopathy. The left ventricle is dilated, and is functioning poorly; the posterior leaflet (PML) is abnormally far from the endocardium during diastole as a result of the dilated, more spherical left ventricular cavity. Echoes from the anterior and posterior leaflet remain separated during systole. Mild mitral regurgitation did exist but there was no prolapse of the mitral valve. RS = right side of septum, LS = left side of septum, AML = anterior mitral leaflet, PLV = posterior left ventricle.

the presence of a prolapsed mitral leaflet indicates the need for indefinite bacterial endocarditis prophylaxis.

Ruptured chordae tendineae of the posterior leaflet is suggested by persistent separation of the anterior and posterior leaflets during systole in addition to increased amplitude of motion and a paradoxic anterior motion of the posterior leaflet in early diastole (4). The common finding in patients with torn anterior chorade is a chaotic, coarse, flapping motion during diastole which can be distinguished easily from the fluttering caused by aortic regurgitation (14). It is important to distinguish the separation of the echoes during systole, which may have a posterior sagging motion, or either leaflet may be thrust back to the left atrial wall throughout systole. This must not be confused with the double or multiple C to D echoes commonly seen in normal individuals. This normal accumulation of echoes during systole run parallel to each other between the normal C and D points. These echoes are apparently caused when the ultrasound beam strikes the leaflets at an angle, causing multiple echoes to be reflected from more than one area encompassed by the beam. The thickness of these layered echoes are normal in contrast to the dense conglomerate of echoes caused by thickened, calcific leaflets.

The echoes from the anterior and posterior leaflets may be separated throughout systole in patients with a cardiomyopathy (Figure 19-7) (39). The mechanism is most likely due to papillary muscle dysfunction or distortion of mitral supporting structures, causing valve prolapse or failure of leaflets to coapt because the shape of the left ventricle has changed.

Abnormal Mitral Valve Motion in Absence of Mitral Valve Disease

A number of conditions may produce reduced mitral valve slope (E to F) and mimic the slow diastolic velocity of the anterior leaflet in mitral stenosis. These include aortic valve disease, idiopathic hypertrophic subaortic stenosis, cardiomyopathy with reduced cardiac output and abnormal left ventricular compliance, left atrial myxoma, primary pulmonary hypertension, and Ebstein's malformation (22, 36, 50, 52). Other abnormal echographic findings characteristic for these diseases make it possible to distinguish them easily from mitral stenosis.

Analyzed further, mitral valve motion can provide valuable information of the dynamics of the left ventricle. The decreased opening velocity of the anterior mitral leaflet (D-E slope) correlates with elevated diastolic pressure in the left ventricle (34). There is good evidence that this reduction in mitral valve slope reflects the rate of early ventricular filling as well as abnormalities of the left ventricular pressure-volume relationship at end-diastole (24, 48). The amplitude of the A-wave may be increased in the presence of elevated left ventricular end-diastolic pressure, however sometimes the relative height of the A wave appears greater because the amplitude of the E point is diminished or obliterated due to slowed D-E slope or marked flutter secondary to aortic insufficiency (Figure 19-8). The rate at which the mitral valve closes after atrial contraction is determined by the velocity of the A-C slope, however since the A-C interval is a function of atrioventricular conduction, this interval must be subtracted from the P-R interval on the electrocardiogram. Konecke *et al.* (34) reported a PR-AC interval greater than 0.06 second in 19 patients with a left ventricular end-diastolic pressure (LVEDP) less than 20 mm Hg in contrast to a PR-AC interval of less than 0.06 second in 14 patients with an LVEDP greater than

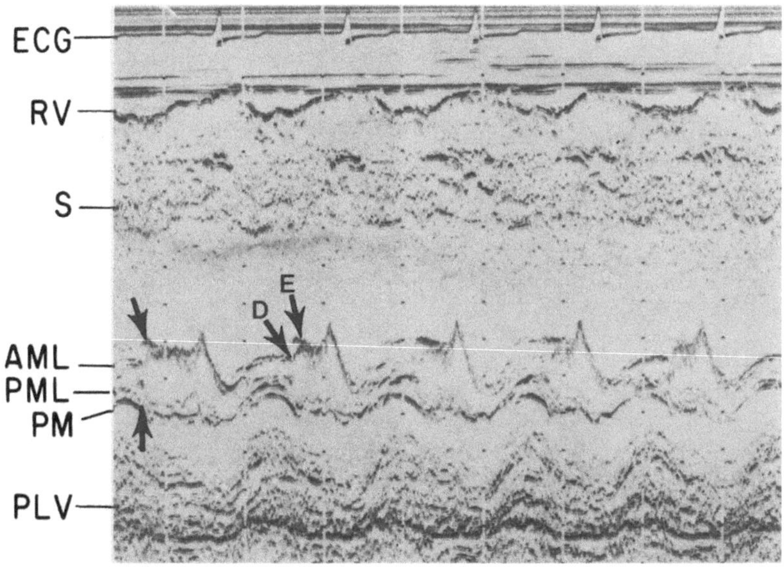

Fig. 19-8. Abnormal mitral valve recording in a 59-year-old man with chronic, severe aortic insufficiency secondary to bacterial endocarditis fifteen years earlier. The top arrow on the left is pointing out the fluttering of the anterior mitral leaflet. The bottom arrow on the left is pointing to the prominent echo from hypertrophied papillary muscle (PM), immediately anterior to that echo is a faint recording of a normal posterior mitral leaflet (PML). The other two arrows are pointing to the D and E points showing both decreased opening velocity (D to E slope) as well as a markedly shortened E point due to the severe aortic insufficiency. RV = right ventricular wall, S = septum, AML = anterior mitral leaflet, PLV = posterior left ventricle.

20 mm Hg. Although this index is not sensitive enough to reflect mild to moderate changes in LVEDP, it does provide a valuable noninvasive addition to evaluate left ventricular function in certain patients.

The echocardiogram is very useful to differentiate the diastolic rumble of mitral stenosis from the Austin Flint rumble of aortic insufficiency (Figure 19-9). The fluttering of the mitral valve is a sensitive indicator of aortic insufficiency and is commonly seen in the absence of an audible Austin Flint murmur (57). This fluttering motion does not, however, provide useful information to quantitate the severity of aortic insufficiency. The mitral valve does not close prematurely in chronic severe aortic insufficiency, however, we have observed such premature closure in 4 successive cases with acute, florid aortic regurgitation caused by bacterial endocarditis (Figure 19-10A). Partial premature closure of the mitral valve may also be caused by first degree atrioventricular block.

Idiopathic Hypertrophic Subaortic Stenosis

One of the most valuable clinical applications of echocardiography is the diagnosis of idiopathic hypertrophic subaortic stenosis. Although the systolic anterior motion of the anterior mitral leaflet has been considered pathognomonic for idiopathic

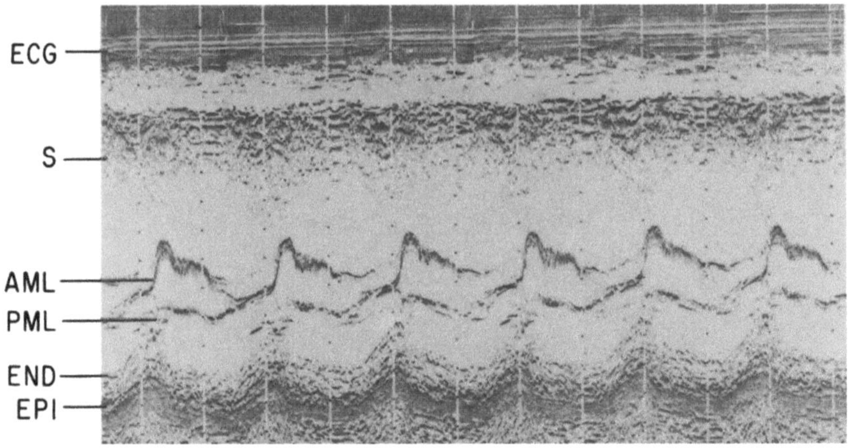

Fig. 19-9. Flutter of the anterior mitral leaflet (AML) in a 60-year-old patient with significant aortic insufficiency and secondary diastolic rumble at the apex. Echocardiogram shows a normal posterior mitral leaflet (PML) and no evidence of mitral stenosis. S = septum, END = endocardium, EPI = epicardium.

hypertrophic subaortic stenosis, it is possible to have echoes from the mitral valve bulging anterior during systole in the presence of severe aortic valvular stenosis or nonobstructive cardiomyopathy; in either case the posterior left ventricular wall is significantly hypertrophied (Figure 19-11). This is presumably caused by distortion of the supporting structures of the mitral valve and the underlying markedly hypertrophied ventricular wall. Henry and his associates (29, 57) reported that the echocardiogram is extremely reliable for diagnosing both idiopathic hypertrophic subaortic stenosis and asymmetric septal hypertrophy. These investigators were able to quantitate the severity of outflow obstruction by measuring the area encompassed by the systolic anterior motion during systole and determining the length of time the interventricular septum and anterior mitral leaflet were in contact during ejection. These authors define asymmetric septal hypertrophy as a disproportionately thickened septum, compared to the posterior left ventricular free wall, by a ratio greater than 1.3 to 1. Generally, this is a very reliable index for the diagnosis of asymmetric septal hypertrophy or idiopathic hypertrophic subaortic stenosis. However, in rare circumstances, disproportionate septal thickening may occur in patients with severe pulmonic stenosis or pulmonary hypertension (27). Such patients should easily be distinguished on the basis of other clinical information. Measurement of septal thickness may be very difficult in some patients since it becomes a technical problem to record distinct echoes from the right side of the septum in some individuals. To avoid false-positive diagnoses of idiopathic hypertrophic subaortic stenosis from an abnormal mitral valve echo, definite evidence of the disproportionately thickened septum should be present. The echocardiogram of a 14-year-old girl with severe idiopathic hypertrophic subaortic stenosis is shown in Figure 19-12A together with an echogram taken from the girl's father (Figure 19-12B), demonstrating asymmetric septal hypertrophy without outflow obstruction. Since most patients with idiopathic hypertrophic subaortic stenosis are treated

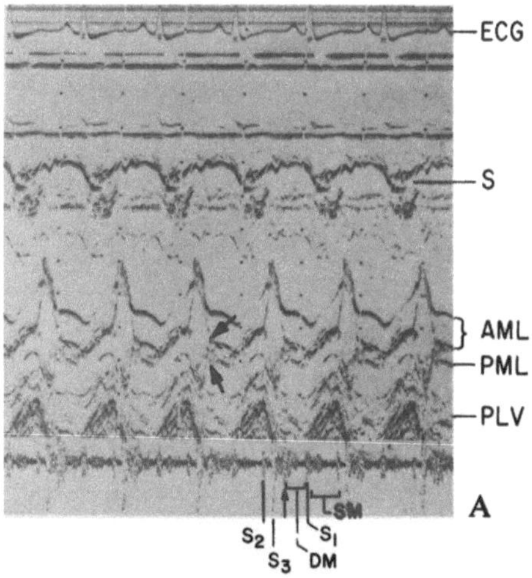

Fig. 19-10A. Premature closure of both anterior and posterior mitral leaflets in early diastole (arrows). The phonocardiogram at the bottom shows systolic and diastolic murmurs, a prominent S_3 followed by a loud sound (arrow), caused by premature closure of the mitral valve, and later a soft S_1 at the beginning of systole, which can be missed on auscultation and thereby lead to confusion as to what represents systole and diastole at the time of physical examination. DM = diastolic murmur; SM = systolic murmur.

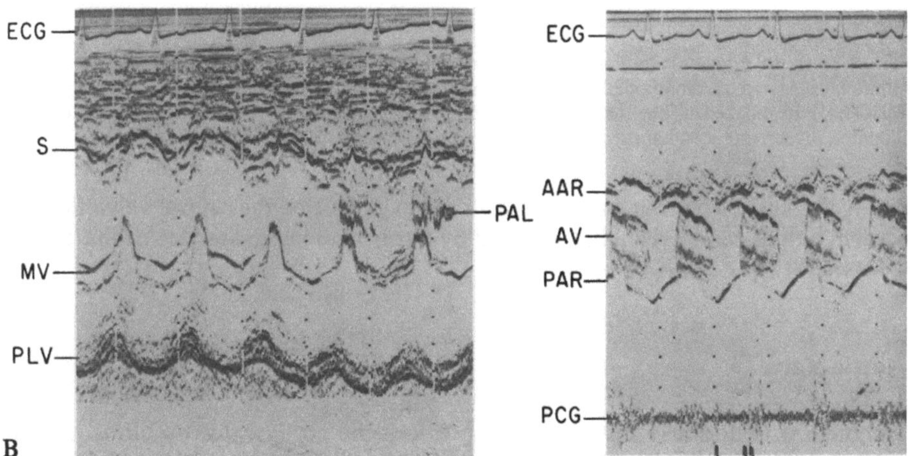

B. A prolapsed aortic valve leaflet (PAL) in the left ventricular outflow tract, confirmed at the time of aortic valve replacement. To the right is the aortic root showing a massive accumulation of echoes during diastole from a severely regurgitant aortic valve in a young adult with bacterial endocarditis. S = septum, AML = anterior mitral leaflet, PML = posterior mitral leaflet, PLV = posterior left ventricular wall, AAR = anterior aortic root, AV = aortic valve, PAR = posterior aortic root, PCG = phonocardiogram, MV = mitral valve.

medically, with or without propanolol, serial echocardiograms over the years may be beneficial in the follow-up evaluation of these patients. Shah and his associates (51) found no significant differences in echocardiograms from patients treated with propanolol as compared with those from patients who were not treated with this drug.

Although mitral valve flow, left ventricular stroke volume, and cardiac output can be determined by echocardiography, these are areas in which more clinical investiga-

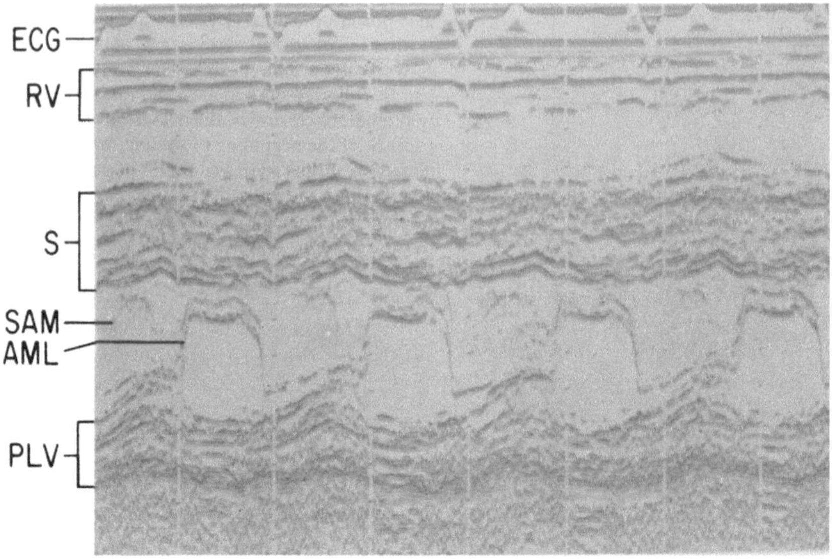

Fig. 19-11. Systolic anterior motion (SAM) of the anterior mitral leaflet (AML) in a 48-year-old man with nonobstructive cardiomyopathy. Both the interventricular septum (S) and posterior left ventricular wall (PLV) are thickened, but there is no disproportionate thickening of the spetum nor evidence of idiopathic hypertrophic subaortic stenosis at the time of cardiac catheterization.

tion is needed. Two groups of investigators have reported that mitral valve flow and cardiac output can be reliably estimated by ultrasound in the absence of mitral valve disease (19, 33).

Aortic Valve

Although it is normally an easy task to record the aortic valve by ultrasound, the echocardiogram is less sensitive technique to diagnose or quantitate specific aortic valve abnormalities than it is for evaluating the mitral valve.

Aortic Root

If the proper technique is employed, the diameter of the aortic root or annulus can be measured (21). The internal diameter ranged from 17 to 33 mm (mean: 23.7) in our group of 159 normal adult subjects. In males the mean diameter was 25 mm compared to 22.4 in females. Aortic root size did not correlate with body surface area. When surgeons replace an aortic valve with a free homograft, they require a preoperative estimate of the diameter of the aortic annulus so that a homograft of the proper size will be available. Preoperative echocardiograms of the aortic root are very reliable for predicting its size. Nanda *et al.* (41) reported on the value of echocardiography for the diagnosis of aortic root dissection, however I have been

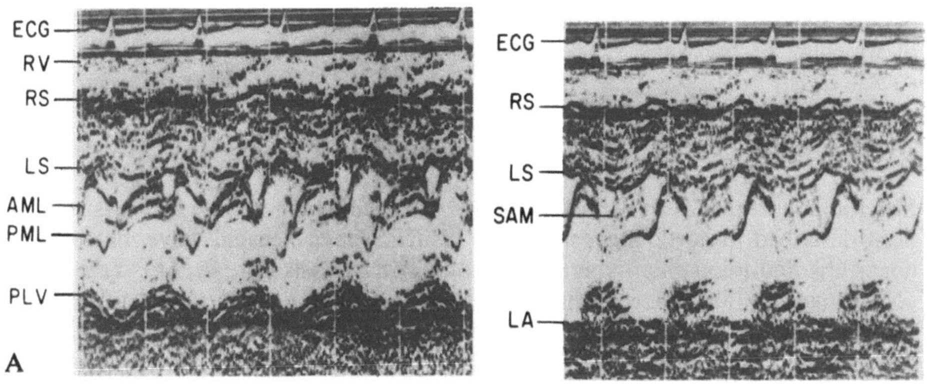

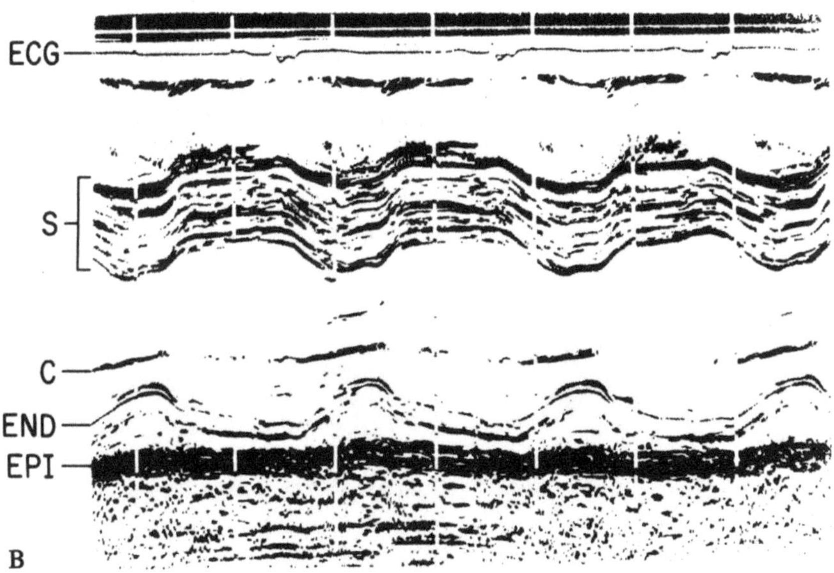

Fig. 19-12. A. Echocardiographic features of severe idiopathic hypertrophic subaortic stenosis in a 14-year-old girl, showing a disproportionately thickened septum, the systolic anterior motion (SAM) of the anterior mitral leaflet (AML) in contact with the left side of the septum (LS), slowed velocity of the AML, and normal motion of the posterior mitral leaflet (PML). There was a resting subvalvular gradient of 100 mm Hg at cardiac catheterization. RV = right ventricular wall, RS = right side of septum, PLV = posterior left ventricular wall, LA = left atrial wall.
B. A markedly thickened septum (S) due to asymmetric septal hypertrophy is shown in a middle-aged man, the father of the girl in Figure 19-12A. The recording of this patient's mitral valve was normal. C = chordae tendineae, END = endocardium, EPI = epicardium.

less impressed with the reliability of the technique. It is very easy to obtain additional parallel echoes from the anterior or posterior aortic root and give a false impression of widening of the walls.

Aortic Stenosis

Specific abnormalities of echoes from the valve leaflets in systole and diastole have been described in aortic stenosis, aortic insufficiency, bicuspid valve, bacterial endocarditis and idiopathic hypertrophic subaortic stenosis (24, 40, 56). Yeh and his coinvestigators (58) reported that the dimensions of the aortic valve orifice can be measured in nearly all patients with aortic stenosis and that a reduction in these dimensions correlated closely with the peak gradient across the valve, measured at cardiac catheterization (26). Experience in our laboratory does not agree with this finding; we have often found it difficult to record the leaflets sufficiently well during systole to measure the dimensions of the valve orifice. In the presence of a significantly calcified aortic valve, frequently only a dense mass of echoes can be recorded in the vicinity of the valve. The presence of a normal aortic valve echogram is sufficient evidence to exclude severe valvular aortic stenosis. Although Nanda and his associates (40) reported the echocardiographic features of a bicuspid aortic valve, we have not found the technique very reliable for predicting the existence of a bicuspid valve in patients with aortic stenosis who have undergone cardiac catheterization and valve replacement.

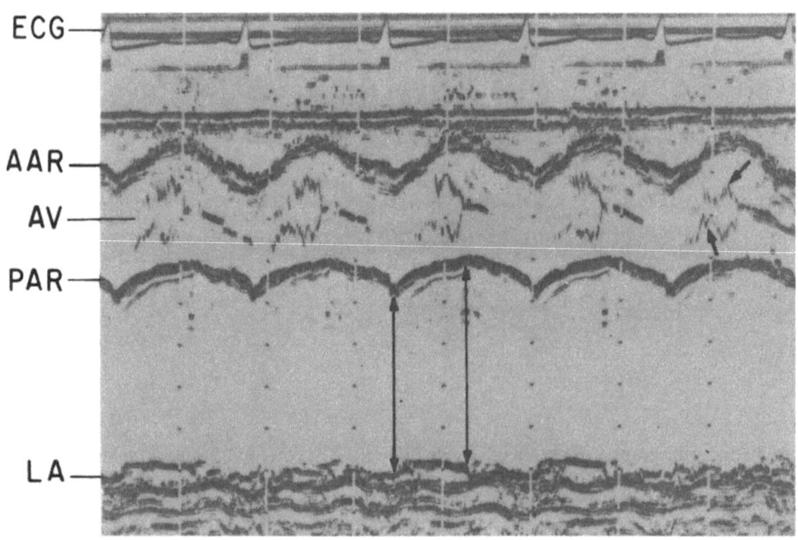

Fig. 19-13. Abnormal echographic recording of the aortic valve as seen in patients with severe idiopathic hypertrophic subaortic stenosis. The leaflets move close together (bottom arrow) in early systole due to subvalvular obstruction and resultant decreased flow, then open wider in late systole (top arrow). Left atrial enlargement can also be appreciated in this recording; arrows show dimensions of left atrium at end-diastole and end-systole. AAR = anterior aortic root, AV = aortic valve, PAR = posterior aortic root, LA = left atrial wall.

Aortic Insufficiency

Echoes from the aortic valve usually appear normal in isolated aortic insufficiency. We have observed two distinct echographic abnormalities of the aortic valve in patients with acute, severe, aortic regurgitation from bacterial endocarditis, i.e., multiple, chaotic accumulation of echoes from the valve during diastole (24), and prolapse of one of the cusps into the left ventricular outflow tract during diastole (Figure 19-10B).

A reflection of aortic valve flow can be appreciated when echoes from the valve leaflets are recorded well throughout systole. Although frequently no abnormality of the aortic valve is demonstrated by the echogram in idiopathic hypertrophic subaortic stenosis, a characteristic feature may be noted in which the valve opening is suddenly reduced in early systole by the subvalvular obstruction, then partially reopens later in systole (Figure 19-13).

The principal factor limiting the clinical usefulness of echograms of the aortic valve is the difficulty the examiner encounters in recording complete motion of the leaflets during systole.

Tricuspid and Pulmonic Valves

It is difficult to record the tricuspid and pulmonic valves in adults, and when they are recorded, the valves are rarely seen as well as the mitral and aortic valves. This is not a significant problem since there is no abnormality of these valves in most adult patients who are being evaluated for rheumatic or coronary heart disease. Adequate recordings of the tricuspid valve can usually be obtained in certain clinical settings when it is relevant, such as tricuspid stenosis in the presence of rheumatic heart disease (Figure 19-14). The tricuspid valve is easily recorded in the presence of right ventricular enlargement due to right-sided volume overload conditions or pressure overload from pulmonic stenosis or pulmonary hypertension.

Very little information is available in the literature in which the pulmonic valve has been studied by echocardiography in adults. Gramiak and his associates (23) reported that the valve could be detected in approximately 25 percent of those adults studied. The technique is not sensitive enough to reliably identify pulmonic stenosis.

The situation is quite different when studying infants in whom the tricuspid valve can be recorded routinely as easily as the mitral valve. We have been able to record the pulmonic valve in 80 percent of normal newborn infants (25). The value of recording both tricuspid and pulmonic valves is very important in infants and children who are being evaluated for various forms of congenital heart disease.

Left Ventricle

A significant amount of clinically useful information can be obtained from echocardiographic measurements of the left ventricle. An extensive amount of work reported by several investigators, indicates that echocardiography can provide an excellent

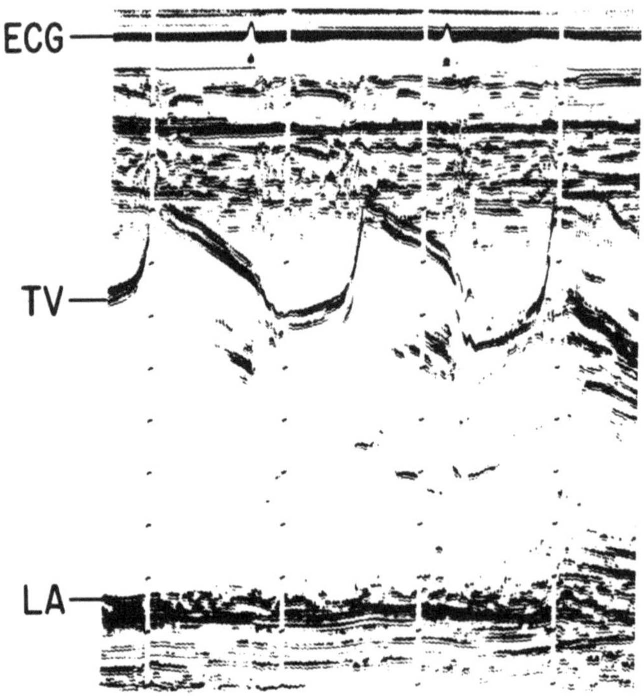

Fig. 19-14. Echocardiogram showing tricuspid stenosis in a lady with rheumatic heart disease and triple valve involvement. TV = tricuspid valve, LA = left atrial wall.

noninvasive method for the evaluation of left ventricular function. Specific parameters of left ventricular size and function, which can be determined by the echocardiogram, include internal dimensions, anterior and posterior wall thickness, posterior wall velocity, interventricular septal motion, end-systolic and end-diastolic volumes, ejection fraction, stroke volume, and wall motion abnormalities. Certain rules have to be followed for determining the measurements of the left ventricle. The transducer beam should be directed posteriorly in the third, fourth, or fifth intercostal space along the left sternal border to identify the mitral valve, then the transducer is directed slightly interior and lateral in order that the beam passes through the ventricle at the level of the chordae tendineae. The chordae are used as the landmarks where the end-systolic and end-diastolic measurements are obtained. Scanning the transducer toward the apex reveals that the distance between the left side of the interventricular septum and the endocardium of the posterior left ventricular wall is shorter in the region of the posterior papillary muscle, and still shorter as the beam is directed toward the apex. When searching for the endocardial echo, the examiner must be careful to avoid mistaking echoes from the papillary muscle or chordae tendineae. It must also be remembered that frequently more than a single echo is reflected from the endocardium due to the trabeculations. Another important reason for measuring the dimensions of the left ventricle at the level of the chordae tendinae is to insure that the echo beam intersects the interventricular septum at a point inferior to the pivot area. It is essential to take these measurements from the posterior endocardium to the left side of the septum below this pivot area to insure that proper

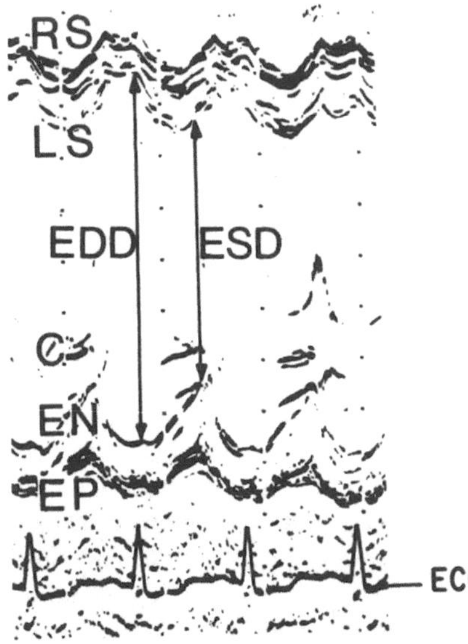

Fig. 19-15. Arrows mark the end-systolic dimension (ESD) and end-diastolic dimension (EDD) of the left ventricle. RS = right side of septum, LS = left side of septum, C = chordae tendineae, EN = endocardium, EP = epicardium.

septal motion is being measured. We have shown previously in our laboratory that the septal motion is flat or variable during systole in the pivot area and that during systole the septum moves anterior, superior to that point (26). Some of the investigators, 3 to 4 years ago, were measuring from the septum to epicardial echo of the posterior left ventricular wall. It is now well accepted that the endocardial echo must be used for accurate measurements.

The end-systolic dimension is determined echocardiographically by selecting the most anterior point of the posterior endocardial echo and drawing a straight line anterior to a point where it intersects the left side of the septum (Figure 19-15). Usually this will strike the septum at its most posterior peak and represent the shortest distance within the ventricle during systole and diastole. The septal peak does not always coincide with the endocardial peak of the posterior wall, and when this occurs, there is not uniform agreement among authorities as to how to determine the end systolic dimension. Cooper and his associates (8) define the end systolic dimension as the smallest distance separating the endocardial surfaces of the septum and left ventricular posterior wall and if the two endocardial surfaces do not peak simultaneously a line is extended from the septal endocardium to intersect the line drawn from the peak of the left ventricular endocardium. Although most investigators define the end systolic dimension in the same manner, they do not discuss how the measurement is determined when the endocardial peaks do not coincide simultaneously (43-45, 54). Some authors measure the end systolic dimension by extending a line downward from the peak of the septal surface to the point where it intersects the endocardium of the posterior wall (2, 18). The timing of the end-diastolic dimension is defined by most investigators as the R-wave on the electrocardiogram. However when calculations are made for ejection time from the echocardiogram 50 msec should be subtracted to allow for isovolumic contraction time (8). When the continuous recording technique instead of Polaroid exposures is used, the resolution of the endocardial echo is sufficiently better that the beginning of ejection can usually be identified from the echocardiogram without using the electrocardiogram as a reference. However, clinical studies have yet to confirm the accuracy of this method. Quinones *et al.* (47) used a simultaneous carotid pulse tracing to determine an accurate ejection time (47). Echocardiographic determinations of ejection fraction and mean velocity of circumferential fiber shortening have been shown to correlate well in the basal state with standard cineangiographic estimates and thereby provide a reliable determination of left ventricular performance (8).

McDonald and Feigenbaum (37) showed that measurements of left ventricular dimensions by ultrasound are reproducible. These investigators found the left ventricular end-diastolic dimension in normal subjects to be 4.0 ± 0.28 cm and shortening of 1.57 ± 0.22 cm (35.5 ± 3.9 percent) occurred during systole. The anterior movement of the posterior endocardial surface contributed 1.15 ± 0.17 cm toward this shortening and posterior movement of the septum contributed 0.42 ± 0.22 cm. The thickness of the posterior left ventricular wall at end-diastole averaged 0.90 ± 0.14 cm in those normal subjects and wall thickness increased by 64 percent (1.48 ± 0.30 cm) at the end of ejection. The thickness of the interventricular septum is normally not significantly different from the posterior left ventricular wall.

Danford (9) reported that left ventricular performance is patients with chronic aortic insufficiency can be better evaluated by employing echocardiography to determine the amplitude of systolic excursion of the posterior wall motion and the mean velocity of circumferential fiber shortening (V_{CF}). We found no abnormalities of ejection fraction or V_{CF} by echo in 12 patients with severe aortic insufficiency prior to aortic valve replacement, whereas 7 of these patients had significant abnormalities of these parameters by cineangiography (1). These discrepancies were not surprising since the left ventricular angiograms revealed normal shortening in the minor axis; however reduced or no shortening was consistently present in the longitudinal axis.

Ludbrook and his associates (25) showed that posterior wall velocity is an unreliable index of total left ventricular performance in patients with coronary artery disease, however Quinones and coinvestigators (47) reported that "normalized velocity" of the posterior wall in the absence of asynergy is a valuable method for evaluating left ventricular performance. It must be remembered that if the echo beam passes through areas of segmental wall motion disorders, the resultant calculations of left ventricular function indices may vary significantly from the overall performance as measured from cineangiography. In such circumstances calculations should be made from several locations between the plane of the mitral valve and inferiorly toward the apex. Unfortunately, in some cases the examiner is unable to record satisfactory echoes from the septum and posterior endocardium in more than one location even by altering the patient's position and the angle and location of the transducer. Special attention must be given to recording the location of the transducer and the position of the patient, preferably by the same examiner, in an effort to make the measurements through the same planes of the ventricle and thereby depend upon changes noted in serial evaluations to be actual rather than examiner-induced artifacts of recording.

Although Jacobs and his associates (32) found specific areas of abnormal wall motion by echocardiogram in the anatomic area predicted by the myocardial infarction pattern on electrocardiography in 18 of 20 patients, it is possible to have signifi-

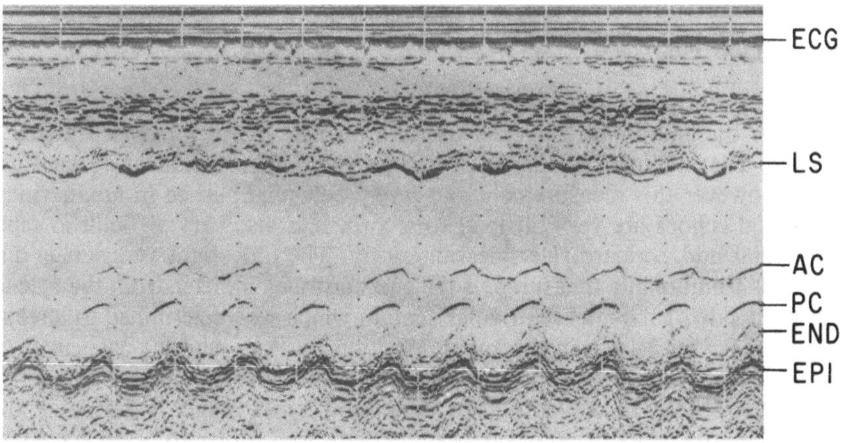

Fig. 19-16. Dilated left ventricle in a patient with congestive heart failure secondary to severe coronary artery disease and previous myocardial infarction. Septal motion is reduced and paradoxic during systole. The posterior left ventricle also shows areas of segmental wall motion disorders. LS = left side of septum, AC = anterior chordae, PC = posterior chordae, END = endocardium, EPI = epicardium.

cant coronary artery disease and reveal no echocardiographic abnormality. The echogram of a patient who suffered an extensive anteroseptal infarction complicated by heart failure is shown in Figure 19-16. The septum is quite abnormal, exhibiting little motion to grossly paradoxic movement in conjunction with a dilated left ventricle. Studies have not yet been reported in which serial long-term echocardiographic evaluations have been made post-operatively in patients who have received coronary saphenous vein bypass grafts. If the echocardiogram proves to be sensitive enough to detect subtle evidence of deteriorating left ventricular function or to detect wall motion abnormalities, which can be correlated to graft closures or progression of disease, this will represent another new, clinically useful, application of the technique.

Patients with a cardiomyopathy have some typical echocardiographic features but they are not specifically diagnostic. The ventricle is dilated and the motion of both septum and posterior left ventricle is reduced. The altered characteristics of the mitral valve have already been discussed (Figure 19-7). Although the typical wall motion abnormalities of coronary artery disease are segmental, the severe forms with heart failure due to "ischemic cardiomyopathy" may have extensive, diffuse abnormalities. Paradoxic septal motion may be present or actual aneurysmal dilatations may be seen.

There are distinct limitations to the practical use of echocardiography for the diagnosis of coronary heart disease and its value for following patients treated either medically or surgically. At present these limitations are twofold: (a) technically satisfactory recordings to assess left ventricular function can be obtained in only 80 percent of all patients with coronary heart disease, and (b) serial long-term studies are needed to assess changing echocardiographic parameters to determine how well they will recognize or quantitate abnormal left ventricular function.

Right Ventricle

The right ventricular chamber or outflow tract is easily recorded by echocardiogram, however the amount of clinically useful information which can be derived is rather limited. The thickness of the anterior right ventricular wall is easily measured in infants however this measurement can rarely be accomplished in adults since the endocardial echoes are very difficult to record. It is also very difficult to separate the epicardial and pericardial echoes anteriorly. The only right ventricular dimension, which is traditionally measured, is the end-diastolic diameter from the epicardium to the right side of the interventricular septum which was determined to have a normal range of 0.5 to 2.1 cm in the supine position by Popp and his associates (46). The upper limits of normal of the right ventricular dimension index is approximately 1.2 cm/M^2. The right ventricular dimension index (right ventricular dimension divided by the patient's body surface area) has been shown to be an accurate method for diagnosing right ventricular volume overload due to atrial septal defect or tricuspid insufficiency (11). The right ventricular dimension index is usually normal in patients with right ventricular pressure overload except in individuals with severe forms of pulmonic stenosis or pulmonary hypertension. The dilated right ventricle in a patient with a large (3 to 1 left-to-right shunt) atrial septal defect is shown in Figure 19-17A).

Left Atrium

Determination of left atrial dimension by ultrasound is technically very easy to perform, and correlation with the size of the left atrium, as determined by cineangiography is excellent (30). These authors found a range of 1.8 to 4.0 cm in

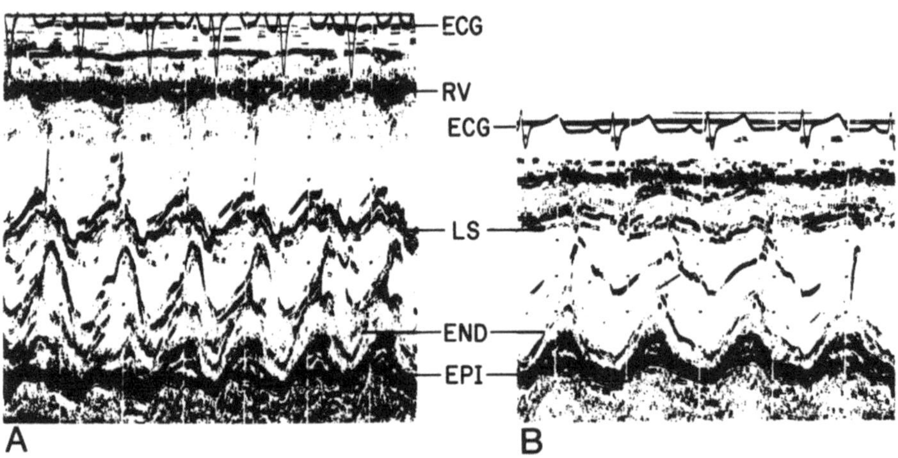

Fig. 19-17. A. Dilated right ventricle and paradoxic septal motion in a patient with a large atrial septal defect. B. Same patient after surgical closure of atrial septal defect, septal motion is still abnormal but less paradoxic. RV = right ventricular wall, LS = left side of septum, END = endocardium; EPI = epicardium.

normal subjects. However, it should be noted that these measurements were taken at the maximum distance near end-systole and were measured from the internal surface of the atrioventricular wall, which appeared to be the same echocardiographic structure as the posterior aortic root. Brown and his associates (3) reported a more sensitive method to determine left atrial enlargement by measuring the left atrial aortic root ratio. It has not been clearly established whether left atrial diameter should be measured at end-diastole or end-systole (Figure 19-13). In a study of 200 normal adults, we found that the normal range is 7 to 30 mm (mean: 19) at end-diastole and 16 to 40 mm (mean: 28.5) at end-systole (20). There is a significant difference in mean left atrial dimension between males and females (males: 20:7 and females: 18.3) but poor correlation with body surface area.

Although it is quite easy to diagnose a left atrial myxoma by echocardiogram, the recognition of thrombi are much more difficult. This is not surprising since there are "blind" areas within the left atrium adjacent to the interatrial septum and the left atrial appendage, which cannot be scanned by the ultrasound beam.

Pericardial Effusion

One of the long-standing clinical applications of echocardiography has been the detection of pericardial effusion. Despite the technical difficulties which may be encountered, the echocardiogram has become the procedure of choice for detecting or excluding pericardial effusion. Horowitz and his associates (31) confirmed that echocardiography is usually sensitive enough to detect only 15 ml of fluid. These investigators proposed a method for estimating pericardial volume using the difference between the cubed diameters at end-diastole of the pericardium and epicardium. The

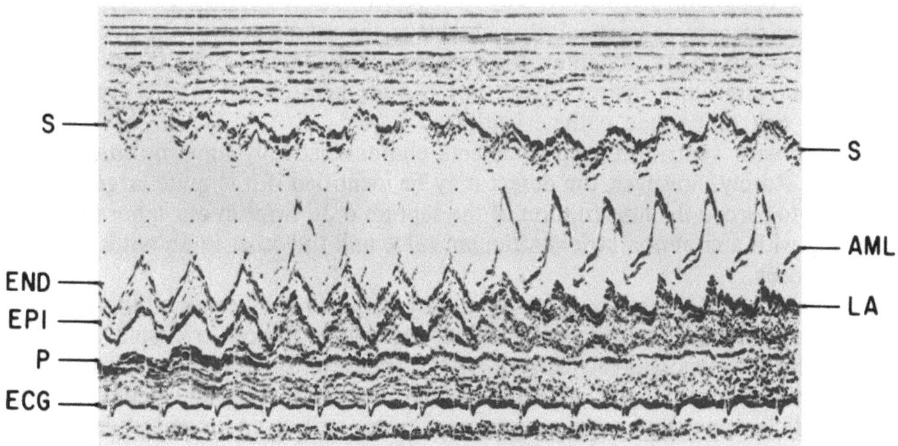

Fig. 19-18. Pericardial effusion is present posterior to the left ventricular wall but is not seen behind the left atrium. The gain setting has been reduced at the left side of the recording which identifies the extent of epicardial-pericardial separation more clearly. S = septum, END = endocardium, EPI = epicardium, P = pericardium, AML = anterior mitral leaflet, LA = left atrium.

method is not very accurate for quantitating small amounts of fluid (< 100 ml), however in 10 patients with greater than 200 ml of pericardial effusion the correlation between calculated and measured volume at surgery was good ($r = 0.86$). It is usually very difficult to identify pericardial fluid anteriorly except in cases with large effusions. One must be very cautious about making a diagnosis of fluid from a small anterior echo-free space, since this is often seen in normal subjects as the contracting right ventricle moves away from the stationary echoes of the chest wall. Effusions are often not seen posterior to the left atrium, therefore it is essential to direct the ultrasound beam through the left ventricle while appropriate gain or reject adjustments are made on the machine (Figure 19-18).

Congenital Heart Disease

One of the most valuable clinical applications of echocardiography is the evaluation of newborn infants and children with suspected congenital heart disease. It is usually easier to obtain technically good echographic recordings in infants or children than in adults. An extensive amount of information, available in the literature, discusses the echocardiographic features of most types of congenital cardiac malformations. It is not possible to discuss all of them within this chapter.

The most commonly encountered form of congenital heart disease in adult patients referred for cardiac consultation is atrial septal defect. Although the echocardiogram is not as sensitive as previously reported for the detection of right side, volume overload conditions (17), the identification of paradoxic septal motion is quite reliable for the diagnosis of large atrial septal defects which have shunts greater than 2 to 1 left-to-right (26). We have observed the right ventricular dimension to decrease in patients following surgical closure of the atrial septal defect, however septal motion is variable postoperatively, with some returning to normal and others remaining paradoxic, but to a lesser degree (Figure 19-17).

Echocardiography is particularly valuable in the assessment of the cyanotic newborn infant. The ability to demonstrate normal cardiac anatomy in infants suffering from acute respiratory distress syndrome is quite helpful and may prevent the unnecessary risk of cardiac catheterization.

Patients with ventricular septal defects characteristically have normal echocardiograms. Rarely, however, the defect may be identified if it is quite large. We have been able to record the interruption of the septum only twice in our laboratory, once in a child with a common atrioventricular valve and the other in an adult with truncus arteriosus.

The diagnosis of Ebstein's anomaly is easy to confirm by echocardiography. The most specific feature is the simultaneous recording of both tricuspid and mitral valves, which shows delayed closure of the tricuspid valve (Figure 19-19). Other echographic features of the anomaly, which have been reported, include a dilated right ventricle, type B paradoxic septal motion, as well as an increased velocity and amplitude of the anterior tricuspid leaflet (53).

Other forms of congenital heart disease diagnosed by the echocardiogram include: hypoplastic left heart syndrome, aortic atresia, tricuspid atresia, single ventricle, endocardial cushion defect, truncus arteriosus, transposition of the great arteries, and

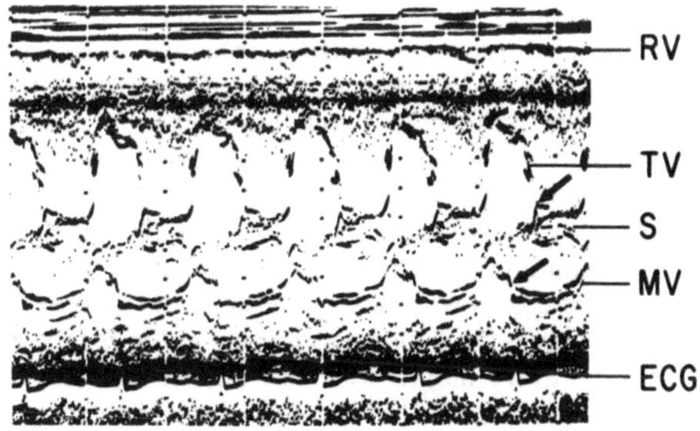

Fig. 19-19. A 52-year-old women with Ebstein's anomaly. Closure of the tricuspid valve is significantly delayed (top arrow) compared to mitral valve closure (bottom arrow). Additional abnormal features include a dilated right ventricular dimension, increased amplitude of the tricuspid valve, paradoxic septal motion, and decreased velocity of anterior mitral leaflet. RV = right ventricular wall, TV = tricuspid valve, S = septum, MV = mitral valve.

double-outlet right ventricle (5–7, 12, 38, 56). The characteristic features in a patient with tetralogy of Fallot are shown in Figure 19-20.

Since normal values have been established for velocity of circumferential fiber shortening in newborns, serial echocardiograms of infants with congenital heart disease should be valuable for the assessment of left ventricular performance (49).

Summary

During the past decade echocardiography has been used extensively in clinical cardiology and has become an accepted, extremely valuable noninvasive technique for the routine evaluation and management of patients with heart disease. Its

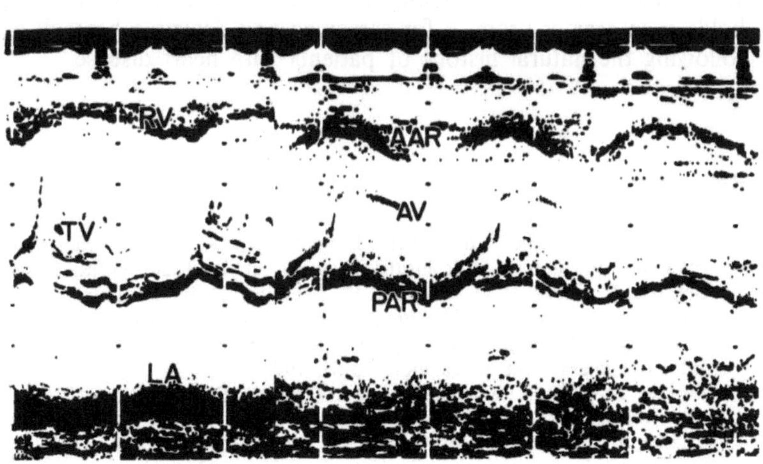

Fig. 19-20. A 21-year-old woman with tetralogy of Fallot. The left side of the recording shows a markedly enlarged right ventricle. The right side shows an enlarged aortic root displaced anteriorly with resultant disruption between the interventricular septum (S) and the anterior aortic root (AAR). The posterior aortic root (PAR) is not continuous with the septum. The two areas were recorded in different transducer positions and placed together for purposes of photography. TV = tricuspid valve, LA = left atrium, AV = aortic valve.

overwhelming popularity with clinicians and its widespread application by inexperienced or poorly trained physicians have not infrequently led to faulty interpretations and incorrect cardiac diagnoses. Difficulty in maintaining quality control in the performance and interpretation of echocardiograms is not limited to physicians employing echocardiography. It is not a difficult task to interpret a high quality echographic recording, the real challenge comes with obtaining complete, technically satisfactory recordings in all patients. The most significant problem today limiting the practical value of echocardiography for the average clinician treating patients with heart disease is the lack of adequately trained cardiovascular technicians. Numerous investigators in the field are literally bombarding the medical literature every month with new applications and further refinements in the use of cardiac ultrasound. It is the obligation of the medical communities and training institutions to provide more programs to produce the type of sophisticated cardiovascular technicians needed. Without these highly trained personnel, echocardiography is at risk, in any given hospital or office, of falling into disrepute and becoming only an instrument for economic gain.

New engineering developments are also needed in ultrasonic equipment to help overcome technical problems in some patients. Hopefully the combination of single-crystal reflected ultrasound together with improved imaging by multiple-crystal and sector-scanning systems will enhance the overall detail of cardiac anatomy and function.

I have tried to review the most important and clinically useful applications of echocardiography in acquired and in congenital heart disease. In addition, I have discussed some of the limitations of the technique as well as some of the controversies among investigators. Space does not allow an in-depth discussion and certainly the section on congenital heart disease was only superficially addressed.

As a result of the rapid growth of new information in this field during recent years, and with new technology and automation, the future of echocardiography holds even greater promise for screening and detecting heart disease as well as for following the natural history of patients with heart disease.

References

1. Alpert, J. S., Francis, G. S., Ockene, I., and Hagan, A. D. Echocardiographic assessment of left ventricular function in aortic insufficiency. Circulation (Supplement), in press, 1975.
2. Belenkie, I., Nutter, D. O., Clark, D. W., McGraw, D. B., and Raizner, A. E. Assessment of left ventricular dimensions and function by echocardiography. Am. J. Cardiol., 31:755, 1973.
3. Brown, O. R., Harrison, D. C., and Popp, R. L. An improved method for echographic detection of left atrial enlargement. Circulation, 50:58, 1974.
4. Burgess, J., Clark, R., Kamigaki, M., and Cohn, K. Echocardiographic findings in different types of mitral regurgitation. Circulation, 48:97, 1973.
5. Chesler, E., Joffe, H. S., Beck, W., and Schrire, V. Echocardiographic recognition of mitral-semilunar valve discontinuity. Circulation, 43:725, 1971.
6. —— Joffe, H. S., Vecht, R., Beck, W., and Schrire, V. Ultrasound cardiography in single ventricle and the hypoplastic left and right heart syndrome. Circulation, 42:123, 1970.
7. Chung, K. J., Alexson, C. G., Manning, J. A., and Gramiak, R. Echocardiography in truncus arteriosus. Circulation, 48:281, 1973.
8. Cooper, R. H., O'Rourke, R. A., Karliner, J. S., Peterson, K. L., and Leopold, G. R. Comparison of ultrasound and cineangiographic measurements of the mean rate of circumferential fiber shortening in man. Circulation, 46:914, 1972.

9. Danford, H. G., Danford, D. A., Mielke, J. E., and Peterson, L. F. Echocardiographic evaluation of the hemodynamic effects of chronic aortic insufficiency with observations on left ventricular performance. Circulation, 48:253, 1973.
10. DeMaria, A. N., King, J. F., Bogren, H. G., Lies, J. E., and Mason, D. T. The variable spectrum of echocardiographic manifestations of the mitral valve prolapse syndrome. Circulation, 50:33, 1974.
11. Diamond, M. A., Dillon, J. C., Haine, C. L., Chang, S., and Feigenbaum, H. Echocardiographic features of atrial septal defect. Circulation, 43:129, 1971.
12. Dillon, J. C., Feigenbaum, H., Konecke, L. L., Keutel, J., Hurwitz, R. A., Davis, R. H., and Chang, S. Echocardiographic manifestations of d-transposition of the great vessels. Am. J. Cardiol., 32:74, 1973.
13. Duchak, J. M., Jr., Chang, S., and Feigenbaum, H. The posterior mitral valve echo and the echocardiographic diagnosis of mitral stenosis. Am. J. Cardiol., 29:628, 1972.
14. —— —— —— Echocardiographic features of torn chordae tendineae. Am. J. Cardiol., 29:260, 1972.
15. Edler, I. Diagnostic use of ultrasound in heart disease. Acta Med. Scand. 308:32, 1955.
16. —— and Hertz, C. H. Use of ultrasonic reflectoscope for continuous recording of movements of heart walls. Kungl. Fysiogr. Sallsk. Lund. Forhandl 24:5, 1954.
17. Feigenbaum, H. Echocardiography, Chap. 4. Philadelphia, Lea and Febiger, 1972, pp. 43–49.
18. —— Clinical applications of echocardiography. Prog. Cardiovasc. Dis., 14:531, 1972.
19. Fischer, J. C., Chang, S., Konecke, L. L., Feigenbaum, H. Echocardiographic determination of mitral valve flow. Am. J. Cardiol., 29:262, 1972.
20. Francis, G. S. and Hagan, A. D. Echocardiographic criteria of normal left atrial size in adults. Catheterization and Cardiovascular Diagnosis, in press, 1975.
21. —— —— O'Rourke, R. A., Oury, J. The accuracy of echocardiography for assessing aortic root diameter. Br. Heart J., 37:376, 1975.
22. Goodman, D. J., Harrison, D. C., Popp, R. L. Echocardiographic feature of primary pulmonary hypertension. Am. J. Cardiol., 33:438, 1974.
23. Gramiak, R., Nanda, N. C., and Shah, P. M. Echocardiographic detection of the pulmonary valve. Radiology, 102:153, 1972.
24. Hagan, A. D. and Vieweg, W. V. R. Ultrasound evaluation of acute aortic regurgitation due to bacterial endocarditis: a case report. Milit. Med., 139:725, 1974.
25. —— Deely, W. J., Sahn, D., and Friedman, W. F. Echocardiographic criteria for normal newborn infants. Circulation, 48:1221, 1973.
26. —— Francis, G. S., Sahn, D. J., Karliner, J. S., Friedman, W. F., and O'Rourke, R. A. Ultrasound evaluation of systolic anterior septal motion in patients with and without right ventricular volume overload. Circulation, 50:248, 1974.
27. Henry, W. L., Clark, C. E., and Epstein, S. E. Asymmetric septal hypertrophy (ASH): The unifying link in the IHSS disease spectrum. Circulation, 47:827, 1973.
28. —— —— —— Asymmetric septal hypertrophy: Echocardiographic identification of the pathognomonic anatomic abnormality of IHSS. Circulation, 47:225, 1973.
29. —— —— Glancy, D. L., and Epstein, S. E. Echocardiographic measurement of the left ventricular outflow gradient in idiopathic hypertrophic subaortic stenosis. N. Engl. J. Med., 288:989, 1973.
30. Hirata, T., Wolve, S. B., Popp, R. L., Helmen, C. H., and Feigenbaum, H. Estimation of left atrial size using ultrasound. Am. Heart J., 78:43, 1969.
31. Horowitz, M. S., Schultz, C. S., Stinson, E. B., Harrison, D. C., and Popp, R. L. Sensitivity and specificity of echocardiographic diagnosis of pericardial effusion. Circulation, 50:239, 1974.
32. Jacobs, J. J., Feigenbaum, H., Corya, B. C., and Phillips, J. F. Detection of left ventricular asynergy by echocardiography. Circulation, 48:263, 1973.
33. Keefe, J., Theodosiou, G., Noggar, C., Flessas, A., and Ryan, T. J. Ultrasonic determination of cardiac output from the mitral valve tracing. Circulation, 48: Suppl 4:185, 1973.
34. Konecke, L. L., Feigenbaum, H., Chang, S., Corya, B. C., and Fischer, J. C. Abnormal mitral valve motion in patients with elevated left ventricular diastolic pressures. Circulation, 47:989, 1973.
35. Ludbrook, P., Karliner, J. S., London, A., Peterson, K. L., Leopold, G. R., and O'Rourke, R. A. Posterior wall velocity: An unreliable index of total left ventricular performance in patients with coronary artery disease. Am. J. Cardiol., 33:475, 1974.
36. Martinez, E. C., Giles, T. D., and Burch, G. E. Echocardiographic diagnosis of left atrial myxoma. Am. J. Cardiol., 33:281, 1974.
37. McDonald, I. G., Feigenbaum, H., and Chang, S. Analysis of left ventricular wall motion by reflected ultrasound. Circulation, 46:14, 1972.

38. Meyer, R. A. and Kaplan, S. Echocardiography in the diagnosis of hypoplasia of the left or right ventricles in the neonate. Circulation, 46:55, 1972.
39. Millward, D. K., McLaurin, L. P., and Craige, E. Echocardiographic studies of the mitral valve in patients with congestive cardiomyopathy and mitral regurgitation. Am. Heart J., 85:413, 1973.
40. Nanda, N. C., Gramiak, R., Manning, J., Mahoney, E. B., Lipchik, E. O., and DeWeese, J. A. Echocardiographic recognition of the congenital bicuspid aortic valve. Circulation, 49:870, 1974.
41. —— —— Shah, P. M. Diagnosis of aortic root dissection by echocardiography. Circulation, 48:506, 1973.
42. —— —— —— Lipchik, E. D. Ultrasound evaluation of mitral valve calcification. Circulation, 46: Suppl 2:20, 1972.
43. Paraskos, J. A., Grossman, W., Saltz, S., Dalen, J. E., and Dexter, L. A noninvasive technique for the determination of velocity of circumferential fiber shortening in man. Circ. Res., 29:610, 1971.
44. Pombo, J. F., Troy, B. L., and Russell, R. O., Jr. Left ventricular volumes and ejection fraction by echocardiography. Circulation, 43:480, 1971.
45. Popp, R. L. and Harrison, D. C. Ultrasonic cardiac echography for determining stroke volume and valvular regurgitation. Circulation, 41:493, 1970.
46. —— Wolfe, S. B., Hirata, T., and Feigenbaum, H. Estimation of right and left ventricular size by ultrasound. Am. J. Cardiol., 24:523, 1969.
47. Quinones, M. A., Gaasch, W. H., and Alexander, J. K. Echocardiographic assessment of left ventricular function. Circulation, 50:42, 1974.
48. —— Gaasch, W. H., Waisser, E., and Alexander, J. K. Reduction in the rate of diastolic descent of the mitral valve echogram in patients with altered left ventricular diastolic pressure-volume relations. Circulation, 49:246, 1974.
49. Sahn, D. J., Deely, W. J., Hagan, A. D., and Friedman, W. F. Echocardiographic assessment of left ventricular performance in normal newborns. Circulation, 49:232, 1974.
50. Segal, B. L., Konecke, L. L., Kawai, N., Kotler, M. N., and Linhart, J. W. Echocardiography, current concepts and clinical applications. Am. J. Med., 57:267, 1974.
51. Shah, P. M., Gramiak, R., Adelman, A. G., and Wigle, E. D. Echocardiographic assessment of the effects of surgery and propanalol on the dynamics of outflow obstruction in hypertrophic subaortic stenosis. Circulation, 45:516, 1972.
52. —— Gramiak, R., and Kramer, D. H. Ultrasound localization of left ventricular outflow obstruction in hypertrophic obstructive cardiomyopathy. Circulation, 40:3, 1969.
53. Tajik, A. J., Gau, G. T., Giuliani, E. R., Ritter, D. G., and Schattenbert, T. T. Echocardiogram in Ebstein's Anomaly with Wolff-Parkinson-White pre-excitation syndrome, Type B. Circulation, 47:813, 1973.
54. Troy, B. L., Pombo, J., and Rackley, C. E. Measurement of left ventricular wall thickness and mass by echocardiography. Circulation, 45:602, 1972.
55. Ulrich, W. D. Ultrasound dosage for experimental use on human beings. Naval Medical Research Institute, Research Report No. 2, Project M4306.01-1010BXK9, August 19, 1971.
56. Williams, R. G. and Rudd, M. Echocardiographic features of endocardial cushion defects. Circulation, 49:418, 1974.
57. Winsberg, F., Gabar, G. E., Hernberg, J. G., and Weiss, B. Fluttering of the mitral valve in aortic insufficiency. Circulation, 41:225, 1970.
58. Yeh, H., Winsberg, F., and Mercer, E. N. Echographic aortic valve orifice dimension: its use in evaluating aortic stenosis and cardiac output. J. Clin. Ultrasound, 1:182, 1974.

Index

MIX
Papier aus verantwortungsvollen Quellen
Paper from responsible sources
FSC® C105338

If you have any concerns about our products, you can contact us on
ProductSafety@springernature.com

In case Publisher is established outside the EU, the EU authorized representative is:
Springer Nature Customer Service Center GmbH
Europaplatz 3, 69115 Heidelberg, Germany

Printed by Libri Plureos GmbH
in Hamburg, Germany